E. H. Farthmann · C. Meyer · H. A. Richter (Eds.)

Springer

Berlin
Heidelberg
New York
Barcelona
Budapest
Hong Kong
London
Mailand
Paris
Santa Clara
Singapore
Tokio

E. H. Farthmann · C. Meyer · H. A. Richter (Eds.)

Current Aspects of Laparoscopic Colorectal Surgery

Indications – Methods – Results

With 49 Figures and 114 Tables

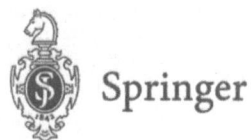 Springer

Prof. Dr. Dr. Dr. h. c. Eduard H. Farthmann
Department of General Surgery
Klinikum Albert-Ludwigs-Universität Freiburg
Hugstetter Strasse 55, D-79106 Freiburg

Prof. Dr. Christian Meyer
Service de Chirurgie Générale et Digestive
Centre de Chirurgie Viscérale et de Transplantation
CHU de Strasbourg-Hautpierre, F-67098 Strasbourg Cedex

Prof. Dr. Hans A. Richter
Department of Surgery
Evangelische Diakonissenanstalt
Groepelinger Heerstrasse 406/408, D-28239 Bremen

ISBN-13: 978-3-642-64381-1   e-ISBN-13: 978-3-642-60382-2
DOI: 10.1007/978-3-642-60382-2

Die Deutsche Bibliothek – CIP-Einheitsaufnahme
Current aspects of laparoscopic colorectal surgery: indications
– methods – results ; with tables / International Workshop
Laparoscopic Colorectal Surgery, Norderstedt, November 27 –
29, 1995. E. H. Farthmann ... (ed.). – Berlin ; Heidelberg ; New
York ; Barcelona ; Budapest ; Hong Kong ; London ; Milan ;
Paris ; Santa Clara ; Singapore ; Tokyo : Springer, 1997
    ISBN-13: 978-3-642-64381-1
NE: Farthmann, Eduard H. [Hrsg.]; International Workshop
    Laparoscopic Colorectal Surgery <1995, Norderstedt>

© Springer-Verlag Berlin Heidelberg 1997
Softcover reprint of the hardcover 1st edition 1997

The use of general descriptive names, registered names, trademarks, etc. in this publication does not imply, even in the absence of a specific statement, that such names are exempt from the relevant protective laws and regulations and therefore free for general use.
Product liability: The publishers cannot guarantee the accuracy of any information about dosage and application contained in this book. In every individual case the user must check such information by consulting the relevant literature.

Coverdesign: de'blik, Berlin
Production: ProduServ GmbH Verlagsservice, Berlin
Typesetting: Fotosatz-Service Köhler OHG, Würzburg
SPIN: 10518576   24/3020 – 5 4 3 2 1 0 – Gedruckt auf säurefreiem Papier

Preface

This publication of the papers presented at the Workshop on Laparoscopic Colorectal Surgery that took place on 27–29 November 1995 in the European Surgical Institute in Norderstedt, Germany, is effectively a snapshot of the current state of knowledge in both the theory and the practice of minimally invasive colon surgery. This snapshot is a mosaic made up of the varied experiences of individual surgeons.

After a long period in which nothing much seemed to be happening, the recent growth in the use of minimally invasive surgery or video-controlled operative procedures in surgery of the abdominal and chest cavities has been unparalleled. More difficult operations have become increasingly possible as more and more new techniques have become available.

Cholecystectomy should be regarded as the pacesetter for video-controlled procedures. Under defined conditions, it has now become the standard operation. Other operative procedures such as appendicectomy, herniorrhaphy, oversewing of a perforated gastric or duodenal ulcer, vagotomy and fundoplication, operations on the spleen or adrenal, staging operations, and thoracic surgical procedures are becoming increasingly widely performed. Minimally invasive operations on the small and large bowel are currently still at the stage of individual reports.

The science of surgery relies on experience and the analysis of that experience. In minimally invasive surgery our experience goes back no more than 6–7 years, less in the case of most procedures, and this means that we are still in the learning phase. To use a metaphor from school, we are just beginning to spell out individual words. This new operative technique should at present be left to surgeons who possess appropriate experience and competence. For surgeons who are still inexperienced in video-controlled surgery, there is no compulsion to follow the new trend. A comprehensive range of proven conventional operations is available for many indications.

Minimally invasive surgery will enrich many conventional procedures and replace them in some cases, but it will not make them redundant. All new operative procedures take place under the protective wing of classical conventional surgery. Mastery of the latter is essential for the testing and introduction of new methods.

Technical solutions to various problems were an important requirement before laparoscopic colorectal procedures could become established. One essential precondition for performing laparoscopic colorectal operations was the ability to fashion a secure intraabdominal anastomosis, for which special instruments had to be developed, and to deliver the operative specimen in a water- and cell-proof specimen bag.

The increased technical demands and the consequent increased costs of laparoscopic colorectal surgery can only be justified if studies can show that the new operative procedure offers the patient a low-risk operation, freedom from complications, increased postoperative comfort, and, above all, long-term results that are at least as good as those after conventional surgery.

The feasibility of minimally invasive colorectal surgery has been demonstrated many times over. However, there are as yet no controlled studies with regard to the long-term results after laparoscopic operations, especially with regard to malignant disease of the bowel. Defined standards need to be drawn up for the near future.

The contributions to this book give an overview of the current state of knowledge and of the technical details of minimally invasive colorectal surgery. It has become clear that the main indications of minimally invasive surgery are benign illnesses such as Crohn's disease, diverticulitits, or rectal prolapse. The feasibility of cancer surgery by the minimally invasive route, from the oncological point of view, is emphasized by several authors. Controlled studies and long-term results will be needed to remove any persisting uncertainty about recurrence. Other authors emphasize the complications of laparoscopic colorectal surgery. These often led to conversion from a minimally invasive to a conventional procedure. In cases where this becomes necessary, the changeover should be made early and in good time for the patient's sake.

The new operative technique involves higher financial costs. However, the reduction of postoperative hospital stay means that these increased costs appear to be economically justifiable. In addition, it should be possible for patients of working age to return to work earlier after surgery, so that a wider economic benefit should also be apparent.

Video-controlled colorectal surgery has opened a new and interesting chapter in surgery. There are still gaps in our knowledge in this area however, and we must try extremely carefully to close these gaps in order to avoid mistakes or errors.

Since we have a great foundation of practical and theoretical knowledge of conventional colorectal surgery on which to build, Sir Karl Popper's words can be applied to the further development of the new technique:
„Advancement of our knowledge consists of the correction, the modification of earlier knowledge."

E. H. Farthmann
C. Meyer
H. A. Richter

I believe that it is worth making an attempt to find out more about the world even if all that emerges from the attempt is no more than the knowledge of how little we know.

Sir Karl Popper, Salzburg, 1979

Contents

List of Authors

C. A. Akle
Nightingale House
90a Harley Street
London W1N 1AF
UK

Ivo Baca
Clinic for General and Casualty Surgery
Central Hospital Bremen-Ost
Züricher Straße 40
28325 Bremen
Germany

L. Bardram
Department of Gastrointestinal Surgery
Hvidovre Hospital
University of Copenhagen
2650 Hvidovre
Denmark

E. Bärlehner
Department of Surgery
Buch Berlin Clinic
Hobrechtsfelder Chaussee 100
13122 Berlin
Germany

U. Baumgartner
University Clinc for Surgery
Department of General Surgery
and Outpatient Clinic
Hugstetterstr. 55
79106 Freiburg
Germany

I. Berki
Department of Surgery
Szt. János Hospital
Semmelweis Medical University
Budapest
Hungary

T. Berselli
Department of General Surgery
S. Agostino Hospital
Modena
Italy

S. Bonilauri
Department of General Surgery
S. Agostino Hospital
Modena
Italy

U. Bonk
Department of Pathology
Central Hospital Bremen-Nord
Hammersbecker Str. 228
28755 Bremen
Germany

E. J. Brennan, Jr.
Department of Surgery
St. Joseph Medical Centre
7620 York Road
Towson, MD 21204
USA

P. Buchmann
Department of Surgery
Wald Municipal Hospital
8037 Zürich
Switzerland

H.-P. Bruch
Department of Surgery
Medical University of Lübeck
Ratzeburger Allee 160
23538 Lübeck
Germany

D. A. Dorsay
University of South Carolina
Dept. of Surgery
Two Richland Medical Parks, Suite 300
USA - Columbia, SC 29203

G. Ehren
Department of General Surgery
Zehlendorf Hospital
Gimpelsteig 3 – 5
14165 Berlin
Germany

J. Faller
Department of Surgery
Szt. János Hospital
Semmelweis Medical University
Diósáeok u. 1.
1125 Budapest
Hungary

O. Firtion
Department of General and Digestive Surgery
Centre for Visceral Surgery
and Transplantation
CHU de Strasbourg-Hautpierre
67098 Strasbourg Cedex
France

A. Franke
Department of Surgery
Evangelischer Diakonissenanstalt
Gröpelinger Heerstr. 406/408
28239 Bremen
Germany

W. Peter Geis
St. Joseph Medical Center
7620 York Road
Towson, MD 21204
USA

V. Götzen
Clinic for General and Casualty Surgery
Central Hospital Bremen-Ost
Züricher Straße 40
28325 Bremen
Germany

F. L. Greene
University of South Carolina
Dept. of Surgery
Two Richland Medical Parks, Suite 300
USA - Columbia, SC 29203

T. Hager
Friesener Str. 41
96317 Kronach
Germany

P. Hanisch
Department of Pathology
Central Hospital Bremen-Nord
Hammersbecker Str. 228
28755 Bremen
Germany

B. M. Helmke
Department of Pathology
Central Hospital Bremen-Nord
Hammersbecker Str. 228
28755 Bremen
Germany

A. Herold
Department of Surgery
Medical University of Lübeck
Ratzeburger Allee 160
23538 Lübeck
Germany

B. Heukrodt
Department of Surgery
Buch Berlin Clinic
Hobrechtsfelder Chaussee 100
13122 Berlin
Germany

U. Hildebrandt
Department of Surgery of the University
of the Saarland
Division of General,
Abdominal and Vascular Surgery
Oskar-Orth-Strasse
66421 Homburg-Saar
Germany

A. Holker
Department of Surgery
Grosshadern Clinic
Ludwig Maximilians University of Munich
Marchioninistrasse 15
81377 Munich
Germany

G. István
Department of Surgery
Szt. Janós Hospital
Semmelweis Medical University
Diósáeok u. 1.
1125 Budapest
Hungary

H. C. Kim
Department of Surgery
St. Joseph Medical Center
7620 York Road
Baltimore, MD 21204
USA

F. Köckerling
Department of Surgery
Krankenhausstraße 12
91054 Erlangen
Germany

J. Konradt
Department of General Surgery
Zehlendorf Hospital
Gimpelsteig 3–5
14165 Berlin
Germany

U. Kunath
Department of General,
Thoracic and Vascular Surgery
Krankenhaus am Urban
Diffenbachstraße 1
10967 Berlin
Germany

A. Kuthe
Hospital SILOAH
Department of Surgery
Roesebeckstr. 15
30449 Hannover
Germany

V. Lange
Department of Surgery
Grosshadern Clinic
Marchioninistr. 15
81377 Munich
Germany

A. Lanzani
Department of General Surgery
S. Agostino Hospital
Modena
Italy

K. Lebrecht
Department of Surgery
Evangelische Diakonissenanstalt
Gröpelinger Heerstr. 406/408
28239 Bremen
Germany

N. de Manzini
Department of General and Digestive Surgery
Centre for Visceral Surgery
and Transplantation
CHU de Strasbourg-Hautpierre
67098 Strasbourg Cedex
France

H. J. Mappes
University Clinic for Surgery
Department of General Surgery
and Outpatient Clinic
Hugstetterstr. 55
79106 Freiburg
Germany

G. Melotti
Department of General Surgery
S. Agostino Hospital
Modena
Italy

G. Meyer
Department of Surgery
Grosshadern Clinic
Marchioninistr. 15
81377 Munich
Germany

C. Meyer
Department of General and Digestive Surgery
Centre for Visceral Surgery
and Transplantation
CHU de Strasbourg-Hautpierre
67098 Strasbourg Cedex
France

A. Nerlich
Department of Pathology
Ludwig Maximilian University of Munich
Munich
Germany

P.-O. Nyström
University Department of Surgery
Hospital Department of Medico-Surgical
Gastroenterology
University Hospital Department of Surgery
58185 Linköping
Sweden

L. Påhlman
Department of Surgery
Colorectal Unit
University Hospital
75185 Uppsala
Sweden

P. P. Petropoulos
Cantonal Hospital
Department of Surgery
Bertigny
1708 Fribourg
Switzerland

M. A. Reymond
Department of Surgery
Krankenhausstraße 12
91054 Erlangen
Germany

H. A. Richter
Department of Surgery
Evangelischer Diakonissenanstalt
Gröpelinger Heerstr. 406/408
28239 Bremen
Germany

S. Rohr
Department of General
and Digestive Surgery
Centre for Visceral Surgery
and Transplantation
CHU de Strasbourg-Hautpierre
67098 Strasbourg Cedex
France

G. Ruf
University Clinic for Surgery
Department of General Surgery
and Outpatient Clinic
Hugstetterstr. 55
79106 Freiburg
Germany

H. M. Schardey
Department of Surgery
Grosshadern Clinic
Ludwig Maximilian University of Munich
Marchioninistr. 15
81377 Munich
Germany

H. Scheidbach
Department of Surgery
Krankenhausstraße 12
91054 Erlangen
Germany

T. Schiedeck
Department of Surgery
Medical University of Lübeck
Ratzeburger Allee 160
23538 Lübeck
Germany

F. W. Schildberg
Department of Surgery
Grosshadern Clinic
Ludwig Maximilian University of Munich
Marchioninistr. 15
81377 Munich
Germany

C. Schneider
Department of Surgery
Krankenhausstraße 12
91054 Erlangen
Germany

R. Schwetling
Department of Surgery
Buch Berlin Clinic
Hobrechtsfelder Chaussee 100
13122 Berlin
Germany

I. Selmi
Department of General Surgery
S. Agostino Hospital
Modena
Italy

S. Skullman
Department of Medicosurgical
Gastroenterology
University Hospital
58185 Linköping
Sweden

W. Steiner
Grosshadern Clinic
Marchioninistr. 15
81377 Munich
Germany

H. O. Steitz
Department of Surgery
Grosshadern Clinic
Ludwig Maximilian University of Munich
Marchioninistr. 15
81377 Munich
Germany

E. Tamborrino
Department of General Surgery
S. Agostino Hospital
Modena
Italy

B. Ulrich
Düsseldorf-Gerresheim Hospital
Gräulinger Str. 120
40625 Düsseldorf
Germany

J. Waninger
Lörrach Regional Hospital
Spitalstr. 25
79539 Lörrach
Germany

A. Woltmann
Department of Surgery
Medical University of Lübeck
Ratzeburger Allee 160
23538 Lübeck
Germany

S. Zeyfang
Department of Surgery
Evangelische Diakonissenanstalt
Gröpelinger Heerstr. 406/408
28239 Bremen
Germany

I Standards

Surgical Treatment of Chronic Inflammatory Bowel Disease

G. Ruf, H. J. Mappes, and U. Baumgartner

Introduction

Despite the appearance of a fair amount of data on the subject the aetiology and pathogenesis of chronic inflammatory bowel diseases (IBD) – ulcerative colitis and Crohn's disease – are still unknown [1]. The diseases occur in a wide spectrum of patients, affecting all age groups, both sexes alike, with a predominance in the young and middle aged. Symptoms are more often chronic than acute. Cardinal symptoms are diarrhoea and rectal bleeding. The diseases follow a chronic relapsing course, with periods of complete absence of symptoms between attacks. On the other hand, chronic continuous disease is seen in some patients. Extracolonic manifestations such as arthritis, iritis, hepatic dysfunction and skin lesions may occur. The factors affecting the recurrence of attacks are only partly known [2, 3].

The highly variable course of IBD makes an interdisciplinary approach essential. Medial treatment is the basic approach. For treatment of mild or moderate attacks, sulphasalazine is useful, as verified in clinical trials [4]. Sulphasalazine also seems to be effective when used to prevent of recurrence also seems to be effective [5, 6]. The pharmacological mechanism of sulphasalazine remains unclear, but some studies seem to show 5-amino-salicylic acid (5-ASA) to be the active moiety [7]. Corticosteroids are beneficial in the first attack, in relapse and also in severe attacks, but have no preventive effect [8]. With medical treatment many patients with chronic IBD can be kept in reasonably good general health, and most moderate attacks will respond to this management. However, in a substantial number of patients medical treatment fails and surgery becomes necessary. Within 20 years of onset of the disease, about 80 % of patients with Crohn's disease and about 40 % with ulcerative colitis have to undergo surgery. These figures indicate the important role of surgery in the treatment of IBD.

Diagnosis

For the management of IBD, whether conservative or surgical, it is essential to distinguish between ulcerative colitis and Crohn's colitis [9]. The features on which the differential diagnosis is based are the clinical symptoms, radiological and endoscopic signs of continuous or discontinuous involvement of the colon, involvement of the terminal ileum and rectum, and the onset of perianal fistula [10]. Taking these together with the histological study, differentiation is possible in up to 85% of cases. "Indeterminate colitis" is diagnosed in up to 15% [11].

The aims of surgical therapy in ulcerative colitis differ totally from those in Crohn's disease. Involvement of the entire gastrointestinal tract in Crohn's disease reduces surgical strategy to treatment of complications of the disease by intestinal-preserving procedures such as minimal surgery, e.g. stricture-plasty and/or limited resection [12–14]. Because of the involvement of colorectal mucosa on the other hand, ulcerative colitis can be cured by radical surgery. Restorative proctocolectomy combines the removal of the mucosa totally with preserving continence [15–17].

Emergency Surgery

Surgical treatment is indicated in order to restore health to patients with chronic disease, prevent the risk of colon cancer, or to save life during a severe attack.

In patients with a severe attack the indications for surgery can be subdivided into fulminant colitis, perforation, toxic colonic dilatation or severe peranal hemorrhage. Fulminant colitis is present when clinical symptoms such as abdominal colic, tenderness and bloody diarrhoea occur together with dehydration, anaemia, fever and tachycardia [18, 19]. Toxic colonic dilatation is defined by radiological measurement of a colonic diameter of 6 cm or more together with a disturbed or absent haustral pattern. Urgent surgery is necessary in patients with a severe attack of ulcerative colitis not responding to medical treatment, in whom the operation may be postponed for 1 or 2 days. Emergency intervention must be performed with immediate surgery in a critically ill patient. Generally, the mortality associated with toxic colonic dilation is 2–5%; with bowel perforation it goes up to 50% [20–22].

In a severe attack one-stage colectomy is best performed either with a closed rectum (Hartmann's procedure) or formation of a mucous sigmoid fistula [23]. In this procedure most of the diseased mucosa is removed, with an eye to the possibility of a secondary reconstructive procedure [24]. Multiple colonic fistulae, as proposed by Turnbull in patients with toxic colonic dilatation, decompress the colon and avoid spontaneous perforation but do not eliminate the diseased mucosa.

Elective Surgery in Crohn's Colitis

Indications for elective surgical treatment are obstructive symptoms caused by strictures, enterocutaneous fistula, side effects of corticosteroids and chronicity of the disease. In right-sided disease the ileal component often dominates the clinical picture. Left-sided colitis can mimic diverticular disease. Another important indication is anorectal disease complicated by stricture, chronic sepsis, a narrow, contracted, inflamed rectum and destroyed sphincters.

Table 1. Surgical therapy in Crohn's colitis (Department of Surgery, University of Freiburg, 1988–1995)

	Surgical procedures *n*	Subsequent ceolectomy *n*
Limited resection	30	6
Strictureplasty	7	
Hemicolectomy	11	3
Subtotal colectomy	4	
Proctocolectomy	9	
	61	9

Depending on the extent and localisation of the disease, stricture plasty, segmental resection, right or left hemicolectomy, subtotal colectomy or proctocolectomy may be performed. In contrast to the standard resection, where the anastomoses are performed in microscopically involved margins, limited resection means anastomosis in macroscopically involved resection margins. The latter is a well-established procedure in the small bowel [13–14]. Sphincter preservation and restoration of intestinal continuity is the most attractive surgical option in Crohn's colitis. Therefore, minimal surgery (limited resection, strictureplasty) can also be used in Crohn's colitis, as shown by our data (Table 1) and others [25–27].

The morbidity of minimal surgery does not differ from that of standard procedures. At the same time the recurrence rate is not increased, as shown by our patients and others (Table 2). If this strategy is adhered to Crohn's colitis, a definitive stoma is only necessary in the minority of the patients (Table 3).

Table 2. Recurrence rates in Crohn's colitis after limited resection and after standard resection

		Recurrence rate (%)		
		Limited resection	Hemicolectomy	Subtotal colectomy
De Dombal [41]	(*n* = 89)		39.3	
Sanfey et al. [25]	(*n* = 16)	44		
Longo et al. [27]	(*n* = 37)	62		67
Goligher [59]	(*n* = 12)	25		71
Our series	(*n* = 35)	20	36.4	22.2

Table 3. Requirement for a definitive ileostomy after limited resection in Crohn's colitis

Sanfey et al. [25]	25%
Stern et al. [26]	40%
Longo et al. [27]	19%
Our series	22%

Elective Surgery in Ulcerative Colitis

Patient Selection

Indications for elective surgical treatment are failure of medical treatment, chronic continuous disease, strictures, burned-out colitis, confirmed dysplasia of the mucosa, side effects of corticosteroids, confirmed cancer and cancer prophylaxis.

Failure of medical treatment over a prolonged period results in a chronic state of morbidity for the patient [18, 29]. The degree of this morbidity is often not appreciated prior to colectomy. Chronic continuous disease with episodes of acute attacks which does not respond to appropriate medical treatment leads to destruction of the mucosa. Irreversible mucosal damage and fibrosis of the wall (burned-out colitis), similar to a third-degree burn injury of the skin, are followed by colorectal dysfunction with very frequent diarrhoea. Even if it does not restore continence, dramatically improves the patient's general health and quality of life.

The risk of colorectal cancer in ulcerative colitis increases up to 5%–7% after the disease has lasted for more than 10 years [30] (Table 4). There is an agreement that the risk of cancer is influenced by the extent of the colitis, the age of the patient and the severity of the first attack [31]. Controversy exists, however, about the malignant potential of polyps and strictures [32]. Recent studies suggest that prophylactic surgery should be recommended if dysplasia is discovered during surveillance in the case of high-grade dysplasia, persistent low-grade dysplasia, dysplastic mass (broad-based elevation) or polypoid dysplastic lesion [33, 34].

A confirmed diagnosis of colorectal cancer also indicates surgical treatment such as colectomy. On the other hand patients found to have a rectal cancer have often been considered to be unsuited to restorative proctocolectomy. Nevertheless, as long as the principles of cancer surgery can be followed, a pelvic pouch need not to be contraindicated. However, it is important that the mid and/or lower rectum are not severely affected by the carcinoma.

Table 4. Cumulative risk of colorectal cancer (%) in patients with extensive ulcerative colitis

No. of patients	Years after onset				References
	15	20	25	30	
234	9.6	24.2	34	–	Kewenter et al. [42]
267	7.0	11.0	20	30	Greenstein et al. [43]
676	–	–	8.0	20	Prior et al. [44]
959	–	5.0	–	–	Maratka et al. [45]
783	1.1	1.4	–	–	Hendriksen et al. [46]
823	3.0	7.2	11.0	16.5	Gyde et al. [47]
401	3.0	5.0	9.0	–	Lenard-Jones et al. [48]
1161	–	–	3.1	–	Langholz et al. [49]
486	–	7.0	–	–	Gillen et al. [50]

Frequent acute attacks of ulcerative colitis or severe extraintestinal manifestations require high doses of corticosteroids to achieve remission [29]. Adverse effects such as corticosteroid-induced osteoporosis, even to the extent of spontaneous vertebra fractures, can be seen especially in younger patients. Morbidity induced by disease or by long-term medical treatment has to be evaluated individually with respect to the postoperative outcome after restorative protocolectomy.

Contraindications for sphincter-saving procedures are the preoperative presence of faecal incontinence and seriously debilitating coexisting medical conditions. However, the age of the patient is not a limiting factor for restorative proctocolectomy; biological age is more important than chronological age.

Surgical Treatment

The current principle of surgical treatment in ulcerative colitis is radical surgery with total removal of the colorectal mucosa. This can be performed by proctocolectomy with a Brooke ileostomy, by colectomy with ileorectal anastomosis and by restorative proctocolectomy with an ileum pouch anal anastomosis.

Total proctocolectomy, either conservative or an intersphincteric protectomy with a Brooke everted end-ileostomy, remains a satisfactory procedure for inflammatory bowel disease. Ileorectal anastomosis can be considered a safe conservative operation in selected patients with ulcerative colitis. It has certain advantages over some of the alternative sphincter-saving procedures. Functional results are comparable with the pelvic pouch procedure [35, 36]. However, disease of tissue is left in place and recurrence of inflammation and the long-term risk of cancer developing in the rectal stump can be a serious problem. During surveillance more than half of the patients require subsequent rectal excision (Table 5).

Restorative proctocolectomy combines the radicality of proctocolectomy with the functional outcome of ileorectal anastomosis [35, 37]. Ileum pouch

Table 5. Mortality, morbidity and failure of ileorectal anastomosis in ulcerative colitis[a]

	No. of patients	Mortality (%)	Leakage (%)	Failure (%)
Aylett [51]	300	6	12	5
Fazio [52]	157	2	1	–
Gruner et al. [53]	57	7	10	–
Oakley et al. [54]	145	0	2	24
Khubchandani et al. [55]	110	0	2	10
Backer et al. [56]	59	0	0	22
Parc et al. [57]	197	–	–	25
Leijonmarck et al. [58]	60	4	2	57

[a] Failure is defined as the necessity for a permanent ileostomy.

anal anastomosis can be performed by two techniques: the two-stage procedure with procto-mucosectomy and hand-sewn anastomosis with temporary
ileostomy [38], and the one-stage procedure with double-stapling in the transitional zone without ileostomy [39]. The latter procedure reduces morbidity
down to 10 % and improves the early functional results as shown by our data
(Tables 6,7). There is no difference between the two techniques as regards late
functional out-come [37, 40] (Table 8).

Table 6. Comparison of morbidity after hand-sewn versus double-stapling ileonal anastomosis in ulcerative colitis (Department of Surgery, University of Freiburg)

	Hand-sewn (1985 – 1989)	Double stapling (1990 – 1995)
No. of Patients affected	8/23 (34,7%)	4/38 (10,5%)
Wound infection	7	4
Obstruction (reoperated)	2 (2)	0
Leakage (reoperated)	3 (2)	2
Pouch dysfunction (reoperated)	4 (4)	0
Pouchitis	5	0
Stenosis	4	1

Table 7. Comparison of early manometric results (mean and range) after hand-sewn and
double-stapling ileoanal anastomosis in ulcerative colitis (Department of Surgery, University
of Freiburg)

	Preoperative ($n = 61$)	Hand-sewn ($n = 23$)	Double stapling ($n\ 4 = 38$)
Maximum resting pressure (mm Hg)	52.5 (20 – 100)	25.0 (10 – 50)	80.0 (60 – 90)
Maximum squeeze pressure (mm Hg)	110.5 (35 – 210)	80.5 (45 – 150)	120 (110 – 180)

Table 8. Comparison of functional results 9 months after hand-sewn versus double-stapling
ileoanal anastomosis in ulcerative colitis (Department of Surgery, University of Freiburg)

	Hand-sewn ($n = 23$)	Double stapling ($n = 38$)
Stools		
Day	4–7	3–7
Night	0–2	0–2
Minor leakage	4	0
Major leakage	0	0
Pad usage (day)	1	0
Pad usage (night)	4	0

Careful preoperative selection of patients and an individualised approach have made restorative proctocolectomy the best surgical option in ulcerative colitis. It is generally accepted that enthusiasm for this method of sphincter preservation should alter neither the indication for nor thresholds to surgery unless we know more about the long-term outcome and the nature of pouchitis, the major complication after restorative procto-colectomy.

References

1. Jewell DP, Lowes JR (1988) Aetiology and pathogenesis of ulcerative colitis and Crohn's disease. Triangle 27:137–141
2. Mee AS, Jewell DP (1978) Factors inducing relapse in inflammatory bowel disease. Br Med J 2:801–802
3. Rampton DDS, McNeil NI, Sarner M (1983) Analgesic ingestion and other factors preceding relapse in ulcerative colitis. Gut 24:187–189
4. Baron JH, Connell AM, Lennard-Jones JE, Avery Jones F (1965) Sulphasalazine and salicylazosulphadimidine in ulcerative colitis. Lancet i:1094–1096
5. Järenot G (1994) New salicylates as maintenance in ulcerative colitis. Gut 35:1155–1158
6. Lichtenstein GR (1994) Medical therapies for inflammatory bowel disease. Curr Opin Gastroenterol 10:390–403
7. Jewell DP, Truelove SC (1988) The first international symposium on olsalazine in the treatment of ulcerative colitis. Scand J Gastroenterol 23 [suppl 148]
8. Lennard-Jones JE, Misiewicz JJ, Connell AM, Baron JH, Avery Jones F (1965) Prednisone as maintenance treatment for ulcerative colitis in remission. Lancet i:188–189
9. Petit S, Irving MH (1992) Non-specific inflammatory bowel disease. Br Med J 304:1367–1379
10. Tanaka M, Riddell RH (1990) The pathological diagnosis and differential diagnosis of Crohn's disease. Hepatogastroenterol 37:18–31
11. Price AB (1978) Overlap in the spectrum of nonspecific inflammatory bowel disease – "colitis indeterminata". J Clin Pathol 31:567–577
12. Lee ECG, Papaioannou N (1982) Minimal surgery for chronic obstruction in patients with extensive or universal Crohn's disease. Ann R Coll Surg Engl 64:229–234
13. Fazio VW, Tjandra JJ (1993) Strictureplasty for Crohn's disease with multiple long strictures. Dis Colon Rectum 36:71–72
14. Alexander-Williams J, Hauynes IG (1985) Conservative operations for Crohn's disease of the small bowel. World J Surg 9:945–951
15. Parks AG, Nicholls RJ (1978) Proctocolectomy without ileostomy for ulcerative colitis. Br Med J 2:85–88
16. Utsunomiya J, Iwama T, Matsuo M, Sawai S, Yaegashi K, Hirayama R (1980) Total colectomy, mucosal proctectomy and ileoanal anatomosis. Dis Colon Rectum 23:459–466
17. Fonkalsrud EW (1987) Update on clinical experience with different surgical techniques of the endorectal pull-through operation for colitis and polyposis. Surg Gynecol Obstet 165:309–316
18. Farmer RG, Hawk WA, Turnbull RB (1976) Indications for surgery in Crohn's disease. Gastroenterology 71:245–250
19. Tytgat GN, Meuwissen S, Huibregtse K, Bartelsmann JF (1981) Colonoscopy in flammatory bowel disease. In: Rechmilewitz D (ed) Inflammatory bowel disease. Nijhoff, The Hayner, pp 217–237
20. Binder SC, Patterson JF, Glotzer DJ (1974) Toxic megacolon in ulcerative colitis. Gastroenterology 66:909–915
21. Fazio VW (1980) Toxic megacolon in ulcerative colitis and Crohn's colitis. Clin Gastroenterol 9:389–407

22. Greenstein AJ, Sachar DB, Gibs A (1985) Outcome of toxic dilatation in ulcerative and Crohn's colitis. J Clin Gastroenterol 7:137–144
23. Frykholm G, Påhlmann L, Enblad P, Krog M, Ejerblad S (1989) Early outcome after emergency and elective surgery for ulcerative colitis. Acta Chir Scand 155:601–605
24. Goligher JC (1954) Primary excisional surgery in the treatment of ulcerative colitis. Ann R Coll Surg Engl 15:316–325
25. Sanfey H, Bayless TM, Cameron JC (1984) Crohn's disease of the colon: is there a role for limited resection? Am J Surg 147:38–42
26. Stern HS, Goldberg SM, Rothenberger DA (1984) Segmental versus total colectomy for large bowel Crohn's disease. World J Surg 8:118–122
27. Longo WE, Ballantyne GH, Cabow CE (1988) Treatment of Crohn's colitis: segmental or total colectomy? Arch Surg 123:588–590
28. Jewell DP (1988) Medical management of severe ulcerative colitis. Int J Colon Dis 3:186–189
29. Truelove SC (1989) Medical treatment of ulcerative colitis and indications for colectomy. World J Surg 12:142–147
30. Farthmann EH, Baumgartner U, Imdahl A, Ruf G (1995) Surgery in ulcerative colitis. In: Fleig WE (ed) Inflammatory bowel diseases. Kluwer, Dordrecht, pp 259–270
31. Ohmann U (1982) Colorectal carcinoma in patients with ulcerative colitis. Am J Surg 144:344–349
32. Gumaste V, Sachar DB, Greenstein AJ (1992) Benign and malignant colorectal strictures in ulcerative colitis. Gut 33:938–941
33. Bernstein CN, Shanahan F, Weinstein WM (1994) Are we telling patients the truth about surveillance colonoscopy in ulcerative colitis? Lancet 243:71–74
34. Vermulapalli R, Lancer P (1994) Cancer surveillance in ulcerative colitis: more of the same or progress? Gastroenterology 107:934–944
35. Pemberton JF, Kelly KA, Beart RA, Dozois RR, Wolff BG, Ilstrup P (1987) Ileal pouch-anal anastomosis for chronic ulcerative colitis: long-term results. Ann Surg 206:504–513
36. Wexner SD, Jensen L, Tothemnberger DA, Wong WD, Goldberg SM (1989) Long-term functional analysis of the ileal reservoir. Dis Colon Rectum 32:275–281
37. Järvinen HJ, Luukkonen P (1991) Comparison of restorative proctocolectomy with and without covering ileostomy in ulcerative colitis. Br J Surg 78:323–325
38. Nicholls RJ, Pezim ME (1985) Restorative protocolectomy with ileal reservoir for ulcerative colitis and familiar adenomatous polyposis. A comparison of three reservoir designs. Br J Surg 72:470–475
39. Keighley MRB, Winslet MC, Yoshioka K, Lightwood R (1987) Discriminations not impaired by excision of the anal transition zone after restorative proctocolectomy. Br J Surg 74:1118–1121
40. O'Connell PR, Pemberton JH, Brown ML, Kelly KA (1987) Determinants of stool frequency after ileal pouch-anal anastomosis. Am J Surg 153:157–162
41. De Dombal FT, Watts JM, Watkinson G, Goligher JC (1966) Local complications of ulcerative colitis: structure, pseudopolypsosis and carcinoma of the colon and rectum. Br Med J 1:1442–1447
42. Kewenter J, Ahlman H, Hulten L (1978) Cancer risk in ulcerative colitis. Ann Surg 15:824–828
43. Greenstein AJ, Sachar DB, Smith H, Pucillo A, Papatestas AE, Kreel I, Geller SA, Janowitz HD, Aufses AH Jr (1979) Cancer in universal and left-sided ulcerative colitis: factors determining risk. Gastroenterology 77:290–294
44. Prior P, Gyde SN, Macartney JC, Thompson H, Waterhouse JAH, Allan RN (1982) Cancer morbidity in ulcerative colitis. Gut 23:490–497
45. Maratka Z, Nedbal J, Kocianova J, Hevelka J, Kudrmann J, Hendl J (1985) Incidence of colorectal cancer in proctocolitis: a retrospective study of 959 cases over 40 years. Gut 26:43–49
46. Hendriksen C, Kreiner S, Binder V (1985) Long term prognosis in ulcerative colitis – based on results from a regional patient group from the county of Copenhagen. Gut 26:158–163

47. Gyde SN, Prior P, Allan RN, Stevens A, Jewell DP, Truelove SC, Lofberg R, Brostrom O, Hellers G (1988) Colorectal cancer in ulcerative colitis: a cohort study of primary referrals from three centers. Gut 29:206–217
48. Lenard-Jones JE, Melville DM, Morson BC, Williams CB (1990) Precancer and cancer in extensive ulcerative colitis: findings among 401 patients over 22 years. Gut 31:800–806
49. Langholz E, Munkholm P, Davidsen M, Binder V (1992) Colorectal cancer risk and mortality in patients with ulcerative colitis. Gastroenterology 103:1444–1451
50. Gillen CD, Walmsley RS, Prior P, Andrews HA, Allan RN (1994) Ulcerative colitis and Crohn's disease: a comparison of the colorectal cancer in extensive colitis. Gut 35:1590–1592
51. Aylett SO (1966) Three hundred cases of diffuse ulcerative colitis treated by total colectomy and ileorectal anastomosis. BMJ 1:1001–1005
52. Fazio VW, Turnbull RB Jr, Goldsmith MG (1975) Ileorectal anastomosis: a safe surgical technique. Dis Colon Rectum 18:107–114
53. Gruner OP, Flamansk A, Naas R et al. (1975) Ileorectal anastomosis and ulcerative colitis. Scand J Gastroenterol 10:641–646
54. Oakley JR, Jagelman DG, Fazio VW et al. (1985) Complications and quality of life after ileorectal anastomosis for ulcerative colitis. Am J Surg 149:23–30
55. Khubchandani IT, Sandfort MR, Rosen L, Sheets JA, Stasik JJ, Riether RD (1985) Current status of ileorectal anastomosis for inflammatory bowel disease. Dis Colon Rectum 32:400–403
56. Backer O, Hjortrup A, Kjaergaard AM (1988) Evaluation of ileorectal anastomosis for the treatment of ulcerative proctitis. J R Soc Med 81:210–211
57. Parc R, Legrand M, Frileux P et al. (1989) Comparative clinical results of ileal-pouch anal anastomosis and ileorectal anastomosis in ulcerative colitis. Hepatogastroenterology. 36:235–239
58. Leijonmarck CE, Persson PG, Hellers G (1990) Factors affecting colostomy rate in ulcerative colitis: an epidemiologic study 31:329–333
59. Goligher JC (1988) Surgical treatment of Crohn's disease affecting mainly or entirely the large bowel. World J Surg 12:186–190

Therapeutic Strategy in Sigmoid Diverticulitis:
A Survey of German Surgical Departments

B. Ulrich

Diverticulitis is one of the most common diseases of the large bowel today and is becoming increasingly prevalent with the alteration in the age profile [26, 27]. In 1973, Reifferscheid [25] spoke of diverticulitis as a public health problem. The disease was first described in detail by Graser [7] in 1899. As a pathologist, he distinguished between diverticulosis as an uncomplicated alteration due to age and diverticulitis with sometimes fatal complications. In order to prevent life-threatening complications, many surgeons argue in favour of early resection for chronically recurring diverticulitis [3, 10, 12, 17, 21, 23, 24]. There is still disagreement about the mode of action in complicated diverticulitis. The choice of the correct operative procedure depends on the indication, the patient's general condition and not least the patient's age. One-, two- or three-stage resection procedures and simple fashioning of a colostomy have been and will be discussed continously. However, a risk adjusted treatment strategy seems necessary and should be clarified by the experiences revealed by the survey of German surgical departments reported below.

Methods

The survey, which covered 1422 general hospital surgical departments contained in the 1991 list of German hospitals or the 1992 list of the Association of German Surgeons e.V., was performed by sending out a questionnaire on the treatment of sigmoid diverticulitis in December 1992. The questionnaire was divided into sections on

(1) conservative management,
(2) operative management and
(3) patients.

With regard to conservative management, questions were asked concerning diagnosis (clinical, contrast studies, colonoscopy) and treatment (parenteral nutrition, antibiotics). The questions about operative treatment included the time of operation and peri-operative management. The main emphasis of the questions was on the procedure chosen in elective surgery and the operative procedures in the various indications for an emergency operation. In answering questions about their own patients, the hospitals could choose between giving estimated and actual numbers of patients with sigmoid diverticulitis.

Results

Replies were received from 749 (52.6%) of the 1422 surgeons to whom the questionnaire was sent. The surgical departments consisted of 20 university hospitals (2.7%), 159 teaching hospitals (TH; 21.5%) and 454 general hospitals (60.6%). The remaining questionnaires had not been stamped by the sender so these hospitals could not be assigned to any of the three groups (15.5%) (Fig. 1).

With reference to the diagnosis, there were no differences between the different types of hospital. Between 81.5% and 100% of the hospitals in each group said that the diagnosis was made clinically. A barium enema was carried out by 23.3% – 35%, 14% being done on admission and 86% at a later time. Data regarding a Gastrografin enema varied between 61.5% and 78%, but this was carried out in 60% at the time of admission. The diagnosis of diverticulitis was confirmed by colonoscopy in 61.3% – 68.3% of the hospitals. An abdominal CT scan was performed in only 0.2% of cases, and ultra sonography contributed to confirmation of the diagnosis in 1.1% – 5% (Table 1).

There were no differences between the different types of hospital with regard to parenteral nutrition and antibiotics either. Ninety percent of the uni-

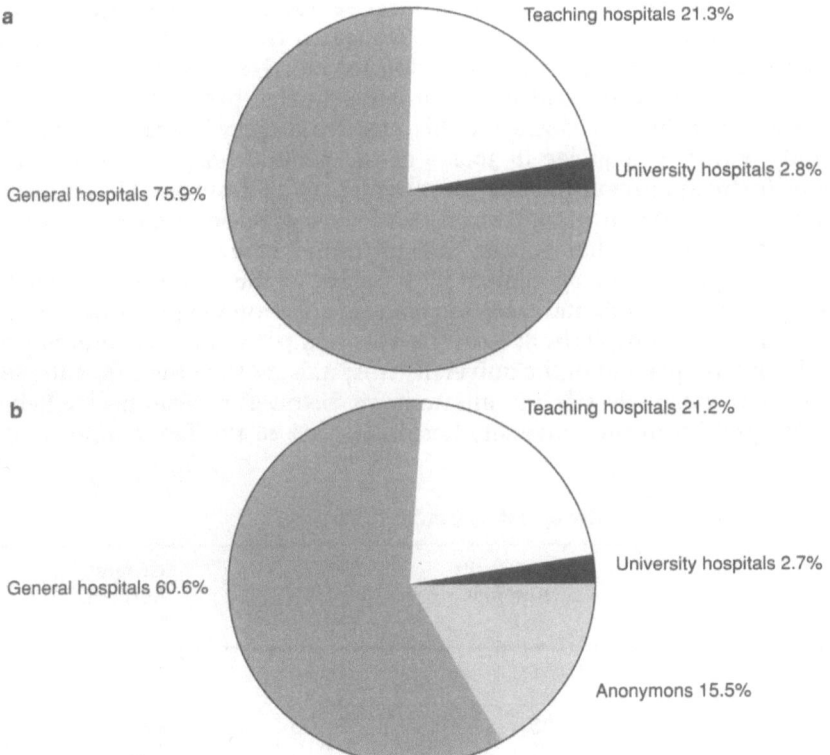

Figure 1. a Distribution of the questionnaires sent to 1422 surgical departments. **b** Distribution of the replies (*n* = 746) received

Table 1. Methods of diagnosis of sigmoid diverticulitis

	University hospitals (%)	THs (%)	General hospitals (%)
Clinical	100	84.9	81.5
Barium enema	35	23.3	34.8
Gastrografin enema	70	78.0	61.5
Colonoscopy	65	61.6	68.3
Ultrasonography	5	3.1	1.1
Abdominal CT	0	0.0	0.2

THs, Teaching hospitals.

versities, 95.6% of the THs and 91.2% of the general hospitals gave parenteral nutrition as part of conservative treatment. The duration of parenteral nutrition was decided according to clinical symptoms in nearly 90% of hospitals. During conservative treatment, antibiotics were administered by 93% overall (80% nitroimidazole, 45% penicillin and approx. 30% cephalosporin).

When asked about the time of the elective operation (Table 2), 65% of the university hospitals and 50% of the THs stated that they regard the second episode of diverticulitis as an indication for elective surgery, while only 5% and 15.1% respectively wait until the late sequelae before they consider an operation indicated. In contrast to this, elective surgery is regarded as indicated only with late sequelae in 30.4% of the general hospitals. Perioperative management appears uniform. Ninety percent of all those questioned perform orthograde irrigation preoperatively and 95% give perioperative antibiotic prophylaxis (60% cephalosporin, 50% nitroimidazole and 30% penicillin).

There appears to be agreement with regard to the operative procedure in elective surgery. Segmental resection without colostomy is performed in 100% of the university hospitals, 87% of the THs and 95% of the general hospitals (Table 3). Fifty percent of the university hospitals, 26% of the THs and 18% of the general hospitals site the anastomosis below the peritoneal reflection. Seventy percent of the university hospitals, 50% of the THs and 40% of the

Table 2. Indication for elective operation (timing of surgery)

	University hospitals (%)	THs (%)	General hospitals (%)
Immediate	15	11.3	9.0
Second episode	65	55.3	42.5
Third episode	15	12.6	13.4
Fourth episode	0	1.9	3.5
When late sequelae occur	5	15.1	30.4

Table 3. Operative procedure in elective surgery

	University hospitals (%)	THs (%)	General hospitals (%)
Segmental resection without colostomy	100	87.5	94.8
Segmental resection with colostomy	5	2.6	10.5
Schloffer operation (three-stage)	0	0.6	0
Hartmann operation	0	0	0.7
Primary colostomy, secondary resection	0	0	0.2
No information	0	7.6	6.6

Multiple entries possible.

general hospitals state that they prefer a hand-sutured anatomosis to a stapled one.

There were also only slight differences with regard to perioperative management in the emergency operations. Orthograde bowel irrigation is not performed preoperatively with an emergency procedure in any of the university hospitals, but is done in 4.5 % of the THs and 3.3 % of the general hospitals. However, 45 % of the university hospitals, 30 % of the THs and 24 % of the general hospitals perform intraoperative lavage.

Perioperative antibiotic prophylaxis is required by 100 % of the university hospitals and 98 % of the other hospitals. The operative strategy in emergency operations is similar only in cases of a bleeding diverticulum, when 85 % of the university hospitals, 87 % of the THs and 76 % of the general hospitals perform a segmental resection without colostomy. In the presence of obstruction or high-grade stenosis, 65 % of the universities but only 42 % of the THs and 33 % of the general hospital do not fashion a protective colostomy along with sigmoid resection. A primary colostomy without resection is performed by 5 % of the universities, 18 % of the THs and 24 % of the general hospitals in cases of obstruction (Table 4).

A segmental resection without colostomy is performed in cases of sealed perforation with local peritonitis in 80 % of university hospitals, but only in 15 % in the event of a free perforation and generalized faecal peritonitis (Tables 5, 6). For the latter, 80 % of the university hospitals and THs prefer a Hartmann procedure. However, 20 % of the THs and 28 % of the general hospitals state that they perform a non-resecting procedure only in the presence of free perforation and generalized peritonitis (e.g. laparotomy and oversewing or construction of a colostomy). This option is not chosen by any of the university hospitals.

With regard to patient numbers, 60 % of the university hospitals, 34 % of the THs and 25 % of the general hospitals stated that they had counted the number of patients. All other and the actual numbers of cases of diverticulitis per year reported by both the university hospitals and the THs and general hospitals. Out of an average of 35 cases of diverticulitis per year in the university hospitals (Fig. 2), 71 % were treated operatively (25 % as emergencies). In the THs

Table 4. Operative procedure in cases of obstruction (ileus)

	University hospitals (%)	THs (%)	General hospitals (%)
Segmental resection without colostomy	65	41.5	32.8
Segmental resection with colostomy	30	31.4	24.9
Schloffer operation (three-stage)	15	11.9	11.7
Hartmann operation	35	20.8	20.7
Laboratomy, oversewing	0	0	0.4
Primary colostomy, secondary resection	5	18.2	24
No information	0	1.3	4.2

Multiple entries possible.

Table 5. Operative procedure in cases of sealed perforation with localized peritonitis

	University hospitals (%)	THs (%)	General hospitals (%)
Segmental resection without colostomy	80	62.3	55.9
Segmental resection with colostomy	10	18.9	21.1
Schloffer operation (three-stage)	0	0.6	3.3
Hartmann operation	25	23.3	15.4
Laboratomy, oversewing	0	2.5	13.7
Primary colostomy, secondary resection	5	2.5	7.5
No information	0	0.6	4.0

Multiple entries possible.

Table 6. Operative procedure in cases of free perforation with generalized or faecal peritonitis

	University hospitals (%)	THs (%)	General hospitals (%)
Segmental resection without colostomy	15	5	6.2
Segmental resection with colostomy	30	13.8	17
Schloffer operation (three-stage)	5	4.4	8.4
Hartmann operation	80	79.2	57.9
Laboratomy, oversewing	0	10.7	11.1
Primary colostomy, secondary resection	0	9.4	17.2
No information	0	0	2

Multiple entries possible.

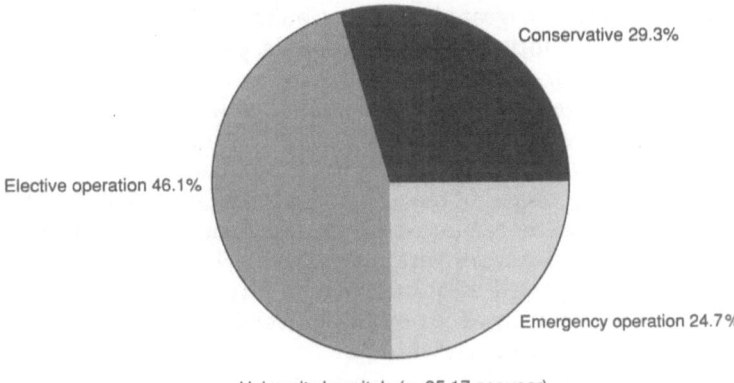

University hospitals (n=35.17 per year)

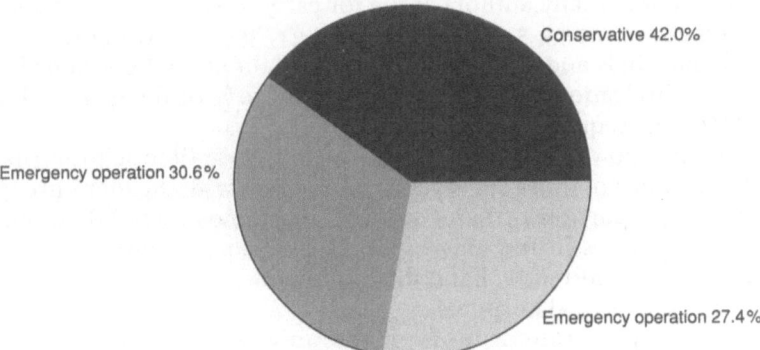

Teaching hospitals (n=44.17 per year)

General hospitals (n=22.3 per year)

Figure 2. Preparation of cases of diverticulitis treated conservatively or by elective or emergency surgery in the different types of hospital

63 % of the 44 cases were treated by operation (23 % as emergencies). Out of 21 patients with diverticulitis in general hospitals, 58 % were treated operatively, (27 % as emergencies).

With regard to the features of patients with diverticulitis, 80 % of those questioned stated that the patients were obese. Twenty percent of the university hospitals, 14.5 % of the THs and 13 % of the general hospitals mentioned Saint's triad. Fifteen percent of the university hospitals, 3 % of the THs and 3 % of the general hospitals noted immunosuppression as a frequent characteristic in patients with complicated diverticulitis. Five percent of the THs and 5 % of the general hospitals stated that patients with diverticulitis had often been on a diet, but this was not observed by the university hospitals. All other symptoms were mentioned only very rarely.

Discussion

Assessing the results of the survey of German surgical departments in regard to the treatment of sigmoid diverticulitis, it is noticeable that there is widespread agreement about diagnostic methods and conservative treatment. Apart from clinical diagnosis, Gastrografin enema in the early acute phase and colonoscopy and barium enema later in the course of the illness play the dominant role in diagnosis (Table 1) [18, 28, 35]. Colonoscopy as a rule does not play an important part in acute diverticulitis. However, it is essential preoperatively in every patient in order to rule out the presence of a coexisting carcinoma either in the previously inflamed area or in another part of the colon.

The low use of ultra sonography in the diagnosis of acute diverticulitis is striking (max. 5 %). Markedly higher rats are quoted in the literature [28, 31, 32, 36]. Hardly any of the hospitals surveyed used abdominal CT to assess the extent of the inflammatory process [2, 8]. With regard to conservative treatment, a treatment plan using parenteral nutrition and antibiotic cover is obviously universal.

In elective surgery, primary segment resection without colostomy is undoubtedly the method of choice. There are differences only with regard to the time of operation. Many authors argue for early resection to avoid life-threatening complications [3, 5, 10, 12, 15, 17, 23, 24, 35]. Accordingly, 65 % of the university hospitals and 55 % of the THs regard the second episode of diverticulitis as an indication for surgery, while only 30 % of the general hospitals consider the late sequelae as indication.

Preoperative bowel irrigation and perioperative antibiotic prophylaxis are employed by most of those surveyed, which agrees with the literature [30].

The large proportion of hand-sutured anastomoses (70 %) compared to stapled anastomoses in the universities is conspicuous. Fifty percent of the anastomoses are sutured by hand during elective operations in the THs and only 40 % in the general hospitals.

In emergency operations, 45 % of the universities prefer intraoperative lavage, compared to 30 % of the THs and 24 % of the general hospitals. Some authors [1, 20] recommend this as standard practice.

In agreement with the literature [14, 15, 16], resection with primary anastomosis and without colostomy is undertaken by all the hospitals in the treatment of a bleeding diverticulum. In the presence of obstruction or a high-grade stenosis, the proportion of resections without colostomy is markedly higher in the university hospitals at 65 % than in the THs (42 %) and the general hospitals (33 %) (Table 4).

We expected to obtain the most important information from the method by which the different hospitals deal with sealed and free perforation.

Despite a clear trend in the literature towards sigmoid resection without colostomy for sealed perforation and localized peritonitis (Table 6), the procedure in the presence of a free perforation with generalized or faecal peritonitis varies very widely [4, 6, 9, 11, 13, 16, 22, 29, 33, 34, 35]. Until the 1970s, emergency surgery for complicated diverticulitis was limited in many hospitals to the fashioning of a colostomy only or oversewing and drainage or a combination of these.

Since the introduction of primary treatment by resection for perforated diverticulitis, with the consequent drop in the number of non-resecting procedures, a dramatic decrease in mortality in the emergency surgical treatment of diverticulitis was recorded [16]. Obviously, there is consensus with regard to the necessity of primary resection to remove the infective focus from the infected peritoneal cavity. The debate about the risk of primary anastomosis with and without a protective colostomy persists in the literature, however. Correspondingly, the survey shows that 80 % of university hospitals and THs compared to 60 % of the general hospitals prefer the Hartmann operation for free perforation with generalized peritonitis, while the general hospitals still prefer a non-resecting procedure in 28 % of such cases.

The advantage of the Hartmann operation is seen by most authors [6, 9, 11, 13, 34] as consisting of the removal of the inflamed and complication-prone segment of bowel while avoiding the risk of a primary anastomosis. The abnormal microcirculation and generalized clinical picture in diffuse purulent or faecal peritonitis are regarded as high risk factors for undisturbed healing of an anastomosis. On the other hand, this procedure necessitates a second operation (with all the risks) to restore bowel continuity, which is why some authors [19, 33] argue in favour of primary resection with primary anastomosis even in complicated sigmoid diverticulitis.

Both this survey of German surgical departments and comparison with the literature demonstrate that the preoperative diagnosis, conservative treatment and elective surgical management of diverticulitis are largely standardized nowadays. The only controversial aspect is the treatment of the sometimes life-threatening complications of diverticulitis. The therapeutic strategy in the operative treatment of this dangerous condition must obviously be assessed individually according to risk and benefit, a careful overview, the severity and extent of the local findings, and on the basis of the patient's general condition and age. Our survey, coupled with review of the literature, shows the following risk adjusted treatment strategies for sigmoid diverticulitis:

1. Conservative management in cases of uncomplicated diverticulitis.
2. Elective resection during an inflammation-free interval after the second inflammatory episode or in high-risk patients.

3. Resection and primary anastomosis for sealed or free perforation with localized peritonitis or for diverticular haemorrhage.
4. Hartmann operation for free perforation with generalised or faecal peritonitis.

References

1. Allen-Mersh TG (1993) Should primary anastomosis and on-table colonic lavage be standard treatment for left colon emergencies? Ann R Coll Surg Engl 75:195
2. Ambrosetti P, Robert J et al. (1992) Prognostic factors form computed tomography in acute left colonic diverticulitis. Br J Surg 79:117
3. Brückner R (1977) Kolondivertikulitis – Indikation zur Operation und Ergebnisse. Leber Magen Darm 7:108
4. Bryne JJ, Hennessy V Jr (1972) Diverticulitis of the colon. Surg Clin North Am 4:991
5. Elfink RJ, Midema BW (1992) Colonic diverticula. Postgrd Med 92:97
6. Gall F (1989) Akute Divertikultis mit diffuser Peritonitis – Kann man sich dem Plädoyer für die einzeitige Resektion mit primärer Anastomose vorbehaltlos anschließen? Langenbecks Arch Chir 374:257
7. Graser E (1899) Entzündliche Stenose des Dickdarms bedingt durch Perforation multipler falscher Divertikel. Zentralbl Chir 25:40
8. Hachigian MP, Salvati EP et al. (1992) Computed tomography in the initial management of acute left-sided diverticulitis. Dis Colon Rectum 35:1123
9. Hesterberg R, Zoedler T, Schmidt U, Wellmann K (1988) Operative Behandlung der akuten Sigmadivertikulitis. Langenbecks Arch Chir [Suppl II] (Proceedings volume):593
10. Hohenberger W, Husemann B, Hemming F (1988) Komplikationen der Divertikulitis: Rechtzeitig zur Operation entscheiden. Notfallmed 8:739
11. Hold M, Denck H, Bull P (1990) Surgical management of perforating diverticular disease in Austria. Int J Colorectal Dis 5:195
12. Hollender LF, Meyer C, Bur F, Marie A (1974) Plädoyer für die Frühresektion der Sigmadivertikulitis Symposium Aachen 1973. In: Reifferscheid M (ed) Colondivertikulitis. Thieme, Stuttgart
13. Hollender LF, Meyer C et al. (1987) Tactique opératoire face aux complications aignës des diverticules du sigmoïd. Chirurgie 113:237
14. Huber MA, Woisetschläger, H Sulzbacher H, Wayand W (1991) Die operative Therapie der komplizierten Divertikelerkrankung. Zentralbl Chir 116:999
15. Jones D (1992) Diverticular disease. BMJ 304:1435
16. Karavias Th, Hager K, Ernst M, Dollinger U (1993) Wandel in der Chirurgie der Divertikulitis. Zentralbl Chir 118:76
17. Kümmerle F, Brückner R, Fuchs HF, Ottenjahn R, Painter NS, Reilly M (1980) Klinik und Therapie der Divertikulitis des Dickdarms. Dtsch Med Wochenschr 105:661
18. McKee RF, Deignan RW, Krukowski ZH (1993) Radiological investigations in acute diverticulitis. Br J Surg 80:560
19. Medina VA, Papanicolaou GK et al. (1991) Acute perforated diverticulitis primary resection and anastomosis? Conn Med 258
20. Murray JJ, Schoetz DJ et al. (1991) Intraoperative colonic lavage an primary anastomosis in nonelective colon resection. Dis Colon Rectum 34:527
21. Nordmann O (1926) Die Entwicklung der Darmchirurgie in den letzten 25 Jahren. Langenbecks Arch Chir 142:312
22. Peoples JB, Vilk DR, Maguire JP, Elliot DW (1990) Reassessment of primary resection of the perforated segment of severe colonic diverticulitis. Am J Surg 159:291
23. Philipp J (1978) Behandlung der Divertikelerkrankung des Kolon. Dtsch Med Wochenschr 103:995
24. Reifferscheid M (1967) Pathogenese der Sigmadivertikulitis und Indikation zur Resektionsbehandlung. Langenbecks Arch Chir 318:134

25. Reifferscheid M (ed) (1974) Vorwort – Kolondivertikulitis – Aktuelle Probleme der Diagnostik und Therapie. Symposium Aachen 1973, Thieme Stuttgart
26. Reifferscheid M (1982) Kolondivertikel. In: Vosschulte (ed) Lehrbuch der Chirurgie. Thieme Stuttgart
27. Riemann JF, Hoerder K, Rödl W (1983) Diverticulose. Intern Welt 58:91
28. Riemann JF (1990) Kolondivertikulitis. Ergeb der Gastroenterologie 25:104
29. Rodkey GV, Welch CE (1974) Coloic diverticular disease with surgical treatment. A study of 338 cases. Surg Clin North Am 54:665
30. Schwenk W, Böhm B, Stock W (1992) Perioperative Behandlung von elektiven kolorektalen Resektionen in Deutschland. Zentralbl Chir 117:403
31. Schwerck WB, Schwarz S, Rothmund M (1992) Sonography in acute colonic diverticulitis. Dis Colon Rectum 35:1077
32. Schwerck WB, Schwarz S, Rothmund M, Arnold R (1993) Kolondivertikulitis: bildgebende Diagnostik mit Ultraschall – eine prospektive Studie. Z Gastroeneterol 294
33. Wedell J, Banzhaf G, Mrohs A, Fischer R (1989) Plädoyer für die primäre Resektion mit primärer Anastomose bei der komplizierten Sigmadivertikulitis. Langenbecks Arch Chir 374:259
34. Wherli H, Sulser T, Akovbiantz A (1993) Notfalleingriffe bei komplizierten Kolondivertikulose. Zentralbl Chir 112:1538
35. Wehrli H (1991) Die Divertikelkrankheit: Wann soll operiert werden? Ther Umsch 48:480
36. Wilson StR, Toi A (1990) The value of sonography in the diagnosis of acute diverticulitis of the colon. AJR Am J Roentgenol 154:1199

Changing Standards in Our Practice of Rectal Cancer Surgery

J. Faller, G. István, and I. Berki

Although sphincter-saving procedures were developed a century ago, Miles abdomino-perineal excision became the "gold standard" in rectal cancer surgery. Recent advances in mechanical sutures and surgical techniques together with improved understanding of the loco-regional spread of rectal neoplasms has led to marked changes in the field of rectal cancer surgery. Restorative resections have proved to be as safe as abdomino-perineal excision in terms of operative mortality, morbidity and long-term oncological results. The sphincter-saving procedures have extended downward, being currently adopted not only for cancers of the middle third, but also proving their feasibility in tumors of the distal third of the rectum.

Considering that in our own department the rate of sphincter preservation was only 44 % in 1989 and 21 % in 1990, with virtually all distal tumors treated by abdomino-perineal excision until 1991, and knowing that the rate of sphincter preservation was only 36 % among the total of 811 rectal cancers resected in Hungary in 1992, one is forced to suspect that the „gold standard" was respected a little bit too much.

Since the early 1990s we have been making continuous efforts to change our treatment policy in accordance with modern international standards. The aim of the present study was to evaluate the effectiveness of these efforts, exclusively form the point of view of sphincter preservation.

The records of all patients who have had rectal cancer surgically removed in the Surgical Department of the Szt. János Hospital between January 1989 and October 1995 were reviewed. The surgical procedures used were analysed according to the site of the tumor.

The number of rectal cancers we operated on each year was around 20 (Fig. 1). The relatively small number can be explained by the fact that our department is one of 15 surgical departments in Budapest, all of them dealing in some way with rectal surgery. It seems evident that a concentration of rectal cancer patients in specialized surgical units with greater experience would be of benefit.

The techniques used are summarized in Table 1. 1990 was a "black" year for anal sphincters, with 19 abdomino-perineal excisions against only 4 anterior resections. After this disaster, a continuous decrease in the rate of abdominal perineal excisions is seen. The great change occurred in 1994; the year we adopted two new procedures: the low anterior resection whit coloanal anastomosis, either by the endoanal or abdominal (double stapling) approach, and the abdomino-transsphincteric resection. I shall make further comments on this second procedure later.

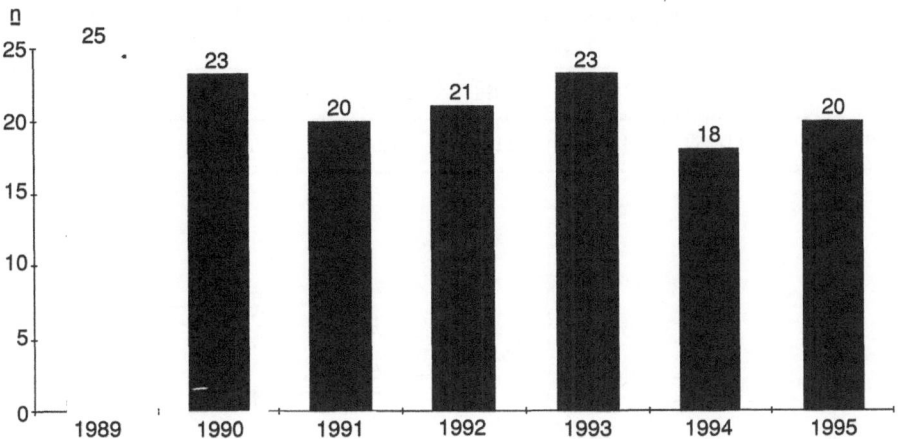

Figure 1. Number of surgically removed rectal carcinomas in the years 1989 to 1995 (Szt. János Hospital, Budapest)

Table 1. Surgical treatment of rectal cancer: techniques used in our department

	1989	1990	1991	1992	1993	1994	1995
Abdominoperineal excision	14	19	9	9	8	6	4
Local excision	2	–	3	1	1	2	–
Anterior resection	9	4	8	11	14	6	9
Low anterior resection (CAA)	–	–	–	–	–	2	2
Abdomino-transsphincteric resection	–	–	–	–	–	2	5
Total	25	23	20	21	23	18	20

Table 2 and Fig. 2 present the rates of sphincter preservation in each year of the period studied. We feel that the progress made is evident and the rate of 16/20 sphincters preserved this years seems acceptable. Furthermore, two of the four abdominoperineal excisions performed this year are prepared of the "gracilis neosphincter" procedure.

Table 3 and Fig. 3 show the same data broken down according to the three thirds of the rectum. It can be seen that restorative resection gradually "conquered" the middle, then the lower third. No abdomino-perineal excision has been performed for tumor of the proximal third in the last 3 years.

One of the most important factors that makes these low resections possible is the suture technique. Table 4 presents the types of sutures used. The biggest change is the introduction of Knigth and Griffen's double stapling technique.

Table 2. Sphincter-saving procedures as a proportion of total number of surgically treated cases of rectal cancer

	1989	1990	1991	1992	1993	1994	1995
SSP/Total	11/25	4/19	11/20	12/21	15/23	12/18	16/20

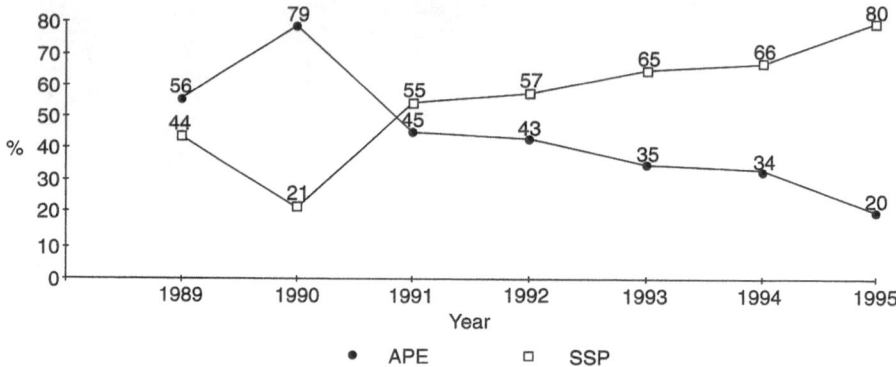

Figure 2. Development over time of percentages of sphincter-saving procedures (SSP, *open squares*) versus abdominal-perineal excisions (APE, *closed circles*) performed in the treatment of rectal carcinoma

The late appearance of this procedure in our practice must also be viewed through the (dark) glasses of the price of the staplers ...

We will now mention some aspects of the abdomino-transsphincteric resection. We perform this operation according to the description of Lazorthes of Toulouse. The patient lies in right lateral position with the left leg elevated. The abdominal approach is performed through an oblique left inferior incision, and the dissection of the rectum is performed as in anterior resection. The unusual position of the patient does not in any way affect the feasibility of the dissection. The operation is then continued by an ano-sacral incision, followed by removal of the coocyx and division of the levator ani muscle. The external sphincters are also divided. Through this wide perineal route the dissection of the inferior third of the rectum and that of the anal canal can be performed with great accuracy and safety. The colo-anal anastomosis, either straight or on the colonic pouch, can be performed by hand-sewn or stapled suture. The sphincters and the pelvic floor are restored and the anastomosis is protected by a loop colostomy for 6–8 weeks. The small experience we have with this procedure suggests that it is a safe way to perform sphincter-saving resection for tumors of the distal rectum when low anterior resection is technically impossible. The functional results are also good.

Finally, we must assure the reader that – of course – preservation of the sphincter is not our ultimate aim. The most important thing remains the cure

Table 3. Sphincter-saving procedures as a proportion of total numbers of surgically treated cases of cancer in the different parts of the rectum

	1989	1990	1991	1992	1993	1994	1995
Proximal third	8/9	4/7	6/7	7/8	10/10	4/4	5/5
Middle third	3/9	0/8	4/10	4/6	4/5	4/4	4/4
Distal third	0/7	0/8	1/3	1/7	1/8	4/10	7/11

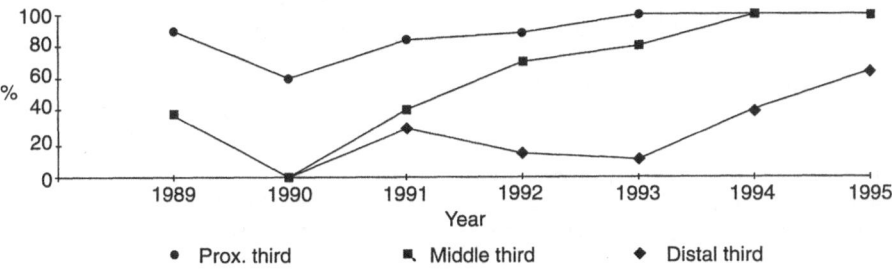

Figure 3. Development over time of rats of sphincter preservation in the surgical treatment of cancer in the different parts of the rectum

Table 4. Changes in suturing technique after rectal resection in our department

	1989	1990	1991	1992	1993	1994	1995
Manual	3	1	1	2	3	3	1
Stapling	6	3	7	10	10	3	6
Double stapling	–	–	–	–	1	4	9
Total resections	9	4	8	12	14	11	16

of the patient's cancer. Our supposition is that technical details of sphincter-saving resections, such as high ligation of the inferior mesenteric vessels and total mesorectal excision, support this aim. We hope that when the time comes to present the long-term results of treatment by these new standards, they will be equal to the international ones.

Standards in the Treatment of Colorectal Carcinoma: A German View

J. Waninger

Introduction

Against the background of new laparoscopic techniques it seems desirable to point up the surgical principles for the treatment of colorectal carcinoma [17]. According to American figures, with 152 000 new cases and 57 000 deaths every year due to colorectal cancer, we are dealing with a major health problem [15].

In regard to tumor site, the incidence increases from proximal to distal, with almost two-third of tumors occurring in the sigmoid colon and rectum. The disease stage at diagnosis determines the outcome; 35 % of the patients already have lymph node involvement and 13 % metastases of the liver, while 35 % have a stage T3 or T4 tumor without lymph node involvement, leaving only 17 % with probably curable disease [7].

Diagnosis

Diagnosis in the case of patients presenting with symptoms typical of color- ectal cancer may be easy. Tumors in the ascending colon, however, are some- times more difficult to diagnose if the patients only present with atypical symptoms and iron deficiency. Goodman and Irvin [8] found a delay of 48 weeks in diagnosis of one-third of the study group because the physicians failed to iden- tify the cancer correctly.

A complete work-up and endoscopic examination of the entire colon, including histology, must be performed before the patient is prepared for sur- gery. Thorough cleansing of the bowel with prophylactic antibiotics is routine. Examination of the entire colon is necessary because of the high incidence of secondary lesions: synchronous adenomas are found in 27 % – 60 % and car- cinomas in 2 % – 11 % of patients [5, 19].

Brullet et al. [1] reported on a group of 65 patients in whom colonoscopy was performed intraoperatively because it had not been done preoperatively, for various reasons. In addition to the primary tumor they found a normal colon in 55 %, polyps located outside the planned resection in 36 %, and a secondary carcinoma in 9 %.

Principles of Surgery

The aim of surgical treatment is complete excision of all tumor tissue. A col- ostomy should be avoided whenever possible, and preoperative morbidity should be kept as low as possible.

Table 1. Principles of surgical technique in colorectal cancer

- Ligation of lymphovascular bundle
- Dissection along planes
- No dissemination of viable tumor cells
- Meticulous control of bleeding
- En-bloc resection
- Use of cytocidal agents
- Careful anastomotic technique

T1 tumors of the colon are cured when they have been removed endoscopically with a clear margin. Histological study should document a high-grade tumor with no vascular or lymphatic invasion. T1 and T2 tumors in the rectum can be removed transanally under similar conditions. Suspect lymph nodes should be checked by endoscopic ultrasonography [11].

Surgical technique is the main element of treatment (Table 1). Following the no-touch isolation technique, favoured by many colorectal surgeons, the lymphovascular bundle is first ligated near its origin [21]. Dissection is along anatomical planes, allowing a bloodless procedure. The entire colon segment is resected en bloc with the lymphatic drainage attached. Use of a cytocidal solution may destroy exfoliated tumor cells and reduce the rate of anastomotic recurrence of the disease.

Dissemination of tumor cells caused by squeezing and rupture of the tumor while dissecting should be avoided at all costs, as this has been shown to lead to a worse outcome [12].

The standard type of resection follows the anatomical blood supply of the colon. Right and transverse colectomies include ligation of the right colic artery and iliocolic artery or the median colic artery. Left hemicolectomy includes ligation of the left colic artery or inferior mesenteric artery, the same vessel as is ligated of anterior resection [11]. The high-tie technique removes the left colic artery; with the low-tie technique it is preserved [4].

The procedure is extended when the tumor is located between two segments with a different lymphovascular supplies, when a second carcinoma is present, when T4 disease is present, or when a marginal liver metastasis has to be removed.

Tumors that have invaded adjacent organs should be removed en bloc. Tumors with inflammatory adhesions to adjacent organs were found to contain carcinoma in 33.8 % of cases and therefore should be removed in the same way [3].

In the deep anterior resections Gall [6] found a local recurrence rate of 46 % when the margin measured 1 cm, but a rate of 14.3 % only when the margin measured 3 cm (Table 2). Heald et al. [9] therefore recommended complete mesorectal excision, and indeed achieved a better outcome this way (Table 3). Local recurrence is due not only to mesorectal spread but also to tumor invasion of the lateral ligaments [18].

Several studies, especially form Japanese surgeons, document a better outcome when lymph nodes were removed supraradically. Iliac lymph drainage

Table 2. Resection margins and local recurrence

Resection (cm)	Number of patients	Local recurrence (%)
1	19	46
1.1–2	91	33
2.1–3	131	30.5
>3	265	14.3

Table 3. Recurrences after complete mesorectal excision in 50 patients with a minimum follow-up of 2 years [9]

Site of recurrence	%
Pelvic wall	None
Suture line	None
Liver	8
Lung, liver, bone	4

was included in anterior resections. However, these patients had a higher morbidity than those who underwent standard resections [14]. Preservation of the autonomic nerve plexus will reduce urinary and sexual complications [20].

Experienced surgeons will achieve similar results whether they perform hand-sewn or stapled anastomosis. However, there is no doubt that stapling is easier in very deep anastomoses.

However, meticulous the technique, the deeper the anastomosis, the higher the risk of leakage [13] (Table 4).

A number of different conditions may be adequately treated with a limited surgical procedure. In cases of large bowel obstruction, high comorbidity, or multiple metastases of the liver, employment of the standard procedure will not lead to better results. A review of the procedures performed when various factors were taken into account showed that elective procedures were performed in 90% of cases, Ro resections in 80%, standard resections in 58%, a multivisceral resection in 20%, a limited resection in 17% and no resection in 5% [7].

Table 4. Anastomotic leakage rates in 495 cases of colonic resection [13]

Procedure	Leakage rate (%)
Right hemicolectomy	2.5
Left hemicolectomy	5.5
Anterior resection	10.1

The Surgeon as a Prognostic Factor

Many recently published studies have shown that the surgeon is the most important factor influencing survival rate and recurrence-free rate [2, 12, 16]. From this it may be assumed that there is great variability in the application of surgical principles for colorectal cancer. The German colorectal study group calculated a significant difference in outcome between surgical centres [12]. Similar results were reported by McArdle and Hole [16], who compared surgeons and found significant differences not only in outcome, but also in the rates of curative resection, wound infection and anastomotic leakage.

Since surgery alone still remains the most effective treatment for colorectal cancer, the principles of surgery should be strictly adhered to in order to achieve the best results possible.

References

1. Brullet E, Montané JM, Bombardo J, Bonfill X, Noguè M, Bordas JM (1992) Intraoperative colonoscopy in patients with colorectal cancer. Br J Surg 79:1376–1378
2. Consultant surgeons and pathologists of the Lothian and Borders Health Boards (1995) Br J Surg 82:888–890
3. Eisenberg SB, Kraybill WG, Lopez MJ (1990) Long term results of surgical resection of locally advanced colorectal carcinoma. Surgery 108:779–786
4. Farthmann EH, Kirchner R, Kirste G (1994) Kolon und Rektumtumoren. In: Farthmann (ed) Breitner Chirurgische Operationslehre, vol 4: Chirurgie des Abdomens, Dünndarm und Dickdarm. Urban & Schwarzenberg, Munich, pp 55–101
5. Finan PJ, Ritchie JK, Hawley PR (1987) Synchronous and early metachronous carcinomas of the colon and rectum. Br J Surg 74:945–947
6. Gall FP (1989) Tiefsitzendes Rektumkarzinom: Auswahl der Operationsmethoden in Abhängigkeit von Lokalization und Ausdehnung. Langenbecks Arch Chir [Suppl II] 669–673
7. Gall FP, Hermanek P (1992) Wandel und derzeitiger Stand in der chirurgischen Behandlung des colorectalen Carcinoms. Chirurg 63:227–234
8. Goodman D, Irvin TT (1993) Delay in the diagnosis of carcinoma of the right colon. Br J Surg 80:1327–1329
9. Heald RJ, Husband EM, Ryall RDH (1982) The mesorectum in rectal cancer surgery – the clue to pelvic recurrence? Br J Surg 69:613–616
10. Herfarth C, Hohenberger P (1989) Lymphadenektomie bei der Primärtherapie colorectaler Carzinome. Chirurg 60:139–147
11. Herfarth C, Hohenberg P (1992) Radikalität mit eingeschränkter Resektion in der Carcinomchirurgie des Gastrointestinaltrakts. Chirurg 63:235–241
12. Hermanek P Jr, Wiebelt H, Staimmer D, Hermanek P (1994) Langzeitergebnisse der chirurgischen Therapie des Coloncarzinoms. Ergebnisse der Studiengruppe Kolorektales Karzinom (SGKRK). Chirurg 65:287–297
13. Hesterberg R, Schmidt WU, Müller F, Röher HD (1991) Therapie und Letalität der Anastomoseninsuffizienz nach elektiver Darmresektion wegen eines kolorektalen Karzinoms. Langenbecks Arch Chir [Suppl] 174
14. Hojo K, Sawada T, Moriya Y (1989) An analysis of survival and voiding, sexual function after wide iliopelvic lymphadenectomy in patients with carcinoma of the rectum, compared with conventional lymphadenectomy. Dis Colon Rectum 32:128–133
15. Lichtmann SM, Mandel F, Hoexter B, Goldman IS, Budman DR, Labow S, Moseson M, Stiel L, McKinley M (1994) Prospective analysis of colorectal carcinoma. Dis Colon Rectum 37:1286–1290

16. McArdle CS, Hole D (1991) Impact of variability among surgeons on postoperative morbidity and mortality and ultimate survival. BMJ 302:1501–1505
17. O'Rourke NA, Heald RJ (1993) Laparsocopic surgery for colorectal cancer. Br J Surg 80: 1229–1230
18. Quirke P, Durdey P, Dixon MF, Williams NS (1986) Local recurrence of rectal adenocarcinoma due to inadequate surgical resection. Histopathological study of lateral tumor spread and surgical excision. Lancet II:996–999
19. Tate JJT, Rawlinson J, Royle GT, Brunton FJ, Taylor I (1988) Preoperative or postoperative colonic examination for synchronous lesions in colorectal cancer. Br J Surg 75:1016–1018
20. Scholefield JH, Northover JMA (1995) Surgical management of rectal Cancer. Br J Surg 82: 745–748
21. Turnbull RB, Kyle K, Watson FR, Spratt J (1967) Cancer of the colon: the influence of the no-touch isolation technique on survival rates. Ann Surg 166:420–428

Surgical Principles in the Treatment of Colorectal Cancer: A French View

C. Meyer, N. de Manzini, S. Rohr, and O. Firtion

Cancer of the colon is the most common neoplasm of the digestive system. Its incidence is progressively rising in economically well developed countries [1] For more than half a century surgical excision has been the only effective treatment; only recently has adjuvant chemotherapy been shown to be useful [2]. As for radiotherapy, it is only indicated for cancer of the rectum [3, 4].

Aims of Surgical Treatment

Surgical excision of a colorectal tumor must abide by certain oncological principles. The first of these is wide resection of the colonic segment at a distance from the apparent limits of the tumor, if necessary with excision of nearby organs which may be infiltrated by the tumor [5, 6]. The extent of logoregional surgery should be such as to prevent local recurrence of the tumor. If the distal and proximal tumor spreading are well known, as is the case with a rectal tumor, the limits of distal spread permit adequate margins of resection, often allowing an excision that both observes oncological principles and spares the sphincter [7].

The second main principle relates to the lymph nodes. While excision of mesocolic lymph nodes has a certain value in the staging of colorectal cancer, its role as curative therapy in extensive disease needs to be assessed. The staging of colorectal cancer is essentially based on evaluation of the degree of visceral and lymph node invasion [8]. The 5-year prognosis is determined by this staging. Staging permits comparison of the results obtained by different surgical techniques, it also allows verification of the validity of surgical interventions involving resection of greater or less extent. In the past few years adjuvant chemotherapy has appeared on the scene; the practice of lymphadenectomy should be encouraged in order to have a worldwide standard of surgical treatment and to be able property to compare the results of chemotherapy trials.

Rigorous adenectomy should be accompanied by careful anatomopathological examination, the risk of missing lymph node invasion being inversely proportional to the number of nodes excised and examined [9]. From the therapeutic point of view, the role of lymphadenectomy is more controversial. Although it is relatively simple to resect a series of nodes along the main blood vessels of the tumor-bearing segment of the colon, the value in terms of 5-year survival of continuing resection to the aorticocaval nodes remains to be proven [10].

Diagnosis

An early sub-clinical diagnosis of colorectal cancer may be made on the basis
of mass screening; the most sensitive method is the faecal occult blood test.
Its sensitivity and specificity are just high enough to be acceptable for a noninvasive diagnostic test; the number of A-stage cancers or pre-cancerous
lesions discovered during a screening campaign certainly seems significant
[11], even though some studies have failed to confirm the value of early
diagnosis of colorectal cancer in terms of better survival [12]. However, the
limited compliance in public screening campaigns, together with the incomplete evaluation of their costs (publicity, mass information), have weakened
enthusiasm for this method, on which there is as yet no general consensus of
opinion [13].

The diagnosis of symptomatic colorectal cancer calls first for an endoscopic examination which permits identification of the lesion, its location
and its anatomopathological nature together with the location of associated
lesions. The role of conventional radiology seems to be limited, its indication
being confined to the rare failures of endoscopy in diagnosing the lesion,
although the latter may be accomplished intraoperatively if complete
examination of the colon was not possible preoperatively [14]. At the rectal
level, digital rectal palpation allows a better appreciation of the lower pole of
the tumor in nearly 60 % – 70 % of patients, and an estimation of its fixity.
The limitations of this examination relate to the site of the lesion, patient
morphotype, and the painful nature of the examination. Endorectal ultrasonography allows assessment of the parietal extension of the tumor, with a
sensitivity of 90 %, over-staging being generally linked to intra-tumoral
oedema [15, 16]. Endorectal sonographic estimation of nodal involvement
has a low sensitivity, 80 %, but this is still higher than corresponding results
by CT or MRI [17] or even lymphoscintigraphy, which is no longer a current
method of diagnosis [18]. CT and MRI seem, however, to contribute greatly
to the estimation of the operability of large tumors, making intravenous
urography obsolete.

Once the diagnosis has been established, tumor extension is assessed with
hepatic ultrasonography and a chest X-ray in order to find distant metastases.
CT has not proved useful in these investigations. A blood sample is taken for
tumor markers, in order to have a pretreatment reference value.

The preoperative assessment is relatively simple and is based on the evaluation of cardiac, respiratory and metabolic functions of the patient [19].
Advanced age is not a contraindication in regard to surgery or the type of
operation [20]. Preparation for any type of colorectal intervention, except
in emergencies, involves orthograde washing of the colon by oral administration of a polyethylene-glycol solution, which reduces the bacterial level
without deleterious effects on the hydro-electrolytic balance [21]. Antibiotic
prophylaxis is necessary and is provided by a cephalosporin active against
aerobic and anaerobic bacteria, possibly combined with a nitro-imidazolie
[22]. Prophylactic treatment for deep venous thrombosis is recommended as
well.

Surgical Techniques

The classical method of surgery for colorectal cancer is by a median laparotomy, particularly for excision of cancers of the left colon and of the rectum, which involve both rectal resection and mobilisation of the left colic angle. On the other hand, tumors of the right colon and the transverse colon can be operated on via a transverse laparotomy, which requires less retraction and induces fewer respiratory repercussions and a lower risk of eventration.

The intraoperative assessment includes the following:

- Locoregional examination of tumor resectability, tanking into account the tumor's relation to the abdominal or pelvic walls, the major retroperitoneal blood vessels and adjacent organs.
- Palpation of the colon, in order to look for associated lesions which may affect the resectability.
- Manual and, especially, sonographic examination of the liver, since intraoperative ultrasonography is more sensitive than ultrasonography performed preoperatively [23].
- Search for peritoneal carcinosis or, possibly, micro-carcinosis, by abdominal lavage and cytological study.

Oncological Principles in Curative Resection

The no-touch technique – first the vascular approach, followed by ligature of the colonic segment before and after the tumor to reduce the number of vascular embolisms, then colonic lavage with a cytotoxic solution to avoid endoluminal dissemination of tumoral cells – has not been proved to be worthwhile in terms of reduction of metastasis or locoregional relapse or in improving survival [24, 26]. Otherwise, first ligating the blood vessels makes it easier to identify the devacularised colonic segments, and reduces bleeding during surgery, especially when tumor resections is complex or extensive.

Since colonic tumors spread in a proximal direction, the proximal safety margin should be at least 10 – 15 cm, which normally does not pose a problem, the vascular ligature usually causing greater devascularisation. As for the distal safety margin, it should be at least 5 cm for a fixed colonic segment and 2 cm for a rectal cancer, with a larger margin for circumferential or undifferentiated tumors [7].

The lymphadenectomy is generally performed by removing the mesocolon of the segments to be excised, and is normally limited by the origin of the principal vascular pedicle supplying the segment to be excised (the ileo-caeco-appendicular artery for the right colon, the middle and left colic artery for the transverse colon, and the lower mesenteric artery for the sigmoid colon and rectum). This type of lymphadenectomy is the one most often practiced by surgical teams; the number of nodes excised should be ten, for this amount allows reliable staging [7, 9]. Of course, lymphadenectomy of two pedicles may be carried out for tumors drained by two lymphatic territories (for example, the right colic angle with the ileo-caecal-appendicular pedicle and the middle colic artery) [8].

Therapeutic Value of Lymphadenectomy

Lumbo-aortic lymphadenectomy for cancer of the left colon and the rectum has been recognised as beneficial by some authors on the basis of better long-term result; but this opinion is not universal and requires confirmation in prospective studies. Lymphadenectomy poses specific problems in the case of rectal cancer, and although proximal lymphadenectomy follows the same rules and is just as debatable as that of the left colon, some authors advocate maximal extension of lymphadenectomy in the cranial direction [10], while others have failed to find a significant difference in survival according to whether the lower mesenteric artery is ligated above or below the issue of the left superior colic artery [27, 28].

Lymphadenectomy in cancer of the rectum has certain special aspects. Nodal involvement in the mesorectum and the hypogastrium makes complete excision of the mesorectum advisable, as this reduces the risk of pelvic recurrence of the tumor [29]. For vascular reasons however, this requires very low section of the rectum, bringing a theoretical increased risk of anastomotic leak as well as functional sequelae. It is worth noting that distal nodal invasion of the mesorectum has not been observed to go further than 2 cm beyond the lower pole of the tumor; if the same margin as for "nodal safety" could be applied to "visceral safety", this would mean that complete resection of the mesorectum is unwarranted for cancers of the upper rectum [30]. As for lateral lymphatic spread, certain Japanese authors have reported hypogastric nodal invasion to be sometimes as high as 20 %, justifying systematic hypogastric lymphadenectomy, gaining a hypothetical improvement of survival at a prohibitive cost in grave urinary and sexual sequelae [31]. Therefore, adoption of a technique of hypogastric lymphadenectomy with preservation of the autonomic pelvic innervation is likely to reduce the functional sequelae at the same time as allowing hypogastric lymphadenectomy [32]. It may be noted that in some European studies, searching for hypogastric nodal invasion not shown any positive nodes, calling into question the utility of such lymphadenectomy [10].

Interventions According to Tumor Site

Cancer of the Caecum and Ascending Colon

A right hemicolectomy is the method of choice, with a ligature at the origin of the ilio-caeco-appendicular and right colic pedicles. During dissection, special care should be taken to avoid injuring the genu inferium of the duodenum or the right ureter. The grate epiploon should not be systematically excised because it possess a lymphatic drainage different to that of the tumor except when adherence are present. The ileo-colic anastomosis may be performed in many different ways, and may be either stapled or hand-sewn.

Transverse Colon

Different options are possible depending on the topography of the tumor and the vascular pedicles that need to be sectioned. Tumors of the first, proximal third require a right hemicolectomy widened to the left, whereas tumors of the middle third require either the same technique or segmental resection with ligation of the middle colic artery. The first is often easier to perform, but with the second it is possible to preserve the function of the ileo-caecal valve. For tumors of the left colic angle, the choice is between subtotal colectomy, left hemicolectomy and segmental resection with ligation of the left superior colic artery. A comparative study has not yet shown any difference in patient survival between these last two types of intervention and the choice remains at the discretion of the surgeon [33].

Descending Colon and Sigmoid Colon

The same considerations as above are valid for tumors in the descending and sigmoid colon. Should a left hemicolectomy or a more limited resection be opted for? This depends on anatomical conditions (length and thickness of mesentery or mesocolon, but equally on the requirements of the principles of visceral resection and nodal excision, keeping in mind that a wide resection makes no difference in terms of survival [33]. However, other reasons may exist to widen the scope of visceral resection, such as diverticular disease associated with major inflammatory changes that would jeopardise the anastomosis.

Rectum

The intervention of choice is anterior resection of the rectum, since it has proved its effectiveness in terms of both short and long-term results. Mortality is currently less than 5%, and the incidence of anastomotic leak is so higher than 5% [34, 35]. This operation is the rule for cancers of the upper and middle rectum, but it is impossible for the lower rectum, for the following reason.

From the oncolocial point of view, the safety margins of resection must be at least 2 cm, and this applies to the mesorectum as elsewhere. If such an excision proves impossible, abdomino-perineal amputation is necessary [36]. In certain cases, the resection may be carried out at the level of the perineal floor. If this option is chosen, it is then impossible to close the rectal stump by stapling or a handsewn suture [37]. It is in this situation that a colo-anal anastomosis by the transanal route is warranted. This technique may be considered if the size and narrowness of the pelvis do to permit placement of the linear stapler; this, however, is a somewhat rare eventuality. From a functional point of view, anterior resection is not justified in the presence of anal incontinence, a terminal colostomy being in this case more comfortable for the patient than an incontinent perineal colostomy. In these cases, and depending on the height of the resection, the intervention consists of performing either Hartmann's operation or an abdomino-perineal amputation. Finally, in certain cases of low-lying cancers, there is the possibility, after abdomino-pelvic amputation of forming a neoanal sphincter using an electrostimulated graciloplasty [38, 39].

Finally, although the general rule is to opt for abdomino-perineal amputation in tumors that do not present adequate safety margins, and this option does provide that maximal guarantee of oncological safety, it can nevertheless be relaxed for tumors of the T1 class. For these, various transanal surgical and radiotherapeutic procedures may be considered, including of course ignoring the question of nodal metastasis, but this still has a good guarantee of safety from the statistical point of view [40, 42].

Special Cases

Intestinal Occlusion

Clinical presentation of intestinal occlusion is not rare in colonic cancers, attaining an estimated incidence of 10 %. Occlusion of the ascending colon does not necessitate any treatment modifications in regard to scheduled surgery except in the rare cases in which the patient's general condition is precarious, and where only an ileostomy should be carried out, at least at first. For neoplastic occlusion of the descending colon, on the other hand, are a variety of alternative tactics, and a number of different elements must be taken into consideration in making a tactical decision: the site of the tumor, the patient's general condition, the dilation of the caecum and whether it has been perforated or not, the existence of distant metastasis, and the condition of the anal sphincter.

The classical form of three-step surgery (colostomy, resection-anastomosis, closing of the colostomy) should be retained especially for patients suffering from major dehydration and those at high risk of perforation; this situation warrants immediate surgical intervention. The inconvenience of this mode of surgery is the long sequence of treatment, the mortality and cumulative morbidity of which are not negligible.

At the other extreme, there are two possibilities of one-step surgery:

- *Subtotal colectomy,* which eliminates the tumor and all of the colon above it, septic and unexplored, at the price of a very wide resection which may in some cases cause diarrhoea, notably when there is a tumor of the lower sigmoid, necessitating an ileo-rectal anastomosis. It is in this kind of case that it is important to know exactly the state of the tonus of the anal sphincter [43].
- *Left segmentary colectomy* after orthograde intraoperative lavage and possibly intraoperative coloscopy, without a protective colostomy. In many experiences, including our own, the mortality and morbidity associated with this technique are very low. Today one-step surgery, has a growing place in the treatment of occlusion in cancer [44].

Perforation

Perforation is a rarer occurrence than occlusion, and its treatment depends on its location. Situated on the caecum, it may occur during an occlusion. The treatment of choice is subtotal colectomy, removing the tumor and the perforation. Depending on the severity of the peritonitis, placement of a protective lileostomy may be considered.

If situated on the tumor, it constitutes a poor prognostic factor from the oncological point of view. Resection is the best operation, for this ruling out the possibility of colostomy-drainage and its frequent complications. The serverity of the peritonitis is the determining factor in deciding whether to perform an immediate anastomosis or not: stercoral contamination of the abdominal cavity argues for Hartman's operation, whereas for a lesser degree of peritonitis, resection-anastomosis with colostomy is advocated. Finally, if peritonitis is localised, colostomy need not be performed. However, in all cases where an anastomosis is performed, it should be accompanied by intraoperative colonic lavage [45].

Palliative Surgery

In three situations palliative surgery may be considered:

- Hepatic metastasis.
- Inoperable tumor.
- Peritoneal carcinosis.

In the first case resection of the tumor, whether colonic or rectal, represents the best possible solution to improve the local evolution. To this may be added oncological considerations in case where the presence of operable hepatic metastasis still allows curative surgery to be attempted. Conversely, if the tumor is not operable, internal or necessary external derivation may be carried out with the aim of avoiding problems of digestive transit.

Most authors regard surgical treatment of peritoneal carcinosis as unpredictable and disappointing in its results. Some attempts at cytoreductive surgery combined with peritoneal chemotherapy in hyperthermy have had results that need to be verified [46].

Laparoscopy in Colorectal Surgery

Laparoscopy has recently been introduced in cancer surgery of the colon and may be applied in many different ways, from video-assisted surgery including the mobilisation of mesentery and mesocolon, and even vascular ligation, to "all-laparoscopic" when, notably, anastomosis is carried out intracorporeally [47].

All the operations performed in open surgery have been reproduced in laparoscopic surgery. A tendency has rapidly appeared concerning right hemi-colectomies: the colon is first mobilised, the ileo-caecal-appendicular artery

ligated and lymphadenectomy performed by laparoscopy, and then the surgical specimen is exteriorised via a mini-laparotomy and the anastomosis performed extracorporally. For the descending colon, the dissection vascular section and lymphadenectomy are performed by laparoscopy and the surgical
specimen is exteriorised by a short suprapubic incision, the anastomosis then
being performed by a double-stapling technique.

First results are promising in terms of mortality and morbidity, with rapid
restoration of bowel movements [48]. At present, a comparative prospective
study of the two techniques needs to be undertaken. Many observations of
parietal graft on the port sites have been reported [49], and this phenomenon
has tempered initial enthusiasm, as has as the fact that the explanations of it
differ. Although experimental models must be established to study this problem, it does appear that an improvement in operative technique may considerably reduce the phenomenon. Laparoscopic cancer surgery of the colon
seems at present to be acceptable for metastatic tumors and for those that do
not affect the serosa (T in situ, T1, T2 tumors) but its oncological value needs
further proof [50].

Adjuvant Treatment

Surgery is no longer the only treatment for colorectal cancer. Chemotherapy
using 5-fluoro-uracil and levamisol or folinic acid improves the 5-year survival
patients with Dukes stage C colonic cancer by the order of 33 % [2]; a lower result
was also obtained for patients with a stage tumor B2 [51]. Several trials are in progress to try to find new combinations of drugs or new ways of administering
them, and improved efficacy without producing side effects or chemoresistance.
Chemotherapy is also indicated for rectal cancer by extrapolation of its effect in
colon cancer. In the same vein, external radiotherapy in rectal cancer reduces the
incidence of local relapse at 5 years; the current consensus is to administer radiotherapy preoperatively to reduce tumoral mass and to limit post-radiotherapy
complications [3, 4]. As for the risk that radiotherapy may lead to understaging
of the operative portion during anatomopathological examination, this may be
avoided by preoperative endoscopic ultrasonography [52].

In summary, the treatment of colorectal cancer remains in the surgical do-
main, but combined with diagnostic, technological, surgical and oncological
procedures in a way that makes the approach to this disease multidisciplinary.

References

1. Faivre J, Klepping C (1981) Epidemiologie des cancers colorectaux. In: Zeitoun P (ed) Progrès en cancerologie: les cancers de l'appareil digestif. Doin, Paris pp 25 – 37
2. Moertel CG, Fleming TR, MacDonald JS et al. (1990) Levamisole and fluorouracil for adjuvant therapy of resected colon carcinoma. N Engl J Med 322:352–358
3. Marks G, Mohiuddin M, Arieh E, Masoni L, Rakinic J (1991) High-dose preoperative
   radiation and radical sphincter-preserving surgery for rectal cancer. Arch Surg 126:
   1534–1540

4. Pahlman L, Gilimelius B (1990) Pre- or postoperative radiotherapy in rectal and rectosigmoid carcinoma. Ann Surg 211:187–195
5. Takahashi T, Mori T, Moossa AR (1991) Tumors of the colon and rectum: clinical features and surgical management. In: Moossa AR, Stephan CS, Martin CR (eds) Comprehensive textbook of oncology, 2nd ed Williams and Wilkins, Baltimore; pp 904–933
6. Izbicki JR, Hosch SB, Knoefel WT, Passlich B, Bloechle C, Broelsch CE (1995) Extended resections are beneficial for patients with locally advanced colorectal cancer. Dis Colon Rectum 38:1251–1256
7. Hermanek P (1982) Evolution and pathology of rectal cancer. World J Surg 6:502
8. Herrera L, Brown MT (1994) Prognostic profile in rectal cancer: Dis Colon Rectum 37 [Suppl]:S1–S5
9. Scott KWM, Grace RH (1989) Detection of lymph node metastases in colorectal carcinoma before and after fat clearance. Br J Surg, 76:1165–1167
10. Leggeri A, Roseano M, Balani A, Turoldo A (1994) Lumboaortic and iliac lymphadenectomy: what is the role today? Dis Colon Rectum 37 [Suppl] S54–S61
11. Hardcastle JD, Farrands PA, Balfour TW, Chamberlain J, Amar SS, Sheldon MG (1983) Controlled trial of faecal occult blood testing in the detection of colorectal cancer. Lancet 2:1–4
12. Ratcliffe R, Kiff RS, Hoare EM, Kingston RD, Walsh SH, Jeacock J (1989) Early diagnosis in colorectal cancer. Still no benefit? Ann Chir 43:570–574
13. Khubchandani IT, Karamchandani MC, Kleckner FS, Sheets JA, Stasik JJ, Rosen L, Riether RD (1989) Mass screening for colorectal cancer. Dis Colon Rectum 32:754–758
14. Brullet E, Montané JM, Bombardo J, Bonfill X, Nogué M, Bordas JM (1992) Intraoperative colonoscopy in patients with colorectal cancer. Br J Surg 79:1376–1378
15. Glaser F, Schlag P, Herfarth C (1990) Endorectal ultrasonography for the assessment of invasion of rectal tumors and lymphnode involvement. Br J Surg 77:883–887
16. Roseau G, Palazzo L, Amouyal P, Amouyal G, Gayet B, Ponsot P, Paolaggi JA (1990) Résultats de l'echoendoscopie dans le bilan pré-opératoire du cancer du rectum. Ann Chir 44:527–530
17. Thaler W, Watzka S, Martin F, La Guardia G, Psenner K, Bonatti G, Fichtel G, Egarter-Vigl E, Marzoli GP (1994) Preoperative staging of rectal cancer by endoluminal ultrasound vs magnetic resonance imaging. Preliminary results of a prospective, comparative study. Dis Colon Rectum 37:1189–1193
18. Arnaud JP, Adloff M, Schloegel M, Haegele P, Grobbe JC (1989) Un progrès dans l'evaluation de l'extension ganglionnaire des cancers du rectum: la lymphoscintigraphie rectale endoscopique. J Chir (Paris) 126:179–182
19. Canivet JL, Damas P, Desaive C, Lamy M (1989) Operative mortality following surgery for colorectal cancer. Br J Surg 76:745–747
20. Adloff M, Ollier JC, Schloegel M, Serrat M (1993) Le cancer colorectal chez les sujets de plus de 80 ans. J Med Strasbourg 24:171–175
21. Cohne SM (1994) A prospective randomized endoscopic double-blind trial comparing precolonoscopy bowel cleansing methods. Dis Colon Rectum 37:689–696
22. Dellinger EP, Gross PA, Barrett TL, Krause PJ, Martone WJ, McGowan JE et al. (1994) Quality standard for antimicrobial prophylaxis in surgical procedures. Clin Infect Dis 18:422–427
23. Rifkin ND, Rosato FE, Branch M et al. (1987) Intraoperative ultrasound of the liver: an important adjunctive tool for decision making in the operative room. Ann Surg 205:466–471
24. Turnbull RB, Kyle K, Watson FR et al. (1967) Cancer of the sigmoid colon. The influence of the no-touch isolation technique on survival rates. Ann Surg 166:420–425
25. Wiggers T (1988) No-touch technique in colon cancer: a controlled prospective trial. Br J Surg 75:409–415
26. Umpleby HC, Fermor B, Symes MO, Williamson RCN (1984) Viability of exfoliated colorectal carcinoma cells. Br J Surg 71:659
27. Glass RE, Ritchie JK, Thompson HR, Mann CV (1985) The result of surgical treatment of cancer of the rectum by radical resection and extended abdominoiliac lymphadenectomy. Br J Surg 72:599

28. Surtees P, Ritchie JK, Phillips RK (1990) High versus low ligation of the inferior mesenteric artery in rectal cancer. Br J Surg 77:618–621
29. Heald RJ, Husband EM, Ryall RD (1982) The mesorectum in rectal cancer surgery – the clue to pelvic recurrence? Br J Surg 69:613–616
30. Morikawa E, Yasutomi M, Shindou K, Matsuda T, Mori N, Hida J, Kubo R, Kitaoka M, Nakamura M, Fujimoto K, Inufusa H, Hatta M, Izumoto G (1994) Distribution of metastatic lymph nodes in colorectal cancer by the modified clearing method. Dis Colon Rectum 37:219–223
31. Hojo K, Sawada T, Moriya Y (1989) An analysis of survival and voiding, sexual function after wide iliopelvic lymphadenectomy in patients with carcinoma of the rectum, compared with conventional lymphadenectomy. Dis Colon Rectum 32:128–133
32. Moriya Y, Sugihara K, Akusu T, Fujita S (1995) Patterns of recurrence afternerve-sparing surgery for rectal adenocarcinoma with special reference to localregional recurrence. Dis Colon Rectum 38:1162–1168
33. The French Association for Surgical Research, Rouffet F, Hay JM, Vacher B, Fingerhut A, Elhadad A, Flamant Y, Mathon C, Gainant A (1994) Curative resection for left colonic carcinoma: hemicolectomy vs segmental colectomy. Dis Colon Rectum 37:651–659
34 Meyer C, Rohr S, Neagu S, de Manzini N, Thiry CL, Hollender LF (1995) Le cancer du rectum: aspects cliniques et thérapeutiques. Quels changements au cours des deux dernières décennies? Chirurgie 120:153–162
35. Leggeri A, Liguori G, de Manzini N, Balani A (1987) La conservation sphinctérienne dans la chirurgie du cancer du rectum. Chirurgie 113:785–792
36. Liguori G, de Manzini N, Balani A, Leggeri A (1989) La place de l'amputation abdomino-périneale dans le traitement chirurgical des cancers du rectum. J Chir (Paris) 126:374–378
37. Cavaliere F, Pemberton JH, Cosimelli M, Fazio VW, Beart RW (1995) Coloanal anastomosis for rectal cancer. Long-term results at the Mayo and Cleveland Clinics. Dis Colon Rectum 38:80–92
38. Williams NS, Patel J, George BD, Hallan RT, Watkins ES (1991) Development of an electrically stimulated neoanal sphincter. Lancet 338:1166–1169
39. Seccia M, Menconi C, Balestri R, Cavina E (1994) Study protocols and functional results in 86 electrostimulated graciloplasties. Dis Colon Rectum 37:897–904
40. Horn A, Halvorsen JF, Morild I (1989) Transanal extirpation for early rectal cancer. Dis Colon Rectum 32:769–772
41. Papillon J, Bérard P (1992) Endocavitary irradiation in the conservative treatment of adenocarcinoma of the low rectum. World J Surg, 16:452–457
42. Said S, Buess G, Huber P (1994) Transanal Endoscopic Surgery. In: Steichen FM, Walter R (eds) Minimally invasive surgery and new technology. Quality Medical Publishing, St Louis, 392–400
43. Brief DK, Brener B, Goldenkranz R, Alpert J, Parsonnet V, Ferrante R, Huston B, Eisenbud D (1991) Defining the role of subtotal colectomy in the treatment of carcinoma of the colon. Ann Surg 213:248–252
44. Meyer C, de Manzini N, Rohr S, Thiry L, Joshi M, Campiglio GL (1994) Les occlusions néoplastiques. La chirurgie en un temps. In: La chirurgie colique d'urgence (course material), 96 Congrès de Chirurgie, Paris, 27–40
45. Meyer C, Hollender LF (1986) Le colon perforé non tramatique. In: Meyer C, Hollender LF (eds) Chirurgie colique d'urgence. Masson, Paris, 41–54
46. Sugarbaker PH (1995) Patient selection and treatment of peritoneal carcinomatosis from colorectal and appendiceal cancer. World J Surg 19:235–240
47. Monson JRI, Darzi A, Carey PD, Guillon PJ (1992) Prospective evaluation of laparoscopic assisted colectomy in an unselected group of patients. Lancet 340:831–833
48. Meyer C, Thiry CL, de Manzini N, Rohr S, Jobard D, Perraud V (1994) La chirurgie colorectale par laparoscopie est-elle licite? A propos de 76 cas. Chir Endosc 3:10–15
49. Cirocco WC, Schwartzman A, Golub RW (1994) Abdominal wall recurrences after laparoscopic colectomy for colon cancer. Surgery 116:842–846

50. Meyer C, Rohr S (1995) Que penser de la chirurgie colo-rectale par voie laparoscopique? Hapato-gastro 5:403–406
51. Wolmark N, Rockette H, Fischer B et al. (1993) Leucovorin-modulated 5-FU (LV-FU) as adjuvant therapy for primary colon cancer: NSABP C-03. Proc Am Soc Clin Oncol 12:197
52. Napoleon B, Pujol B, Berger F, Valette PJ, Gerard JP, Souquet JC (1991) Accuracy of endosonography in the staging of rectal cancer treated by radiotherapy. Br J Surg 78:785

II   Indications

Laparoscopic Sigmoid Resection in Diverticulitis

T. Schiedeck, A. Herold, and H.-P. Bruch

Introduction

After the first laparoscopic colon resection was performed by Jacobs in 1991, tremendous hope was generated in the new approach. However, while the laparoscopic technique is at present in cholecystectomy widespread, in colorectal surgery it is well established only in a few specialized centres. After treating cancer patients laparoscopically, surgeons were soon confronted with early recurrence rates and port-site metastases, so in these patients laparoscopic surgery is still under debate.

In addition to these problems, there are some general drawbacks to minimally invasive colorectal surgery. Because of the limited, two-dimensional view, intra-abdominal ligation and suturing are often time-consuming procedures. The loss of the tactile sense makes anatomical orientation and identification of important structures or landmarks often very difficult. Especially in conditions of acute inflammation (diverticulitis, Crohn's disease, or endometriosis), the laparoscopic surgeon often has to face insurmountable technical problems and may in the end be compelled to convert to standard open surgery. In view of all this, it is not difficult to understand why the laparoscopic technique is not as widely accepted in colorectal surgery as in cholecystectomy at present.

On the other hand, the great advantages of the laparoscopic procedure are obvious in the postoperative period. Apart from better cosmesis, patient convalescence is quicker, patients suffer less pain, and bowel movements occur earlier. All these together may result in a shortened hospital stay and probably could decrease costs.

Method

Patients

In 1992 we started performing laparoscopic colorectal surgery. So far we have operated on 121 patients. Twenty-four of them, ranging from 47 to 81 years in age, underwent colon resection for diverticular disease. The general indication for surgical intervention was complicated diverticular disease or diverticula and associated lesions (e.g. outlet obstruction or rectal prolapse). The laparoscopic technique was chosen in patients with minor or recurrent bleeding, stenosis without ileus and recurrent diverticulitis or inflammatory mass. Patients with perforation with faecal or purulent peritonitis or abscess, and major bloodloss underwent open laparotomy. In these cases the laparoscopic technique was thought to be contraindicated.

Preoperatively patients were assessed by proctorectoscopy, total colonoscopy and/or contrast enema. In patients with constipation and outlet obstruction, defecography and measurement of transit time were also performed.

The bowel was prepared before surgery by orthograde cleansing with Golytely solution. Additionally, in patients with acute inflammation we would recommend splinting the left ureter. At the start of the operation every patient was given prophylactic antibiotics (single-shot cefotaxime and metronidazole). To prevent deep vein thrombosis, low-molecular-weight heparins were administered.

Surgical Procedure

The operation is performed with the patient in the Lloyd-Davies position. Exposure of the descending colon is facilitated by a slight tilt to the right. For preparation we only use bipolar coagulation tweezers, scissors and atraumatic swabs. A 12-mm trocar is placed through a small paraumbilical incision and after CO_2 insufflation a 30° telescope is inserted. We use three more 12-mm ports placed in the lower abdomen, describing a semicircle. In a few cases an additional 5-mm trocar may be needed in the left abdomen.

We start with the incision of the secondary fusion line. To prevent inadvertent injury the left ureter is generally identified, but it remains covered by Gerota's fascia. Then the peritoneum of the mesosigmoid is incised and if necessary the splenic flexure is mobilised. Next follows the tunneling of the colon. We use a atraumatic Endoretract for this. The bowel is then elevated to the anterior abdominal wall and held under slight tension. In this way the sigmoid colon and the rectum are mobilised down to the pelvic floor. The lower lateral ligaments and the median haemorrhoidal vessels are preserved. Then a 4- to 5-cm-long crosswise approach is performed using the port incision in the left lower abdomen. Under cautious traction the sigmoid bowel is exteriorized through the abdominal wall. The sigmoid colon is then resected, preserving the lower and upper colic artery (tubular resection). Anastomosis is performed by a hand-sewn running suture. The bowel is then replaced and the incision closed. The operation is completed laparoscopically. In general the peritoneal incisions are closed by running sutures.

Results

We had a typical learning curve with our 24 patients, and operating time went from 360 to 130 min as our experience grew. The majority of patients could be treated by sigmoid resection, but in two a left hemicolectomy was performed. For this we had to mobilise the splenic flexure of the colon. The length bowel resected ranged between 26 and 57 cm (Table 1). The postoperative hospital stay was between 10 and 27 days.

Table 1. Summary of operative data in 24 patients undergoing laparoscopic-assisted colon resection for diverticulitis

	n	Range
Age of patients (years)	65	41–87
Duration of surgery (min)	253	130–360
Resected bowel length (cm)	32	26–57
Blood transfusion requirement (u)	1.0	0–4
Intensive care stay (days)	0.9	0–2
Postop. hospital stay (days)	145	10–27

Our conversionrate is 12.5% (3 of 24). In one patient with perforated diverticulitis we were forced to convert by local peritonitis. In another extremely obese patient, secure identification of anatomical landmarks was not possible so we had to change to standard open surgery. In one case conversion was caused by problems connected with the anesthesia.

We have six complications to report:

- A minor complication was bleeding from the urethra after ureter splinting.
- One retroperitoneal haematoma was managed by CT-guided puncture and drainage.
- In another patient, bleeding from a small artery of the mesosigmoid prompted laparotomy.
- Local abscess 12 days postoperatively led to anastomotic leakage with peritonitis. In this case a Hartmann operation was carried out combined with etappenlavage for 2 days. Because of the long time spent on mechanical ventilation the patient developed an ARDS (acute respiratory distress syndrome) and died 3 weeks later. At this time the abdomen was closed and the peritonitis cured.
- Two weeks after surgery one patient showed an ileus caused by adhesions, so we had to perform a laparotomy for adhesiolysis.
- In one case we saw an incarcerated hernia at the trocar incision, which was treated by segmental resection of the small bowel.

Discussion

Like colorectal laparoscopic surgery in general laparoscopic treatment of diverticular disease needs great experience. As published by other groups, one has to learn to master certain technical difficulties, which gives rise to a typical learning curve. In our case, operation time went from 6 h down to about 2 hours. The extent of resection (32–57 cm) was similar to that in open surgery. The complication rate of 25% is very high, but two of our six complications were minor ones which could be handled conservatively or by simple percutaneous puncture and drainage. Nevertheless, four complications resulted in laparotomy and in one of these cases the patient died. On the other hand, this severe complication is not typical of laparoscopic procedure as such: local abscess and peritonitis may of course occur in standard open surgery as well.

Three times we had to convert. This may be due to our selection of patients for surgery. One patient with acute diverticulitis had local abscess and another one was very fat. Other surgeons would rule these patients out for laparoscopic surgery in the first place. Our method of management is different. In our opinion laparoscopic treatment may help to minimise surgical trauma to the patient, so generally we try to perform the procedure laparoscopically. However, one should of course not attach undue importance to the method, and conversion must anyway not be a sign of failure but of responsible patient care.

In two patients the extent of diverticula required a left hemicolectomy, so we had to mobilise the splenic flexure. This procedure, especially in fat patients or those with acute inflammation, can be very difficult and so operation time often is prolonged. In open surgery it could often be performed much faster. So in these patients an open technique may sometimes be the better choice. Nevertheless, as in open surgery, operation time depends on training, and with increasing familiarity with the laparoscopic technique, exposure of the splenic flexure, and the whole dissection itself, may become much quicker even under difficult conditions.

In one patient we saw an incisional hernia. To prevent the same happening again, every incision of the fascia more than 5 mm is now closed by a direct suture or with special suturing devices (e. g. Reverdin needle).

To sum up we believe that laparoscopic surgery is a technically feasible method in diverticular disease. However, especially in acute or chronic inflammation, dissection may be very difficult and one should not hesitate to convert. Faecal or purulent peritonitis in general is a contraindication for laparoscopic surgery. Successful laparoscopic treatment requires a well-trained operation team, but with growing experience the same results could be reached as in open surgery.

References

Baca I, Gotzen V, Schultz C (1995) Laparoscopic interventions in acute and chronic diverticulitis. Zentralbl Chir 120:396–399

Beart RWJ (1994) Laparoscopic colectomy: status of the art. Dis Colon Rectum 37:S47–S49

Darzi A, Super P, Guillou, PJ, Monson JR (1994) Laparoscopic sigmoid colectomy: total laparoscopic approach. Dis Colon Rectum 37:268–271

Elftmann TD, Nelson H, Ota DM, Pemberton JH, Beart RWJ (1994) Laparoscopic-assisted segmental colectomy: surgical techniques. Mayo Clin Proc 69:825–833

Franklin ME Jr, Ramos R, Rosenthal D, Schuessler W (1993) Laparoscopic colonic procedures. World J Surg 17:51–56

Jacobs M, Plasencia G (1994) Laparoscopic colon surgery: some helpful hints. Int Surg 79:233–234

Jansen A (1994) Laparoscopic-assisted colon resection. Evolution from an experimental technique to a standardized surgical procedure. Ann Chir Gynaecol 83:86–91

Köckerling F, Gastinger I, Schneider B, Krause W, Gall FP (1993) Laparoscopic abdominaperineal excision of the rectum with high ligation of the inferior mesenteric artery in the management of rectal carcinoma. Endosc Surg Allied Technol 1:16–19

Lebrecht K, Richter HA, Franke A (1995) Laparoskopische Kontinuitätsresektion am Sigma und Rektum. Chir Gastroenterol 11:178–182

Monson JR, Hill AD, Darzi A (1995) Laparoscopic colonic surgery. Br J Surg 82:150–157

Plasencia G, Jacobs M, Verdeja JC, Viamonte M (1994) Laparoscopic-assisted sigmoid colectomy and low anterior resection. Dis Colon Rectum 37:829–833

Scoggin SD, Frazee RC, Snyder SK, Hendricks JC, Roberts JW, Symmonds RE, Smith RW (1993) Laparoscopic-assisted bowel surgery. Dis Colon Rectum 36:747–750

Simons AJ, Anthone GJ, Ortega AE, Franklin M, Fleshman J, Geis WP, Beart RWJ (1995) Laparoscopic-assisted colectomy learning curve. Dis Colon Rectum 38:600–603

Wood C, Maher P, Hill D (1993) Laparoscopic removal of endometriosis in the pouch of Douglas. Aust N Z J Obstet Gynaecol 33:295–299

Indications for Laparoscopic Sigmoid Resection in Diverticulitis

U. Kunath

Any discussion of the indications for surgery in a particular disease must take account of its natural course and sequelae. In discussions of laparoscopic procedures, technical problems are to the fore. Both of the elements are addressed in the present paper.

Pathogenesis of Diverticulosis

Diverticula of the colon are initially relatively harmless changes. How do they occur?

In simple terms, the colon consists of an outer muscular tube and an inner mucosal tube (Fig. 1). The inner mucosal tubes stretches with the outer muscular tube, causing the mucosa, which is arranged in transverse folds, to smoothen out. The intestinal contents cause this stretching and smoothening out of the mucosal folds. The colon is now prepared for voluminous contents.

A low-fibre diet, which is particularly usual in Western societies, reduces the intestinal contents. Parks [2] demonstrated that this causes the passage of intestinal contents to be slowed down and the excitability of the colon which is under reduced stress to become increased. The colon enters a state of permanent contraction and works in an uncoordinated manner. The musculature of the taeniae becomes particularly hypertrophic, the colon segment shortens and a bundle of telescopic circular muscles may be seen histologically [5]. The contacted colon is no longer able to perform rapid peristalsis, but can only work slowly in small steps.

Intestinal contents which are only slowly pushed forwards can no longer smoothen out the mucosal folds in the contracted muscular tube. They push themselves through performed gaps. These gaps in the muscular tube are present where the blood vessels pierce the intestinal wall at a slant. Diverticula known as false diverticula occur.

Follow-up of patients with diverticulosis [1] shows that diverticulitis occurs in approx. 10 % of cases in the 5 years after the change has been diagnosed. This percentage rises in a further 5 years to 25 %. Diverticulosis for 20 years and more is associated with a diverticulitis rate of 40 %.

Pathogenesis of Diverticulitis

Inflammation of the diverticula occurs in the following manner. The neck of the diverticula is narrowed by the contracted musculature. The inflammation

Fig. 1. Pathogenesis of diver
ticulitis (From [5])

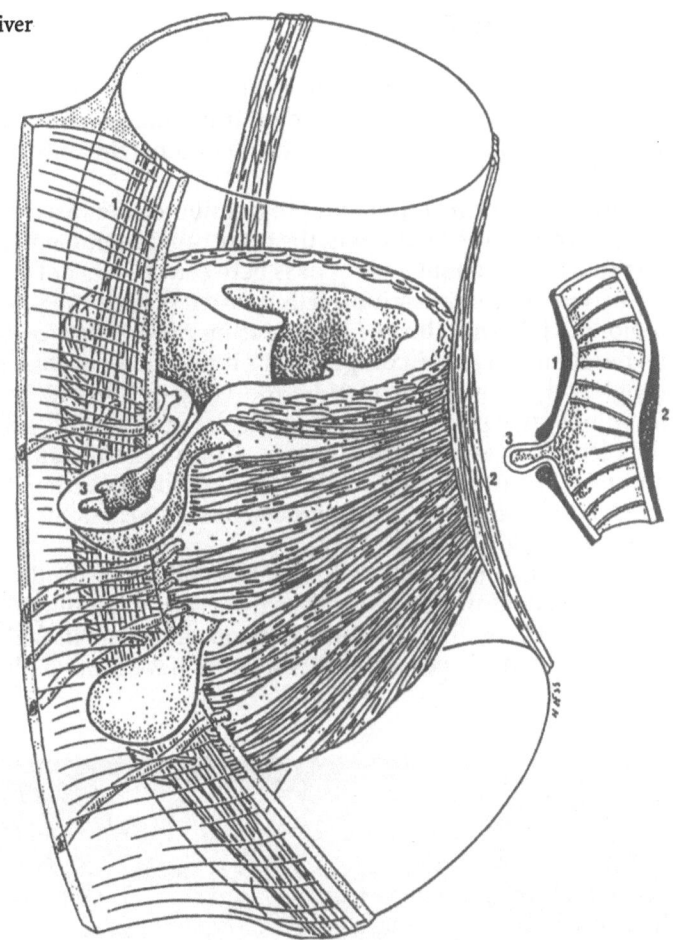

which flares up in the diverticula due to pressure from the stagnating intestinal contents, is not supplied with the blood it needs. Thus the irreversible, destructive stage of the disease process begins: due to the concomitant oedema, hyperaemia does not occur, causing the inflammation to progress rapidly to tissue necrosis and to advance. The diverticulitis becomes peridiverticulitis and finally parietal phlegmon. The necrotic musculature of the inflammation is replaced by fibrotic scar tissue. This means that the muscle spasm cannot be relaxed. The permanent spasm of the taeniae persists, and so on in a vicious circle. The advanced stage of this process is called pericolitis.

Another phenomenon also characterizes this disease: in rare cases, free perforation of the inflamed diverticula occurs. This is because the diverticula are embedded in the epiploic appendages or the migration process is covered the serosa of the neighboring organs (bowel, urinary bladder, uterus, posterior fornix).

Indications for Surgery

Bearing in mind that diverticular inflammation cannot heal and does not heal, but rather progresses to a chronic inflammatory process which slowly advances in to the surrounding area and organs, the only treatment can be *early resection*.

Inflammatory reaction and progression of the disease are closely connected. The younger the patient is, the more rapid their course. If the patient is over 60 years of age, about 2 years pass between the start of the complaints and the occurrence of complications. If the patient is under 50 years of age, it takes only 6 months [1]. This chronic smouldering process few complaints and only becomes manifest in the complications it produces, such as stenosis, fistulae and conglomerate tumor. It may be too early or too late to rectify these manifestations by laparoscopy. A diverticular tumor with calloused adherence to the bladder, uterus or small intestine or all these cannot be clearly detached and resected with laparoscopy (Fig. 2). Only diverticulitis in the early stage, when adhesions are not yet vascularized, is accessible by laparoscopic resection (Figs. 3, 4).

It is true that the first attack of diverticulitis may be the last. However, one in three diverticulitis patients suffers from recurrent inflammatory episodes. The aim should be to identify these patients at a stage in which Reifferscheid and Raguse [4] already advise early resection. If we think of the pathomechanics of

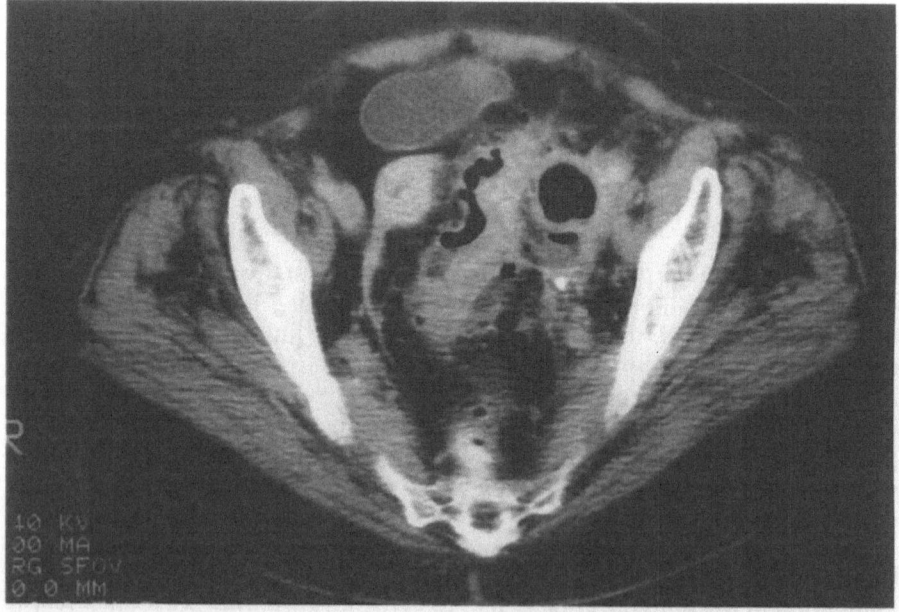

Fig. 2. 75-year-old female patient with diverticulitic conglomerate tumor and formation of abscesses in the true pelvis. The attempt at laparoscopic resection failed

Fig. 3. Stenosing sigmoid diverticulitis in a 52-year-old man

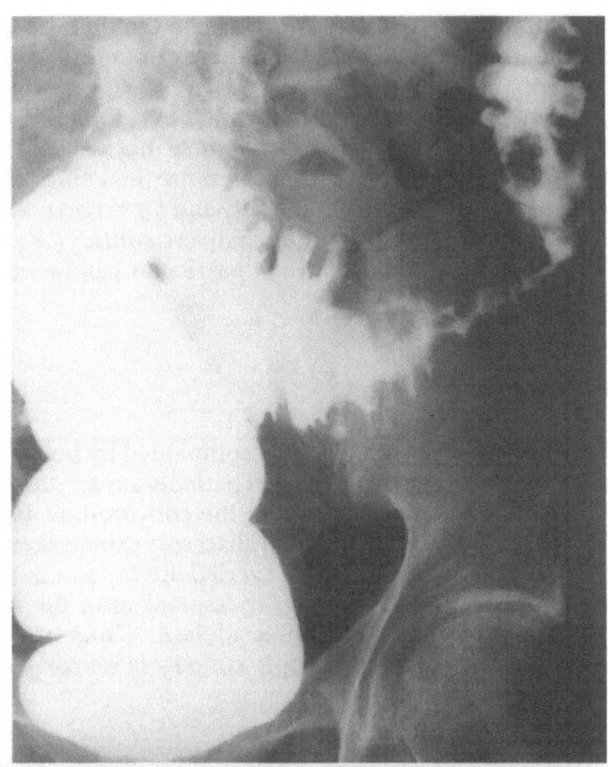

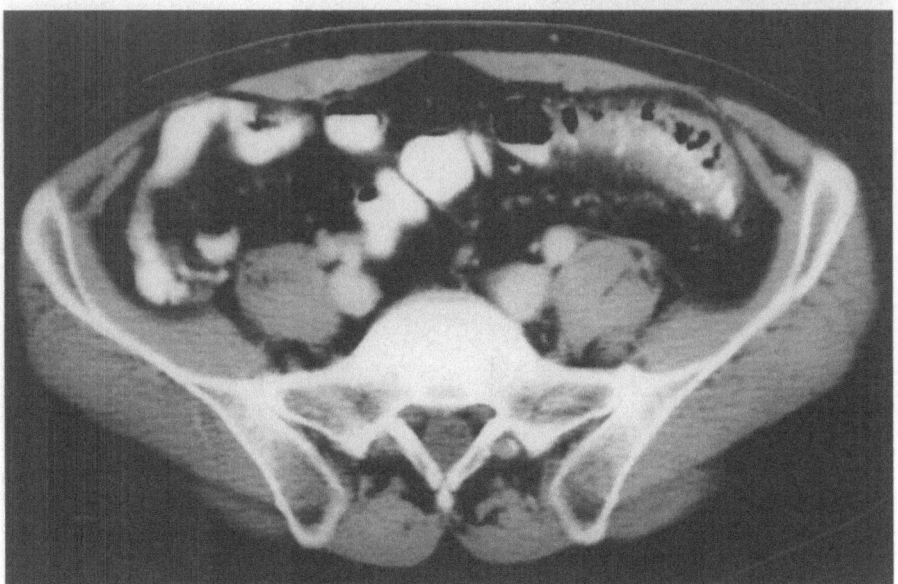

Fig. 4. CT scan of the patient in Fig. 3. The thickening of the wall of the sigmoid colon can be clearly seen. Laparoscopic resection was successful

the inflammatory process, it is easy to see that the first inflammatory episode ends with partial recovery and the pathognetic principle – contracture of the taeniae – is reinforced.

Parks and Cannell [3], reporting on 297 patients who were treated conservatively over period of 2–6 years, show that 2% died due to complications, 42% were treated on an in-patient basis more than one, 30% were still suffering complaints even at the end of the study and 6.7% had eventually to undergo surgery.

The plea for early resection in diverticulitis [4, 6] is still not heeded enough. The laparoscopic procedure in particular can be used to reduce stress on the patients.

Principles of Treatment

Acute lower abdominal pain accompanied by fever must now be regarded as a possible sign of diverticulitis in patients as early as in their 40 s. Thickening of the wall of the sigmoid colon, the concomitant inflammatory reaction and sometimes formation of small abscesses can be seen on the CT scan (Fig. 5).

Conservative treatment is carried out for 10–14 days (reduced food intake, antibiotics and mild laxative measures) until the acute signs have subsided. Then laparoscopic resection is advised. While fresh inflammatory adhesions can be detached, laparoscopic surgery is no longer possible on a hard conglomerate tumor.

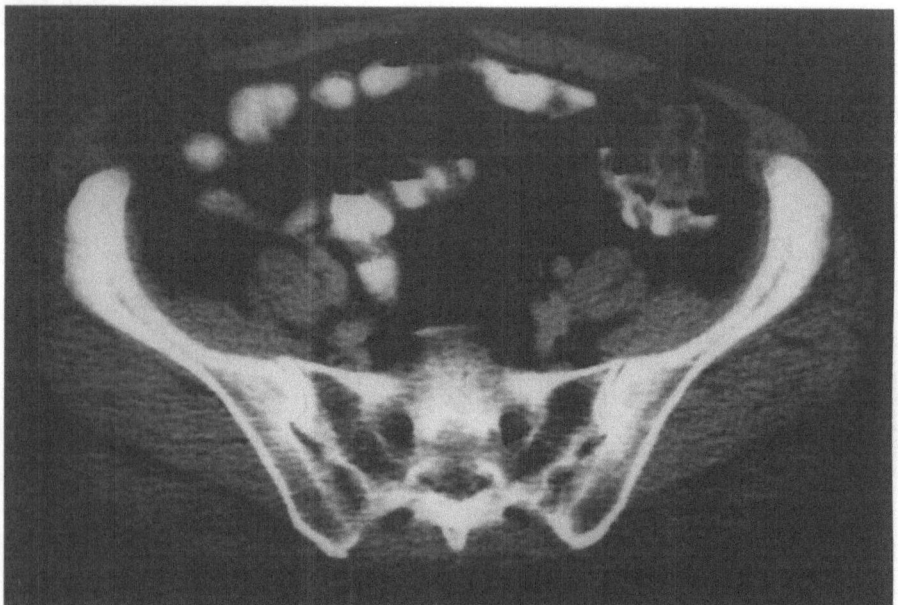

Fig. 5. 50-year-old female patient with peridiverticulitis. Laparoscopic resection was performed without difficulty

It would be a mistake to let the matter rest once the inflammatory episode has subsided with conservative treatment. Fistulae or stenosis often appear to occur spontaneously later on, but are in fact the results of unnoticed chronic inflammation.

Experience at the Krankenhaus am Urban

Between January 1991 and 31 July 1995, 127 patients underwent surgery for diverticulitis of the sigmoid colon in the Surgical Department of the Krankenhaus am Urban. The fact that 64 patients required only surgery by laparotomy at once gives an impression of the severity of the clinical picture and of the patient population, which was not very health-conscious. Fifty-one patients underwent surgery several times or as an emergency measure. In only 10 patients was the diverticulitis in a stage at which laparoscopic resection (available since April 1992) was possible. In one female patient, the procedure had to be changed during the operation. There were no fatalities in the 10 patients who were operated on laparoscopically, whereas mortality in patients operated on in the conventional manner was 16.5%. The average age of the patients operated on conventionally was 66 years versus 49 years for those operated by laparoscopy.

Summary

Diverticulitis is a disease whose severity – i.e. degree of danger and likelihood of complications – is still largely underestimated by those who treat it conservatively. If the practice of medicine is also to be interpreted as disease prophylaxis, then early resection is indicated in diverticulitis. The early stage of diverticulitis (uncomplicated, confined perforation) is best suited to the laparoscopic procedure. For technical reasons and due to the lack of clarity on the subject, complicated diverticulitis does not yet constitute an indication for minimally invasive surgery. There is no effective conservative treatment.

References

1. Parks TG (1969) Natural history of diverticular disease of the colon. A review of 521 cases. Br Med J 4:639
2. Parks TG (1974) Diet and diverticular disease. Proc R Soc Med 67:1037
3. Parks TG, Connell AM (1970) The outcome in 455 patients admitted for treatment of diverticular disease of the colon. Br J Surg 57:775
4. Reifferscheid M, Raguse T (1977) Die chirurgische Behandlung der Diverticulitis. Chirurg 48:577
5. Stelzner F, Lierse W (1976) Über die Entwicklung der Diverticulose und der Diverticulitis. Langenbecks Arch Chir 341:271
6. Thiede A (1993) Behandlung der unkomplizierten und komplizierten Diverticulitis. Prospektive Studie aus chirurgischer Sicht. Chri Praxis 46:253

Laparoscopic Colorectal Surgery: Indications and Design of a Multicentre Study

F. Köckerling, C. Schneider, H. Scheidbach, M.A. Reymond, C. Wittekind, W. Hohenberger, and the Laparoscopic Colorectal Surgery Study Group [1]

Introduction

Numerous problems accompany the introduction of laparoscopic colorectal surgery into clinical practice. A number of publications have reported on the practicability, complication rate, mortality, short-term results and costs of laparoscopic colorectal surgery [9, 15, 16, 21, 25, 33, 34]. Opinions as to the use of laparoscopic operative procedures in colorectal carcinoma differ greatly in these reports. First, the effectiveness of laparoscopic colorectal surgery for carcinoma has not yet been confirmed by long-term results, and secondly, there are reports of metastases in the trocar entry sites and specimen delivery incisions [1, 3, 24, 26]. General adoption of laparoscopic operative procedures can therefore not be recommended for colorectal carcinoma. The value of these new operative procedures must be confirmed by appropriate studies. Special clinical studies should include histopathological examination of the resected tumors by reference to the oncological criteria of a wider study programme such as that of the German Tumor Centres Study Group [14].

Diagnostic and Palliative Operations in Colorectal Carcinoma

There are no oncological reasons not to use laparoscopy to search for peritoneal or liver metastases. Non-resecting procedures, e.g. bypass operations in

[1] J. Witte, A. Heiss (Augsburg); E. Bärlehner, B. Heukrodt (Berlin); H.J. Buhr, C.-T. Germer (Berlin); J. Konradt (Berlin); G. Szinicz, S. Beller, K.P. Henle (Bregenz); I. Baca, V. Götzen (Bremen); H.A. Richter (Bremen); H.D. Saeger, U. Wehrmann (Dresden); K. Ludwig, G. Hellmich (Dresden); F. Köckerling, C. Schneider, H. Scheidbach, M. Reymond, C. Wittekind, W. Hohenberger (Erlangen); P. Mattes, Zeidan (Esslingen); C. Hottenrott, Menzel (Frankfurt a.M.); W. Bayerl (Gelsenkirchen-Resse); K.H. Muhrer, K. Schnell (Giessen); H.R. Willmen, A. Krebs (Grevenbroich); C.E. Brölsch; C. Zornig (Hamburg); E. Gross (Hamburg); K. Rückert (Hamburg); K. Reichel, A. Kuthe (Hannover); H. Troidl, E. Eypasch (Cologne); T. Hager (Kronach); K.-H. Vestweber, F. Haaf (Leverkusen); H.-P. Bruch, A. Herold (Lübeck); K. Schönleben, F.-U. Zittel, F.-J. Zender (Ludwigshafen); T.M. Raguse (Mühlheim); J.R. Siwert, I. Brune, H. Feussner (Munich); F.W. Schildberg, G. Meyer (Munich); W. Heitland, W. Bittmann (Munich); U. Kleine (Neuruppin); H.-F. Weiser, J. Gerberding (Rotenburg a.d.W.); K. Dommisch, H.-J. Lorenz (Schwerin); J. Lange, J. Nägele (St. Gallen); H. Herwig, I. Gastinger (Suhl); H.D. Becker, K. Manncke (Tübingen); W. Kreuzer (Vienna); A. Fritsch, R. Függer (Vienna); K. Dinstl, K. Dittrich (Vienna); P. Pietsch, W. Dreyer (Wismar); D. Wilker, J. Becker (Wuppertal); A. Thiede, K.-H. Fuchs (Würzburg).

advanced carcinoma of the splenic flexure with diffuse liver metastases, or construction of a transverse or sigmoid colostomy or a loop ileostomy in advanced metastasizing colorectal carcinoma, can be undertaken laparoscopically [11, 20 23, 28]. Palliative colorectal resections or rectal excisions in the presence of diffuse lung or liver metastases can also represent an indication for a laparoscopic procedure. In the palliative operations, the argument of rapid recovery and early discharge of the patient from hospital carries particular weight. When the tumor has a clearly unfavourable prognosis, less traumatic operative techniques ca be preferred to the open procedures.

Curative Laparoscopic Colorectal Procedures in Carcinoma Which Should Not be Analysed in Studies

Individual surgeons experienced in laparoscopy have reported that anterior and low anterior rectal resections and right-sided hemicolectomies for carcinoma are both feasible and of sufficient quality [2, 4, 5, 10, 13, 31].

Our own experimental and clinical experiences with laparoscopic colorectal surgery show that the operations turn out to be more or less difficult depending on the anatomical situation. Dissection following given anatomical planes is entirely possible, and reconstructive procedures can be successfully carried out with technical assistance in easily accessible anatomical regions, but there are some technical and anatomical limits which can be overcome only by making concessions with regard to either the radicality of resection or the safety of the operation. For these reasons, we see no indication for performing low anterior resections of the rectum in a multicentre study. Clean dissection of the mesorectum at the level of transection and distal transection of the rectum with an adequate safety margin from the tumor are very difficult. In contrast to excision of the rectum, in which the low position of the tumor allows dissection to take place in the tumor-free region in the lesser pelvis, in low anterior resection of the rectum the tumor has to be manipulated in the pelvis during dissection. High ligation of the inferior mesenteric artery can be done laparoscopically without difficulty but then demands extensive mobilization of the descending colon, the splenic flexure and the left side of the transverse colon from the lower border of the pancreas and ligation of the inferior mesenteric vein at the lower border of the pancreas – maneuvers that are technically very time-consuming and demanding when performed laparoscopically. Right hemicolectomy or extended colon resections in carcinomas of the flexures are also, in our opinion, too complicated for the laparoscopic method and involve oncological risks. In the first place, searching for the ileocolic artery and the right colic artery or middle colic artery at corresponding exposure of the inferior mesenteric artery. Removal of the greater omentum from the greater curve of the stomach, opening of the omental bursa, mobilisation of the transverse mesocolon and the hepatic flexure from the duodenum and the head of the pancreas are also too difficult in our opinion. Carcinomas of the right colon, which are often quite large, have to be removed through a correspondingly large minilaparotomy.

Technical Feasibility of Laparoscopic Colorectal Procedures in Carcinoma While Adhering to Oncological Principles

In our opinion, techniques and instruments which make laparoscopic colorectal resection technically feasible while adhering to the principles of cancer surgery exist for the treatment of small sigmoid and upper rectal carcinoma and very low rectal carcinoma which can be treated curatively only by abdominoperineal excision [2, 4, 5, 8, 10, 13, 17, 18, 23, 31]. High division of the inferior mesenteric artery is achieved by dissection, exposure and division of the vessel with the linear stapler or PDS clips. The less extreme mobilization of the left colon for sigmoid resection is feasible. Delivery of the resected sigmoid containing a small carcinoma in a specimen bag is oncologically justifiable. Secure intracorporeal anastomosis is achieved by conventional anastomosis techniques using the pursestring suture and circular staplers. Analysis of whether laparoscopic surgery with intent to cure is indicated for T_1, T_2 or small T_3 sigmoid carcinomas which have just infiltrated the fat tissue could therefore be justified within a clinical study. However, proper clinical staging by colonoscopic ultra-sonography is a prerequisite here just as in rectal carcinoma.

Abdominoperineal excision of the rectum for a low rectal carcinoma is fundamentally different from low anterior rectal resection. In this operation, also, the conditions for laparoscopic surgery are more favourable since the pelvic dissection takes place in the region of tumor-free bowel and the actual tumor operation is undertaken from the perineum. It is important to remove the rectum in the anatomical planes of the pelvis, taking the mesorectum and the lateral ligaments at the same time. Dissection must follow the anatomical layers in laparoscopic surgery as considerable bleeding occurs otherwise. The perineal part of the operation is the same as in the conventional procedure. Fashioning of the descending colostomy is better performed laparoscopically, as the integrity of the abdominal wall is preserved, but here, too, range of indications is narrow. The T_1 low-risk tumor is treated nowadays by a rectum-preserving full-thickness excision, because the results are comparable to those after radical resection.

In cases where the tumors are advanced with infiltration of neighboring organs, or there is wide tumor infiltration into the perirectal fat tissue and lymph node clusters, a conventional procedure should of course always be chosen.

Laparoscopic Colorectal Surgery for Benign Lesions

There is much less debate over the possibilities of laparoscopic surgery for benign colorectal lesions. The indications include rectal prolapse, sigmoid volvulus, endometriosis, reversal of Hartmann's procedure, arteriovenous malformations, diverticulitis, Crohn's disease, broad-based adenomas which cannot be removed endoscopically, severe obstruction, iatrogenic, traumatic and spontaneous perforations, faecal incontinence, ulcerative colitis and familial polyposis, and protective stomas in complicated anal fistulas or rectovaginal fistulas, sealed rectal perforations and ischaemic or radiation strictures [6, 7, 9 – 12, 15, 16, 19, 20 – 22, 25, 27, 29, 30, 32 – 34]. Because some of these disorders are quite rare, it is difficult to obtain conclusive data from individual institutions on the complication rate and long-term results, other than a simple statement of feasibility. In addition, there is the large number of possible indications. Multicentre studies are as necessary for the benign indications as for colorectal carcinoma in order to obtain evaluable within an acceptable period of time.

Multicentre Study: Design and Early Results

For the reasons mentioned above, we set up a multicentre observation study and laparoscopic colorectal surgery in the German-speaking countries, starting on 1 August 1995. Forty hospitals in Germany, Austria and Switzerland are now taking part in this study (Table 1) In this study, the cases of all patients who undergo a laparoscopic colorectal operation in theses hospitals are recorded and followed up according to a uniform study protocol and the information is analysed centrally at the Department of Surgery University of Erlangen. Since this is an observation study, the indications for laparoscopic colorectal surgery are determined by the individual hospitals themselves. Technical details are not prescribed, nearly documented. Study participants are advised to exercise restraint with regard to curative intent in colorectal carcinoma. However, if curative operations for colorectal carcinoma are performed, the documentation is in accordance with the extended questionnaire of the German Tumor Centres Study Group. The study is to run for about 2 years. By 15 December 1995, complete documentation was available for 123 patients and has already been analysed. This showed that laparoscopic colorectal surgical procedures were used for widely differing indications (Table 2), mostly for benign disease ($n = 66$) or as a palliative procedures ($n = 23$). In 34 cases, laparoscopic surgery was performed with curative intent. In both the palliative and curative operations, the tumors were mostly in the sigmoid and upper rectum (Table 3). The laparoscopic procedures performed, classified according to benign and malignant disease can be seeing Tables 4 and 5. In 7 cases conversion to open surgery was necessary (Table 6). Intraoperative complications recorded were haemorrhage and bowel injury. (Table 7). The significant postoperative surgical complications were anastomotic leaks ($n = 7$, managed conservatively), secondary haemorrhage ($n = 2$), haematoma ($n = 2$) and disorders of bowel motility ($n = 5$) (Table 8). The other postoperative complications delayed wound healing, fever, general complications) are listed in Table 9.

We hope that this multicentre study will succeed in accumulating, within a reasonably short space of time, sufficient data to allow soundly based conclusions about the indications for laparoscopic colorectal surgery in practice.

Table 1. Participating institutions in the Laparoscopic Colorectal Surgery Study Group

Institution	Department	Location
Zentralklinikum	Chirurgische Klinik II	Augsburg, FRG
Universitätsklinikum Benjamin Franklin	Chirurgische Klinik	Berlin, FRG
Städtisches Krankenhaus Zehlendorf	Chirurgische Abteilung	Berlin, FRG
Krankenhaus Buch	Allgemeinchirurgie	Berlin, FRG
Krankenhaus der Landeshauptstadt	Chirurgie	Bregenz, Austria
Evangelische Diakonissenanstalt	Chirurgische Klinik	Bremen, FRG
Zentralkrankenhaus Bremen-Ost	Chirurgische Klinik	Bremen, FRG
Klinikum Merheim	Chirurgische Univ.-klinik	Cologne, FRG
Chirurgische Universitätsklinik		Dresden, FRG
Krankenhaus Dresden-Friedrichstadt	Chirurgische Klinik	Dresden, FRG
Chirurgische Universitätsklinik		Erlangen, FRG
Städtische Krankenanstalten	Chirurgische Klinik	Esslingen, FRG
St.-Elisabeth-Krankenhaus	Chirurgische Klinik	Frankfurt Main, FRG
St.-Hedwig-Hospital	Chirurgische Abteilung	Gelsenkrichen-Resse, FRG
Evangelisches Krankenhaus	Chirurgische Abteilung	Giessen, FRG
Kreiskrankenhaus	Allgemein- und Unfall-chirurgie	Grevenbroich, FRG
Universitätsklinikum Eppendorf	Allgemeinchirurgie	Hamburg, FRG
Allgemeines Krankenhaus Ochsenzoll	Chirurgische Abteilung	Hamburg, FRG
Allgemeines Krankenhaus Barmbek	Chirurgische Klinik I	Hamburg, FRG
Krankenhaus Siloah	Chirurgische Klinik	Hannover, FRG
Frankenwaldklinik	Allgemeinchirurgie	Kronach, FRG
Städtisches Krankenhaus	Chirurgische Klinik	Leverkusen, FRG
Chirurgische Universitätsklinik		Lübeck, FRG
Städtisches Klinikum	Chirurgische Klinik	Ludwigshafen, FRG
Evangelisches Krankenhaus	Chirurgische Klinik	Mühlheim, FRG
Klinikum Großhadern	Chirurgische Univ.-klinik	Munich, FRG
Städtisches Krankenhaus Bogenhausen	Chirurgische Abteilung	Munich, FRG
Klinikum rechts der Isar	Chirurgische Univ.-klinik	Munich, FRG
Ruppiner Klinikum GmbH	Klinik f. Allgem.- u. Gefäßchirurgie	Neuruppin, FRG
Evangelisch-Lutherisches Diakoniekrankenhaus	1. Chirurgische Klinik	Rotenburg a.d.W., FRG
Klinikum Schwerin	Klinik für Chirurgie	Schwerin, FRG
Kantonsspital	Klinik für Chirurgie	St. Gallen, Switzerland
Klinikum Suhl	Chirurgische Klinik	Suhl, FRG
Chirurgische Universitätsklinik		Tübingen, FRG
Krankenanstalt Rudolfstifung	1. Chirurgische Abteilung	Vienna, Austria
I. Chirurgische Universitätsklinik		Vienna, Austria
Wilhelminenspital	2. Chirurgische Abteilung	Vienna, Austria
Städtisches Krankenhaus	Chirurgie	Wismar, FRG
Bethesda Krankenhaus	Chirurgische Abteilung	Wuppertal, FRG
Chirurgische Universitätsklinik		Würzburg, FRG

Table 2. Indications of operation in 123 patients

	n
Benign disease (n = 66)	
Colon/rectal adenoma	13
Sigmoid diverticulitis/diverticulosis	23
Reversal of Hartmann procedure	4
Crohn's disease of terminal ileum	5
Rectal prolapse, intussusception	9
Sigmoid megacolon	3
Other	9
Malignant disease (n = 57)	
Curatively resectable colon/rectal carcinoma	34
Noncuratively resectable colon/rectal carcinoma and tumors infiltrating the colon	23

Table 3. Tumor sites (n = 57)

	n
Curative resection (n = 34)	
Lower rectum	8
Upper rectum	9
Sigmoid colon	13
Ascending/descending colon	3
Descending colon	1
Palliative resections (n = 23)	
Upper rectum	13
Sigmoid colon	6
Descending colon	1
Splenic flexure	1
Ascending colon	2

Table 4. Procdures carried out for benign disease ($n = 66$)

	n
Resective procedures ($n = 56$)	
Rectal resection	3
Sigmoid resection	32
Rectopexy and rectosigmoid resection	4
Rectosigmoid resection for prolapse	4
Reversal of Hartmann's procedure	3
Ileocaecal and ascending colon resection	9
Proctocolectomy	1
Non-resective procedures ($n = 10$)	
Rectopexy	4
Creation of stoma	1
Sigmoidopexy	1
Oversewing of colon (after iatrogenic perforation)	1
Exploration of colon (after stab wound)	1
Division of colon adhesions	1
Closure of colostomy after Hartmann procedure	1

Table 5. Procedures carried out for carcinoma ($n = 57$)

	n
Non-curative procedures ($n = 23$)	
Rectal resection	10
Sigmoid resection	4
Segmental resection of descending colon	1
Left hemicolectomy	1
Segmental resection of ascending colon	1
Creation of stoma	6
Curative procedures ($n = 34$)	
Rectal excision	5
Rectal resection	12
Sigmoid resection	13
Hemicolectomy	4

Table 6. Reasons for conversion to laparotomy ($n = 7$)

	n
Adequate safety margin could not be achieved laparoscopically	1
Local findings in a gunshot injury of the splenic flexure	1
Massive adhesions	1
Tumor size 10 cm	1
Paracolic abscess in diverticulitis	1
Tumor lower than preoperative findings	1
Bowel mobilisation for creation of stoma impossible	1

Table 7. Intraoperative complications ($n = 10$)

	n
Vessel injury	3
– Trocar haemorrhage	2
– Presacral venous plexus haemorrhage	1
Bowel injury	5
– small bowel	2
– Large bowel	3
Other	2
– Bladder wall injury	1
– Diffuse bleeding in active diverticulitis	1

Table 8. Postoperative surgical complications ($n = 19$)

	n
Abnormality in motility for more than 3 days	5
Creation of new stoma because of necrosis	1
Subacute obstruction	1
Omental blockage of drain	1
Anastomotic leak, treated conservatively	7
Haematoma	2
Secondary haemorrhage requiring operation	2

Table 9. Other postoperative complications ($n = 49$)

	n
Delayed wound healing ($n = 12$)	
Infection of minilaparotomy incision	7
Wound dehiscence at site of previous stoma	1
Perineal haematoma	1
Delayed healing at a trocar puncture site	2
Delayed perineal healing	1
Postoperative pyrexia ($n = 27$)	
Pyrexia for 1 day	13
Pyrexia for 2 days	11
Pyrexia for >2 days	3
General postoperative complications ($n = 10$)	
Phlebitis at elbow, abscess on forearm	2
Low back pain	1
Depression	1
Cardiac arrhythmia	1
Cystitis, urinary tract infections, urinary retention	3
Acute liver haemorrhage from varices	1
Symptoms of raised intracranial pressure with known varices	1

References

1. Alexander RJT, Jaques BC, Mitchell KG (1993) Laparoscopically assisted colectomy and wound recurrence. Lancet 341:249–250
2. Beart RW Jr (1994) Laparoscopic colectomy: status of the art. Dis Colon Rectum 37: 547–549
3. Berends FJ, Kazemier G, Bonjer H, Lange JF (1994) Subcutaneous metastases after laparoscopic colectomy. Lancet 344:58
4. Bleday R, Babineau T, Forse RA (1993) Laparoscopic surgery for colon and rectal cancer. Semin Surg Oncol 9:59–64
5. Cohen SM, Wexner SD (1993) Laparoscopic colorectal resection for cancer: the Cleveland Clinic Florida experience. Surg Oncol 1:35–42
6. Cuschieri A (1992) The spectrum of laparoscopic surgery. World J Surg 16:1089–1097
7. Cuschieri A, Shimi SM, Vander Velpen G, Bantin S, Wood RAB (1994) Laparoscopic prosthesis fixation rectopexy for complete rectal prolapse. Br J Surg 81:138–139
8. Decanini C, Milsom JW, Böhm B, Fazi VW (1994) Laparoscopic oncologic abdominoperineal resection. Dis Colon Rectum 37:552–558
9. Franklin ME, Ramos R, Rosenthal D, Schüssler W (1993) Laparoscopic colonic procedures. World J Surg 17:51–56
10. Franklin MW Jr, Rosenthal D, Norem RF (1995) Prospective evaluation of laparoscopic colon resection versus open colon resection for adenocarcinoma – a multicenter study. Surg Endosc 9:811–816
11. Fuhrmann GM, Ota DM (1994) Laparoscopic intestinal stomas. Dis Colon Rectum 37: 444–449
12. Gorey TF, O'Connell PR, Waldron D, Cronin K, Kerin M, Fitzpatrick JM (1993) Laparoscopically assisted reversal of Hartmann's procedure. Br J Surg 80:109
13. Gray D, Lee H, Schlinkert R, Beart RW Jr (1994) Adequacy of lymphadenectomy in laparoscopic-assisted colectomy for colorectal cancer: a preliminary report. J Surg Oncol 57: 8–10
14. Hermanek P, Wittekind C (1994) Inwieweit sind laparoskopische Verfahren in der onkologischen Chirurgie vertretbar? Chirurg 65:23–28
15. Hoffman GC, Baker, JW, Fitchett CW, Vansant JH (1994) Laparoscopic-assisted colectomy. Ann Surg 6:732–743
16. Jacobs M, Verdeja JC, Goldstein HS (1991) Minimally invasive colon resection (laparoscopic colectomy). Surg Laparosc Endosc 3:144–150
17. Köckerling F (1994) Laparoscopic abdominoperineal excision with high transection of the inferior mesenteric artery. Surg Oncol Clin North Am 4:731–743
18. Köckerling F, Reck T, Gastiner I (1995) Laparoscopic abdominoperineal rectum extirpation. In: Phillips, EH, Rosenthal RJ (eds) Operative strategies in laparoscopic surgery. Springer, Berlin Heidelberg New York, pp 242–245
19. Köckerling F, Reck R, Gastinger I (1995) Laparoscopic rectopexy. In: Phillips EH, Rosenthal RJ (eds) Operative strategies in laparoscopic surgery. Springer, Berlin Heidelberg New York, pp 246–250
20. Lyerly HK, Mault JR (1994) Laparoscopic ileostomy and colostomy. Ann Surg 219:317–322
21. Milsom JW, Lavery IC, Church JM, Stolfi VM, Fazio VW (1994) Use of laparoscopic techniques in colorectal surgery. Dis Colon Rectum 37:215–218
22. Nezhat C, Nezhat F, Ambroze W, Pennington E (1993) Laparoscopic repair of small bowel and colon. Surg Endosc 7:88–89
23. O'Rourke NA, Heald RJ (1993) Laparoscopic surgery for colorectal cancer. Br J Surg 80: 1229–1230
24. O'Rourke N, Price PM, Kelly S, Sikora K (1993) Tumor inoculation during laparoscopy. Lancet 342:368
25. Phillips EH, Franklin M, Carroll BJ, Fallas MJ, Ramos R, Rosenthal D (1992) Laparoscopic colectomy. Ann Surg 6:703–707

26. Ramos JM, Gupta S, Anthone GJ, Ortega AE, Simons J, Beart RW (1994) Laparoscopy and colon cancer – is the port site at risk? Arch Surg 129:897–900
27. Sackier JM, Berci G, Hiatt JR, Hartunian S (1992) Laparoscopic abdominoperineal resection of the rectum. Br J Surg 79:1207–1208
28. Schlag PM, Hünerbein M, Rau B (1994) Diagnostic and operative laparoscopy in oncology. Onkologie 17:226–232
29. Schmitt SL, Cohen SM, Wexner SD, Nogueras JJ, Jagelman DG (1994) Does laparoscopic-assisted ileal pouch anal anastomosis reduce the length of hospitalization? In J Colorect Dis 9:134–137
30. Sosa JL, Sleeman D, Puente I, McKenney MG, Hartmann R (1994) Laparoscopic-assisted colostomy closure after Hartmann's procedure. Dis Colon Rectum 37:149–152
31. Tate JJT, Kwok S, Dawson JW, Lau WY, Li AKC (1993) Prospective comparison of laparoscopic and conventional anterior resection. Br J Surg 80:1396–1398
32. Wexner SD, Johansen OB, Nogueras JJ, Jagelman DG (1992) Laparoscopic total abdominal colectomy. A prospective trial. Dis Col Rect 35:651–655
33. Wexner SD, Cohen SM, Johansen OB, Nogueras JJ, Jagelman DG (1993) Laparoscopic colorectal surgery: a prospective assessment and current perspective. Br J Surg 80: 1602–1605
34. Zucker KA, Pitcher DE, Martin DT, Ford RS (1994) Laparoscopic-assisted colon resection. Surg Endosc 8:12–18

Laparoscopic Surgery in Crohn's Disease

U. Hildebrandt

Crohn's disease is a chronic inflammatory disease which affects the entire intestinal tract. Between 69 % and 87 % of those who become ill when young can expect to be operated on once in their lives. The illness recurs in most of those operated on, and the probability of reoperation is greatest in the first 5 years after surgery. After 15 year, 40 % – 70 % of those affected have been operated on because of recurrence. The disease cannot be cured surgically, but it has been shown that early surgical intervention results in lower morbidity and mortality. Crohn's patients are well informed about the chronic character of their illness and live with the awareness that an operation may be needed some day. For this reason, we have applied the "minimal access" method to operations for Crohn's disease. It was our intention to give our patients greater comfort by using smaller incisions.

Patient selection

A requirement for selection for surgery is radiologic and endoscopic assessment of the small and large bowel. Exclusion criteria are fever, sepsis, intra-abdominal abscesses, obstruction and external and internal fistulas. Inclusion criteria are stenoses of the small and large bowel and failure to respond to medical treatment. In the period from January 1993 to September 1995, laparoscopic bowel resections were performed in 43 patients, 17 female, and 26 male. Ages ranged from 18 to 67 years, with an average of 33 years. The duration of illness was 1–18 years, with an average of 6 years. Twenty-three of the 43 patients were being treated with steroids at the time of operation. A bowel resection had already been performed in 7 patients for the same illness, one patient had been operated on twice, and all of the operated patients had an ileocaecal resection. The extent of resection was as follows: small bowel resection 9, ileocaecal resection 18, right hemicolectomy 12, subtotal colectomy 2, colectomy 2. With one exception, all of the operations were laparoscopically assisted. Through a mini-incision, the laparoscopically mobilized, devascularised segment of bowel was drawn through the abdominal wall resected, and the anastomosis was except in a few cases performed outside the abdomen.

Operative Technique for Ileocaecal Resection

The line of incision for a gridiron incision is marked on the right lower abdomen. The pneumoperitoneum is produced through the Veress needle, which is subumbilical in position. The first trocar is positioned in the lateral clavicular line in the left upper abdomen. Under camera vision, two further trocars are placed along this line in the left middle and lower abdomen. These serve as access for the operating instruments. Twelve-millimetre trocars are used so that the linear endoscopic stapler can be used from every position. A 10-mm trocar is inserted through the incision line previously marked in the right lower abdomen; it is used for inserting the Babcock forceps with which the terminal ileum is held and removed.

The first stage of the operation consists of lateral mobilisation of the caecum and the ascending colon including the hepatic flexure. The peritoneum is then incised along the caecal pole and over the ileocolic artery. The ileum is grasped close to the caecum with the Babcock forceps and is drawn in the mediocranial direction. The caecum and ascending colon are then mobilised medially using the dissecting swab. Strands of connective tissue are divided with scissors and small bleeding points are coagulated. The ovarian or testicular vessels are pushed laterally and the ureter is identified. If the terminal ileum is adherent to the wall of the pelvis or to the sigmoid colon because of inflammation, mobilisation is performed with small scissor cuts under close view with the camera.

After mobilisation is complete, the ileocolic artery and vein are placed under tension using the Babcock forceps on the caecum, and the cranial window in the mesentery is opened with scissors. On the other side of the vessels, the mesoileum is opened longitudinally, well away from the bowel if there is much inflammatory thickening or contraction. The ileocolic artery and its accompanying vein are divided with the cutting stapler through one of the trocars on the opposite side. The terminal ileum is grasped with the Babcock forceps in the vicinity of the inflammation, the mesentery is opened, and the ileum is divided with the linear stapler. The remaining vessel connections are divided with two or three further applications of the reloadable stapler. The two bowel ends are grasped with two locking Babcock forceps and the pneumoperitoneum is released. The trocar sleeve in the right lower abdomen is removed and the marked gridiron incision is made.

Held by the Babcock forceps, the end of the inflamed bowel is first drawn outside the abdomen. The same is done with the caecum as far as the middle of the ascending colon. Extensive mobilisation of the ascending colon is of great importance, because after division of the ileocolic artery, the perfusion limit proximal to the caecum defines the line of division. After exenteration of the ileum, an all-layer continuous anastomosis is made with 4–0 PDS. The slit in the mesentery can be closed with one or two sutures through the small incision which is held open with two Roux retractors. After replacing the anastomosis inside the abdomen, the abdominal cavity is irrigated copiously. After closing the incision in layers, the pneumoperitoneum is produced again, the operative area is inspected, and a Robinson drain is placed in the pouch of Douglas through the left lower trocar.

Operative Technique for Right Hemicolectomy

The line of incision is marked under the right costal margin. A 12-mm trocar is inserted at a point along its course. The other trocar positions and stages of the operation are the same as those for ileocaecal resection. The resection technique for laparoscopic ileocaecal resection is supplemented by mobilisation of the colon beyond the hepatic flexure. The gastrocolic ligament is partially divided with the linear stapler through the upper right trocar position. This is followed by identification of the right colic artery, keeping the colon stretched, and the artery is divided with the stapler close to the bowel. Opening of the window in the mesentery under the hepatic flexure is an important step since the duodenum runs here. The ascending colon is held under tension with the Babcock forceps through the right upper working channel, parallel to the transverse colon. The optic is moved to the lower left trocar position and this gives an optimum view of the right upper abdomen. Using the scissors, the delicate connections between the hepatic flexure and the C of the duodenum are divided. Small bleeding points are coagulated with the tip of the closed scissors. Right lateral branches of the middle colic artery are closed with clips and divided. After full mobilisation of the Crohn's segment that is to be resected, the ileum and caecum are grasped with locking Babcock forceps. The pneumoperitoneum is released and a 4- to 6-cm incision is made at the previously marked site. Muscles are not divided but are split in their course. The incision is in the right upper abdomen because the ileum can be mobilised up to there outside the abdomen. The ascending colon is first drawn outside the abdomen and if necessary, sections of the greater omentum are resected. After the open resection, the end of the ileum is brought outside the abdomen using Babcock forceps and a continuous all-layer ileotransverse anastomosis is made with 4-0 PDS. The anastomosis is replaced, the abdomen is irrigated, the incision is closed, the pneumoperitoneum is restored, the operative area is inspected under laparoscopic vision, a Robinson drain is placed in the pouch of Douglas, and the trocars are removed.

Results

During the period from January 1993 to September 1995, the operation was begun laparoscopically in 50 patients. Conversion to the conventional procedure was necessary in 7 patients. The reasons for conversion were: inflammatory adhesion that could not be divided (5), abscess (1), and ileosigmoid fistula (1). The operation could be performed laparoscopically in 43 patients. The operating time varied considerably, in particular with ileocaecal resections, and the duration of operation became distinctly shorter in hemicolectomies because of increasing experience. For ileocaecal resection, the operating time varied from 90 to 280 min, for right hemicolectomy from 120 to 240 min, for subtotal colectomy from 280 to 320 min, and for colectomy from 330 to 420 min.

Complications

Intraoperative Complications

Conversion to conventional surgery is not regarded as a complication, but in one case of inflammatory adhesions, perforation of the small bowel with the grasping forceps contributed to the decision to convert. No other intraoperative complications were noted.

Postoperative Complications

One patient developed an acute abdomen with severe lower abdominal pain on the 2nd postoperative day after laparoscopic ileocaecal resection. On conventional laparotomy, haemorrhage of a corpus luteum cyst of the left ovary was found to be the cause. A subhepatic abscess became clinically apparent in one patient on the 6th postoperative day. After ultrasound-guided aspiration and irrigation, the further course was uncomplicated. In two patients, intermittently raised temperatures occurred postoperatively over periods of 9 and 13 days respectively. Both patients were on steroid treatment. The anastomoses after ileocaecal resection and right hemicolectomy were satisfactory on X-ray. One patient was given antibiotics. Apart from the prolonged hospital stay (18 days), no further events were noted. In two patients, there was secondary healing of the mini-incision.

Clinical Course

The postoperative hospital stay was 7–26 days. The first bowel movement was recorded on the 1st – 4th postoperative day. Eating postoperatively commenced between the 3rd and 5th days. The analgesic requirement varied between 0 and 4 injections of piritramide (Dipidolor®). An outstanding advantage compared to conventional operations was the early complete mobilisation of the laparoscopically operated patients.

Discussion

Non-occurrence of remission during medical treatment is the indication for surgical intervention in Crohn's disease. Waiting raises the rate of septic complications, which can be as high as 40 %. The change in attitude towards early surgical intervention has lowered morbidity and mortality. At the time of operation, the physical fitness of Crohn's patients is good with modern assessment of the surgical indications. This results in the possibility of selection for laparoscopic surgery.

The end result of laparoscopic resection in Crohn's disease is the same safety with greater patient comfort. We see a great benefit in the small access route for the patients, the further course of whose illness is unpredictable. The operating times are very long, but with increasing experience of ileocaecal resection and hemicolectomy they are becoming comparable to those of conventional procedures. Complications due to the longer-lasting anaesthesia were not noted.

The operating technique is „laparoscopically assisted." The anastomosis is made outside the abdomen. An incision is required for delivery of the resected specimen, and the length of the incision depends on the degree of inflammation of the specimen. Since inflammatory masses are difficult to separate laparoscopically, and can contain a walled-off abscess, they are a contraindication for laparoscopy. The presence of a mass, an entero-enteric fistula or an abscess cannot always be recognised preoperatively. For this reason, the operation ended conventionally in 7 of the 50 patients. The bowel segments to be anastomosed are mobilised laparoscopically so far that they can be brought outside the abdomen without tension. The incision is made in the quadrant in which the anastomosis will lie. Since the gridiron incision is necessary for removal of the specimen and the anastomosis can be carried out extracorporeally through it, we regard completely intracorporeal anastomotic techniques as unnecessary.

"Laparoscopically assisted" operations in Crohn's disease combine the advantages of conventional anastomotic techniques with the advantage of a small access. If the benefit for the patient is assessed from the modern viewpoint, the chief gain is the early complete mobilisation due to reduced pain. The postoperative hospital stay is unaltered since the time needed for the anastomosis to heal is the same. The uncomplicated course and the small incision have a positive psychological effect on the patients who are aware of the chronic nature of their illness.

References

1. Puntis J, McNeish AS, Allan RN (1984) Long-term prognosis of Crohn's disease with onset in childhood and adolescense. Gut 25:329
2. Lindhager T, Ekelund G, Leandeer L, Hildell J (1983) Crohn's disease in a defined population; course and results of surgical treatment. Acta Chir Scand 149:407
3. Hultén L (1988) Surgical treatment of Crohn's disease of the small bowel or ileocaecum. World J Surg 12:180
4. Goligher JC (1988) Surgical treatment of Crohn's disease affecting mainly or entirely the large bowel. World J Surg 12:186
5. Betzler M, Schürmann G, Herfarth C (1992) Chirurgisches Vorgehen bei Morbus Crohn. Chirurg 63:13
6. Hildebrandt U, Feifel G (1994) Laparoskopische viszerale Chirurgie. Zentralbl Chir 120:345
7. Lindemann W, Kreissler-Haag D, Hildebrandt U, Ecker KW (1994) Laparoskopische Darmresektionen bei Morbus Crohn – Was ist machbar, was ist sinnvoll? Endosk Heute 7:190
8. Asoklis S, Lange O, Hildebrandt U, Mertzlufft F, Lemmermeier P (1994) Effekte laparoskopischer Kolonresektionen (LCR) auf Hämodynamik und Atmungsparameter. Coloproctology 16:400
9. Böhm B, Milsom JW, Fazio VW (1994) Laparoskopische Ileocoecalresektion beim Morbus Crohn. Zentralbl Chir 119:420

Extracorporeal Resection of the Rectum in the Treatment of Prolapse Using the Stapler

B. Ulrich

The rare syndrome of a complete rectal prolapse was described as early as 1500 B. C. (Ebers papyrus). Since the beginning of this century, over 130 operative procedures for the treatment of this syndrome have been described. Convincing results with regard to postoperative continence have not been achieved hitherto. To date, there does not appear to be any uniform treatment plan [8, 10, 20, 23].

Because of the continuing protrusion of the rectum, lackness of the overstretched sphincter develops in most cases so that the condition is complicated by ulceration, small bowel herniation and occasionally by strangulation as well. The patient's state of health plays an important role in the selection of an operative procedure to treat complete rectal prolapse. Usually the patients are elderly and they often have multiple illnesses.

The many operative procedures described for treating rectal prolapse can be divided into three groups:

1. Narrowing of the anal opening
2. Methods of rectopexy
3. Resection operations

Operative procedures which brought about a narrowing of the anal opening were used formerly because it was assumed that the rectal prolapse was a sliding hernia. Thiersch recommended the sublevator wire ring in 1890 and Sarafoff an external scar stenosis (1937 and 1951) [18]. Other procedures aimed to tighten up the slack pelvic floor (Table 1). By means of these procedures, however, the stage of obvious rectal prolapse was merely converted to a latent stage.

Table 1. Options for Surgical treatment of rectal prolapse

I   Narrowing of the anal opening
    - Sublevator wire ring (Thiersch 1890) [2]
    - External stenosis (Sarafoff 1937, 1951) [18]
    - Tightening the pelvic floor musculature

II Rectopexy
    - Anterior rectopexy (Ripstein 1952, modification 1965) [16, 17]
    - Posterior rectopexy – sometimes with implant of plastic material (Wells 1959, Cutait-Kummel 1959) [3, 21]

III Resection
    - Transabdominal, sometimes combined with rectopexy (Frykman – Goldberg 1969) [5]
    - Extracorporeal perineal (Delorme 1901, Altemeier 1971) [1, 4]

A persisting internal hidden prolapse remained. Complications such as wire breakage, perforation of the skin, infections and coprostasis were the order of the day. Even replacement of the silver wire by synthetic materials such as nylon, teflon, polypropylene, Marlex and Dacron did not bring about any improvement. In addition, there was a high rate of recurrence. It is therefore understandable that abdominal procedures have been increasingly preferred in recent decades. Using the transabdominal route, either resection or fixation or a combination of the two procedures was performed. Anterior rectopexy was first described in 1952 by Ripstein and modified in 1965 by means of the use of plastic [16, 17]. Wells and Cutait-Kummel proceeded in 1959 according to the same principle but with posterior rectopexy [3, 21]. The fixation procedure was extended in 1969 by Frykmann and Goldberg by the addition of resection [5].

The Delorme method (1901) occupied an intermediate position between anal procedures and those involving rectal resection; this consisted of peranal resection of mucosa and submucosa over the entire length of the prolapsing rectum, followed by plication of the denuded bowel extracorporeally, in order to construct a kind of muscular pessary above the levators [4].

A regular extracorporeal perineal rectosigmoidectomy was described for the first time in 1889 by Mikulicz and was reintroduced by Miles in 1933 [11]. Altemeier took up this operation again in 1971 and added to the resection an anterior reconstruction of the poburectalis and levator ani muscles and obliteration of the pouch of Douglas [1].

In the abdominal fixation operations of Ripstein and Wells, Teflon or an Ivalon sponge were used. The principle consisted of encircling the rectum with a kind of cuff and fixing it in the vicinity (e. g. to the sacrum). Aseptic inflammation was provoked in this way, leading to consequent fibrosis and eventually to lasting fixation of the rectum in the rectal hollow. The results of the different procedures (Table 2) are very variable and do not allow any procedure to appear as the operative method of choice [1, 6, 7, 9, 12 – 14, 17, 22]. It becomes clear that the recurrence rates after the non-resecting procedures are higher than those after treatments which include resection. In addition, it also ap-

Table 2. Results of different operative procedures for rectal prolapse

	Complications (%)	Mortality (%)	Recurrence (%)	Success (%)
Thiersch (anal cerclage)	12	–	–35	76
Ripstein (anterior rectopexy)	3.7 – 29	0.7 – 2.8	1.5 – 13	90 – 96
Wells (posterior rectopexy)	9 – 39	0 – 1.4	0 – 11.5	80 – 100
Pemberton-Stalker (rectopexy)	30	1 – 4	12.5 – 35	72
Frykmann-Goldberg (resection and rectopexy)	– 50	0 – 1	0 – 3.7	91
Altemeier (perineal resection	12 – 18	–	0 – 2.8	94
Delorme (rectal muscosectomy and plication)	16	0 – 1	0.24	85

pears that the complication rates are higher with the abdominal procedures than with the perineal procedures.

Because of these totally unsatisfactory results with transabdominal procedures, we have decided in favour of the low-complication procedure of extracorporeal resection using a stapler for our usually very old patients with multiple illnesses.

Patients and Methods

Study Design

In the period from 1 April 1988 to 30 April 1995, 18 patients were operated on in our hospital because of a rectal prolapse. The patients or their doctors were questioned about the results after an interval of at least 6 months. If there was the slightest suspicion of a recurrence or the findings were unclear, the patients were re-examined.

Operative procedure

During extracorporeal rectal resection using a stapler for the treatment of rectal prolapse, the prolapsed bowel segment is infiltrated with a diluted 1:100 000 adrenaline in saline solution about 2 cm proximal to the anocutaneous line. It is then incised in a circular fashion using the electrical scalpel. A 3- to 4-cm-long distal cuff of rectum should be preserved as this ensures preservation of sensitivity in the rectoanal transition area. The sigmoid mesocolon or mesorectum of the protruding segment of bowel is divided between two ligatures (Fig. 1). The rectosigmoid is resected until it all appears stretched (it is possible

Fig. 1. Incision lines for rectal prolapse

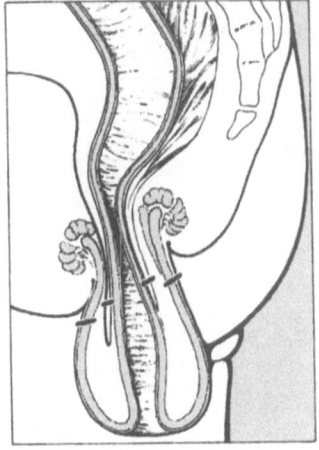

Fig. 2. The rectosigmoid is freed from the sigmoid mesocolon and its peritoneal covering

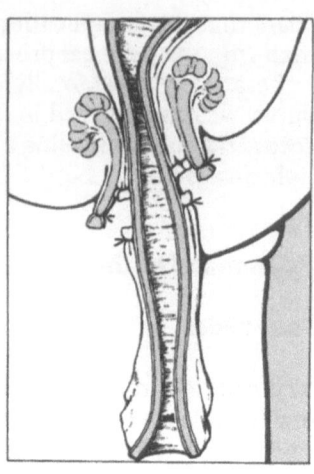

to resect as much as 60 or even 80 cm of bowel). The peritoneal covering of this bowel segment, which lies extra-anally in part, is divided and ligated (Fig. 2). After placing a continuous purse-string suture (Size 1 suture) around the distal rectal cuff, the sigmoid is divided 2–3 cm above the anus. A purse-string suture is placed at this resection margin also. Retaining sutures are placed to assist preparation of the stapled anastomosis. The stapler with the greatest possible magazine diameter (usually ILS-33 or EEA-31) can then be introduced and the purse-string sutures can be tied firmly over the axis of the instrument. The instrument is then released (Fig. 3). After withdrawing the instrument, the tissue rings are inspected for completeness and the intact anastomosis becomes visible and palpable.

Fig. 3. Automatic anastomosis after perineal resection of the rectum and sigmoid

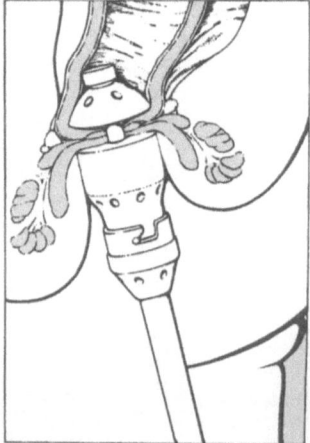

Table 3. Perioperative management of extracorporeal rectal resection

- Preoperative orthograde bowel irrigation
- Perioperative antibiotic prophylaxis
- Anastomosis using a stapler
- 2–3 days parenteral nutrition

Results

In the period referred to above, extracorporeal rectal resection was performed in 18 patients with rectal prolapse. All 18 patients were female and 8 patients (44.4%) had an underlying psychiatric disease. The median age of our patients was 79 years; the youngest patient was 36 and the eldest was 90 years old.

Perioperative management is relatively simple and standardized (Table 3). All patients had preoperative orthograde bowel irrigation and perioperative antibiotic prophylaxis. Initially the patiens received parenteral nutrition for 5 days postoperatively, but oral nutrition in the last three patients began immediately after operation. All of the anastomoses were made exclusively with the stapler. An ILS-33 instrument was used in ten cases and an EEA-31 in eight. The median operating time was 62 min (35–145 min). The operation was done under general anaesthesia in eight patients, and spinal anaesthesia (regional anaesthesia) was sufficient in the last ten patients.

Three patients suffered complications (16.6%). One died on the 3rd postoperative day from a massive pulmonary embolus. There were three systemic complications: urinary tract infection, acute exacerbation of chronic obstructive pulmonary disease and pulmonary embolus. Among the specific complications, we found only one anastomotic leak. This was in a patient who hat a combined rectal and vaginal prolapse. After the usual extracorporeal rectal resection, the gynaecologic procedure of pelvic floor repair was performed. Later in the course, lower abdominal peritonitis occurred with subsequent dehiscence at the rectum. The anastomosis was still intact when the peritonitis occurred. The four complications occurred in three patients. The median postoperative hospitalization was 10 days (range 2–28 days). We did not see any recurrence in the long term. Eleven patients reported a good result; a further six patients were unable to assess the result because of their psychiatric condition. The doctors treating them assured us that no recurrence had occurred. Six of the 18 patients had rectal incontinence preoperatively, as did six postoperatively. However, one patient who had been continent preoperatively was incontinent afterwards and one who was incontinent preoperatively was continent afterwards. The patients were followed up for a median of 18 months.

Discussion

In the literature a ratio of women to men in the incidence of rectal prolapse is given as from 3:1 to 10:1 [6, 20]. In our group of 18 patients, there were only women. The incidence of rectal prolapse associated with underlying psy-

Table 4. Possible complications after operation for rectal prolapse

- All typical complications of transabdominal operations
- Infection of the implant (pelvic sepsis)
- Recurrence after non-resecting procedure

chiatric illness (40 %) described in the literature was confirmed in our series
(44.4 %).

Because of the very unsatisfactory results of surgery for rectal prolapse and
the fact that most patients with a rectal prolapse are already very old and often
have multiple illnesses, and since it is a benign condition, the recommended
treatment method should not only be effective but should also have few complications, i. e. it should be safe. We therefore decided on extracorporeal rectal
resection using a stapler for these patients. The reasons for this can be defined
as in Table 4. All of the typical complications of a transabdominal operation,
such as disturbed wound healing, adhesions, ileus, sacral haemorrhage, im-
potence in the male and injury to other organs, can be avoided by this procedure. In addition, infection of the implant, which may be followed by pelvic infection and sepsis usually fatal is avoided as no foreign body is introduced. The
recurrence rate after the perineal procedure is markedly lower than after the
non-resection procedures (see literature).

The advantages of extracorporeal resection as the treatment for rectal prolapse (Table 5) are that the stress for the patient is minimal. Regional anaesthesia is sufficient. The operating time is comparatively short. The operative
technique, when carried out by a surgeon who is experienced in using the
circular stapler, is unproblematic. The postoperative hospital stay is short
compared to other procedures and can now be estimated as 2 – 3 days.

The question of an improvement in continence can be answered by observ-
ing that in this high-risk patient group removal of the prolapse is the main objective (this is what the patients are conscious of). Although the question of an
additional repair of the levator ani to improve continence [15] is raised increasingly rarely even in young patients, because an improvement of the order of
10 % – 15 % at best can be anticipated, it does not play a part in this group of patients. Here it is only a matter of removing the prolapse and its consequences.
Apart from this, Stelzner [20] reported that a large proportion of younger patients with rectal prolapse were able to regain continence after it was removed
without performing a levator repair.

Table 5. Advantages of extracorporeal resection for rectal prolapse

- Minimal stress for the patient
- Regional anaesthesia is sufficient
- Short operating time
- Simple operative technique
- Short postoperative hospital stay

Because of our good experience with extracorporeal rectal resection to treat rectal prolapse in elderly patients, and because of the advantages listed above, we have since performed it as the procedure of choice not only in patients with a raised operative risk but in all patients. We are of the opinion that the treatment plan for surgical management of a benign condition should be assessed individually by reviewing the general condition of the patient and the therapeutic success to be anticipated. In adopting this treatment plan, the security and time-saving obtained with the automatic stapled anastomosis gave new relevance to the operating method first described by Mikulicz in 1889 and later propagated by Altemeier. Even the increasingly propagated procedure of laparoscopic rectopexy does not seem to be a genuine alternative with regard to its benefit for the elderly patient with multiple illnesses.

References

1. Altemeier WA, Cuthbertson WR, Schowengerdt C, Hunt J (1971) Nineteen years experience with the one-stage perineal repair of rectal prolapse. Ann Surg 173:993–1006
2. Carrasco AB (1934) Contribution des l'étude du prolapsus du rectum. Masson, Paris
3. Cutait D (1959) Sacropromontory fixation of the rectum for complete rectal prolapse. Proc R Soc Med 52:195
4. Delorme E (1901) Communication sur le traitement des prolapsus du rectum totaux, par l'excision de la muqueuse rectale ou recto-colique. Bull Mem Soc Chir Paris 26:499–518
5. Frykmann HM, Goldberg SM (1969) The surgical treatment of rectal procidentia. Surg Gynecol Obstet 129:1255
6. Goligher JC. Prolapse of the rectum. In: Surgery of the anus, rectum and colon, 5th edn. Ballière Tindall, London, pp 246–284
7. Gopal RA, Amsriel AL, Shonberg IL et al. (1984) Rectal procidentia in elderly an debilitated patients: experience with the Altemeier procedure. Dis Colon Rectum 27:376–381
8. Hancke E, Junginger TH (1991) Rektumprolaps. Ätiologie, Klinik und aktueller Stand der chirurgischen Therapie. Med Klin 86:204–208
9. Launer DP, Fazio VW, Weakley FL et al. (1982) The Ripstein procedure: a 16-year experience. Dis Colon Rectum 25:41–45
10. Madoff RO 81992) Treatment of rectal prolapse and intussusception. Saunders, Philadelphia (Seminars in colon and rectal surgery, vol 3.2)
11. Miculicz J (1889) Zur operativen Behandlung des prolapsus recti et coli invaginati. Arch Klin Chir 38:74
12. Moore HD (1964) Complete prolapse of the rectum in the adult. Ann Surg 169:368–375
13. Penfold JCE, Hawley PR (1972) Experience of Ivalon sponge implant of complete rectum prolapse at St Mark's Hospital 1960–1970. Br J Surg 59:845–848
14. Porter N (1962) Collective results of operations for rectal prolapse. Proc R Soc Med 55:1087–1091
15. Ramamugan PS; Venkatesh (1988) Perineal excision of rectal prolapse with posterior levator ani repair in elderly high-risk patients. Dis Colon Rectum 31:701–706
16. Ripstein CB (1952) Treatment of massive rectal prolapse. Am J Surg 83:68
17. Ripstein CB (1965) Surgical care of massive rectal prolapse. Dis Colon Rectum 8:34
18. Sarafoff D (1937) Ein einfaches, ungefährliches Verfahren zur Behandlung des Mastdarmvorfalls. Arch Klin Chir 190:219
19. Stelzner F (1991) Kommentar zur Therapie des Mastdarmvorfalls. Chirurg 62:54
20. Stelzner F (1994) Über die Ursache und die Therapie des Mastdarmvorfalls – Erfahrungen bei 308 Fällen aus den Jahren 1956–1992. Chirurg 65:533–545

21. Wells C (1959) A new approach to the rectal prolapse. Proc R Soc Med 52:603
22. Wells C (1962) Polyvinyl alcohol sponge prosthesis for rectal prolapse. Proc R Soc Med 55:1083
23. Williams JG, Rothenberger DA, Madoff RD, Goldberg SM (1992) Treatment of rectal prolapse in the elderly by perineal rectosigmoidectomy. Dis Colon Rectum 35:830–834

Rectal Prolapse: Rectopexy or Resection?

T. Hager

Rectal prolapse is a serious condition with major consequences for the patient, especially when diagnosed very late. A simple ulcer can occur, without complete anal incontinence. A distinction is made between external and internal rectal prolapse. Many discussions mention only external rectal prolapse, but in our practice we find not only an external prolapse, but an internal one in half of our patients, most of whom are female. Nor is it exclusively a condition of advanced age, as the youngest patient with a rectal prolapse was 19 years old.

The majority of our patients had chronic constipation with considerably prolonged transit time in addition to the rectal prolapse. If there is no external prolapse or internal prolapse with histological evidence of a simple rectal ulcer, which is proof of rectal prolapse, extensive diagnostic procedures are required to diagnose rectal prolapse: defecatogram, colonoscopy, radiology of the large bowel to establish the length, and manometric investigations. The descending perineal syndrome coexists in nearly all of the patients. Surgery is suggested when conservative treatment fails, i.e. changeover to a high-fibre diet, increase in liquid intake, pelvic floor training, avoidance of straining during defecation, and a long explanation especially with regard to toilet habit.

Various procedures have been proposed for the treatment of rectal prolapse. The three main types of operative procedure are those involving the anus, the perineum and abdominal procedures. We do not perform any perianal or anal procedures such as the Delorme method in our hospital, as I am not convinced of the results with regard not only to the rectal prolapse but also to the entire pelvic floor function. Some patients also have a prolapse of the uterus and vagina and bladder incontinence. All of these problems cannot be solved safely from the perineum. We therefore perform abdominal procedures only, of which there are two methods: rectopexy and anterior rectosigmoid resection, extending to left hemicolectomy in patients with chronic constipation with elongated colon. In 1983, after moving from Erlangen University to Kronach, we began to perform the Rippstein-Wells operation for rectal prolapse but were never completely happy with these results either. The recurrence rate, as reported internationally, also seemed to us too high. One of the main problems – chronic constipation – could not be removed. A large number of patients complained about considerable flatulence and increased constipation. We therefore began in 1984 to carry out anterior rectal resection with sigmoid resection and fixation of the rectum in selected patients in parallel with rectopexy in others. A preliminary study of patients operated on in this way yielded clearly better results, and since 1985 we have been performing only rectosigmoid resection. Since the introduction of laparoscopic colon surgery in our hospital in 1993, we have been trying to carry out the resection procedure by the minimally invasive method, which means endoscopically assisted rectosigmoid resection.

So far, 99 patients have been treated for an internal or external rectal prolapse. A rectopexy was done in 16, and resection procedures were performed in all the others (Table 1). Fifty-one patients had an external rectal prolapse, 48 patients an internal, in 25 there was a simple rectal ulcer and in 12 patients we were treating a recurrent prolapse after previous rectopexy (Table 2). Some of our patients had undergone other operations because of the prolapse before admission to our clinic, including removal or rectal polyps. In each case there was misdiagnosis of a simple rectal ulcer, and it is noteworthy that in 18 patients a hemorrhoid operation had been performed in ignorance of the differential diagnosis between haemorrhoids and an external rectal prolapse (Table 3).

During preoperative investigations, it became apparent that two–thirds of the patients had problems with continence; 54, i.e. over half of the patients, were completely incontinent, in some cases for a very long time. Seventy-five

Table 1. Surgical procedures carried out to treat rectal prolapse in 99 patients (Frankenwaldklinik Kronach, January 1983 to May 1995)

	$n = 99$
Rectopexy	16
Rectosigmoid resection	81
Hartmann resection	1
Excision of rectum	1

Table 2. Preoperative patient data ($n = 99$)

Age (range, years)	19–90
Male: female ratio	1:5
Duration of condition (range)	2 months–40 years
External prolapse (n)	51
Internal Prolapse (n)	48
Simple rectal ulcer (n)	25
Recurrent prolapse (n)	12

Table 3. Previous operations undergone by patients

	n
Thiersch ring	2
Rectopexy	9
Sudeck operation (sacral rectopexy)	1
„Rectal polyps"	7
Haemorrhoid operation	18
Gracilis sling	1

patients complained of chronic constipation, 68 of considerable urgency, and 54 of pain in the region of the anus or rectum (Table 4).

Table 5 shows a comparison of the postoperative complications after resection and after rectopexy. It is certain that morbidity is greater with resection, but we believe that this increased morbidity can be regarded as acceptable and the insufficiency rate is relatively low considering how high the resections were (2/81, corresponding to 2.5 %).

At the end of 1994, we followed up the patients operated by us or surveyed them in a detailed questionnaire, and obtained data from 74 %. As expected, there was no recurrence of prolapse in the resected patients; there were four recurrences in the patients who had had rectopexy. One was treated by resection and one patient had a post-anal repair. Two patients did not want any further treatment. However, what was really decisive for us was the evalutation of continence, as this showed continence to have improved considerably in the resected patients compared to the rectopexy patients. With the exception of five patients who remained fully incontinent, all patients achieved considerable improvement in continence some of them complete continence. With rectopexy we did not succeed in improving continence significantly compared to the preoperative situation. In all cases however, the simple rectal ulcer had healed (Table 6).

We also find the patients' opinion with regard to the success of the operation noteworthy. In comparing resection and rectopexy, resection comes off signif-

Table 4. Preoperative continence (*n* = 99)

	n
Full continence	14
Incontinence:	
Grade I	10
Grade II	21
Grade III	54
Other symtoms:	
Constipation	75
Urgency	68
Pain (anal, rectal)	54

Table 5. Postoperative complications after resection vs rectopexy

	Resection (*n* = 81)	Rectopexy (*n* = 16)
Wound infection	3	2
Ileus	2	1
Insufficiency	2	–
Pulmonary complications	9	0
Urinary tract infection	9	0

Table 6. Results of follow up of patients operated on between 1 January 1983 and 31. December 1992 ($n = 74$)

	Resection ($n = 58$)		Rectopexy ($n = 16$)	
	Preop.	Postop.	Preop.	Postop.
Full continence	9	37	3	6
Incontinence:				
Grade I	5	9	2	6
Grade II	13	7	3	1
Grade III	31	5	8	3
Simple rectal ulcer	22	0	3	0
Recurrence	0		4[a]	

[a] One treated by resection, one by post- and repair, Two patients did not want further treatment.

icantly better in patient opinion than rectopexy. Of those who underwent rec-topexy, quite a high proportion – 30 % – stated that they did not regard the operation as successful. Only 5 % of the resected patients stated that they did not see their operation as successful, and only another 5 % regarded their oper-ation as partly successful. These are the patients in whom we failed to improve the incontinence (Table 7).

In summary, we have determined that the treatment for rectal prolapse is not rectopexy but resection of the proximal rectum together with the sigmoid colon or left hemicolectomy in cases of massive chronic constipation, with or without simultaneous tightening of the pelvic floor. Concomitant procedures can also include removal of the prolapse, hysterectomy and correction of blad-der incontinence.

With the introduction of minimally invasive surgery in large bowel surgery, an operative method is available which allows resection for rectal prolapse re-latively quickly, without major stress to the patient, we have been performing rectosigmoid resection for rectal prolapse as a minimally invasive procedure in nearly all patients since 1993.

Table 7. Patients' verdicts on the success of the operation

	Resection ($n = 58$)		Rectopexy ($n = 16$)	
	n	%	n	%
Successful	52	90	8	50
Partially successful	3	5	2	20
Not successful	3	5	6	30

Laparoscopic Surgery for Cancer of the Colon: A Pragmatic Approach

Charles A. Akle

Introduction

The spectacular advent of laparoscopic cholecystectomy onto the surgical scene in 1989 has resulted in an unprecedented demand for the use of minimally invasive techniques in almost every branch of surgery. In general surgery, the lessons learnt from cholecystectomy have been adapted well to appendicectomy as well as to diagnostic procedures, but many lessons have had to be relearnt, particularly in the evolution of laparoscopic hernia repair.

The first reports of laparoscopically assisted colonic surgery appeared in 1990 and a wave of enthusiasm spread through the international surgical community, driven not only by the success of cholecystectomy but also by increasing patient demand for the new technology. Sadly, whilst there were a few good and honest reports of early experience from some centres, a mass of anecdotal cases began to surface which demonstrated that surgical quality had been compromised and many disastrous cases left unreported. Operations were taking so long that an anaesthetist commented that the theatre staff had exchanged the clock for a calendar in the operating room, and the extended duration of surgery brought with it all the attendant consequences for patient morbidity and cost. Bowel and other intra-abdominal injuries were common, particularly late perforation from diathermy injuries, tumor spillage and wound contamination. Disastrous tears in the rectum and anus caused by attempts to perform totally closed operations were seen but not reported. Worse still, wrong segments of bowel were removed leaving the tumor in situ.

Perhaps worst of all, the hard lessons learnt from open surgery relating to the extent of tumor and lymph node resection were forgotten and only very limited segmental resections performed. Reports of tumor deposits in port sites further served to raise concern in the surgical fraternity that we had lost sight of our surgical aims in the treatment of this common condition. A moratorium was advocated especially by the American Society of Colon and Rectal Surgeons, and this has introduced a welcome opportunity to review the situation and chart an acceptable course for the future.

Technical Complexity

The technical demands of colonic surgery are far greater than those of cholecystectomy, substantial skills and powers of innovation and are required even of experienced surgeons. Moreover, there are several recognised operations in colonic surgery with gradations of complexity elegantly defined by Geis et al. [1] and based on the three elements of an intracorporeal procedure: namely, mobilisation, devascularisation and anastomosis. To this should be added the following procedural elements:

- Tumor staging
- Laparoscopic mobilisation
- Laparoscopic devascularisation
- Bowel transection
- Specimen retrieval
- Anastomosis

These describe all the stages involved in a colonic resection and which must be mastered sequentially before a full intracorporeal procedure can be performed. It is clearly logical to build up one's skills by starting with simple appendicectomy, progress to mobilisation for right hemicolectomy and sigmoid colectomy, and then graduate to the more challenging procedures involving devascularisation and intracorporeal anastomosis. There is no doubt that the transverse colon remains a difficult mobilisation, especially if the patient is fat, and in this situation patient selection is important. There are a number of relative contraindications for laparoscopic colonic surgery in the author's experience and these include:

- Any patient unsuited for a long laparoscopic procedure
- Obesity – worse in men – 90 kg and over
- Large and/or fixed tumors
- Abscess formation
- Ureteric involvement or fistula formation
- Acute obstruction, especially with intestinal dilatation
- Dense intestinal adhesions

Most modern colorectal surgeons accept that a "cancer operation" is of benefit in malignant colonic surgery and favour the sort of approach advocated by Turnbull et al. [3] – the "No-Touch Isolation Technique". A more recent and excellent report from the French Association for Surgical Research [2] confirms what many have suspected for some time: namely, that a proper segmental resection gives just as good long-term results as a more radical traditional resection. The study looked at the left colon only and reported a median survival at 10 years. It is likely that the same can be said of the rest of the colon but not the rectum. It is essential to stress that the resection remained a segmental one and not a limited excision, and care was taken to ligate the blood supply early, isolate the tumor-bearing segment, minimise handling of the tumor and take 5 cm distally and at least 15 cm proximally with its contiguous blood and lymphatic supply.

The final element of this jigsaw is the increasing recognition that the size of the incision is far less important than the resulting physiological effect. The message that comes through is that post-operative recovery seems to depend more on the kind of anaesthetic given, the length of time the abdomen is open, the use of retractors and packs, and the extent of handling of the bowel rather than the length of the incision. It also seems generally less painful to use transverse incisions wherever possible supplemented with long-acting local anaesthetic blocks.

Some of the author's personal preferences are highlighted below and are simply an extrapolation of good open surgical practice:

- Handle the tumor as gently as possible – do not use crushing instruments.
- Do not spill the tumor.
- Ligate the draining vessels early if safe.
- Allow a length margin for tumor shedding as well as local infiltration. Seal the ends early. Consider distal limb irrigation.
- Do not leave crushed or dead tissue in the operative field.
- Do not try to remove the specimen through an inadequate hole – even with a bag. Beware damage to the rectum and anus if removing the specimen transanally – better still, do not use this method in cancer.
- Clean the port sites and incision with a tumoricide, e.g. Betadine.
- Do not struggle to achieve an intraperitoneal technique at the cost of safety. Length of incision is not as important as physiological care.
- Know when to convert to conventional surgery.

Innovation is still needed on many fronts to try to overcome a variety of technical handicaps. Improvements in visualisation are needed especially in providing 3-D vision, which dramatically facilitates hand suturing and tying and speeds training. Head-mounted display units are likely to become the norm and will relieve some of the clutter in the theatre. Site access remains a problem as we still rely mainly on gravity for retraction in colonic surgery, and the loss of tactile information can be a huge worry as tumor localisation, nodal assessment, liver palpation and checking for synchronous tumors is then dependent on pre-operative imaging. It is all the more important to ensure imaging of the entire colon and liver before surgery, although intra-operative ultrasound can be helpful.

Dissection modalities need to be perfected and careful haemostasis maintained at all times. The early promise of laser technology has not been fulfilled and lasers are now rarely used. A tool to facilitate safe dissection of the omentum and mesentery is needed, and the Argon Spray diathermy is a step in the right direction.

Most surgeons still find intracorporeal suturing and ligation tedious and further improvements in stapling technology are needed, especially instruments which can angulate so as to transect the lower rectum – the author has not had much difficulty here as instruments for open use can readily be inserted through the small working incision.

Case Experience

Table 1 gives an overview of the author's case experience to date (37 patients; overage age 58.3 years, range 23–88 years; male: female ratio 19:18) which

Table 1. Overview of 37 cases of cancer of the colon treated by laparoscopic procedures

Age (years)	Sex	Diagnosis	Operation	Histology	Survival	LOS	Comments
55	F	CA rectum 11 cm	Anterior resection	C2	48	5	Chemotherapy
40	M	CA descending colon	Left hemicolectomy	B	48	4	
58	M	CA rectosigmoid	Anterior resection	C1	47	4	Inf epigastric bleed/Chemotherapy
75	F	CA rectosigmoid	Reversal of Hartmann's	B (perforated	46	5	
45	F	CA rectosigmoid	Reversal of Hartmann's	B (perforated)	45	5	Died
44	F	CA caecum	R hemicolectomy	B	41	4	
73	F	CA rectum 13 cm	Anterior resection	B	39	26	Int. obstruction +PE
62	M	CA rectosigmoid	Reversal of Hartmann's	B (perforated)	37	4	
44	M	CA caecum	R hemicolectomy	B	37	4	
71	F	CA rectosigmoid	Anterior resection	B	36	5	
83	F	CA rectum	Anterior resection	B	36	5	
32	M	Lymphoma appendix	R hemicolectomy	–	31	4	
71	F	CA hepatic flexure	R hemicolectomy	A	25	5	2nd operation
56	F	CA caecum	R hemicolectomy	B	25	4	
36	M	CA descending colon	L hemicolectomy	A	24	4	Malignant Polyp FH+
59	F	CA sigmoid	L hemicolectomy	B	24	5	
66	F	CA rectum 10 cm	Anterior resection	C1	23	5	Chemotherapy
54	M	CA sigmoid	Anterior resection	B	22	5	
24	M	FAPC	Subtotal colectomy + IRA	FAPC	21	5	
71	F	CA sigmoid	Sigmoid colectomy	B	20	7	Asthma/post-op. chest infection
46	M	CA sigmoid	L hemicolectomy	B	19	5	
50	M	CA caecum	R hemicolectomy	B	18	4	
82	F	CA rectosig + splenic flex, est.	L hemicolectomy	C3	18	14	Ileus/CA ovary
51	M	CA ascending colon	R hemicolectomy	B	17	4	
50	M	CA appendix	R hemicolectomy	A	17	4	
68	M	CA ascending colon	R hemicolectomy	C3	16	5	CEA/CA 19–9 ++
57	F	CA sigmoid	Sigmoid colectomy	B	14	5	
68	F	CA rectosigmoid	Anterior resection	C1	12	6	Chemotherapy

Table 1 (continued)

Age (years)	Sex	Diagnosis	Operation	Histology	Survival	LOS	Comments
23	F	Lymphoma ileum	R hemicolectomy	–	11	6	Chemotherapy
88	M	CA rectum	Anterior resection	C3 + liver mets.	9	7	Post-op. urine retention
73	F	CA sigmoid	Sigmoid colectomy	Liver mets.	8	4	Chemotherapy
68	M	CA caecum	R hemicolectomy	B	7	4	
42	M	FAPC CA R colon x2	Subtotal colectomy +IRA	B/C3	6	4	
55	F	CA ascending colon	R hemicolectomy	B	5	4	
73	M	CA rectum	Laparoscopic colostomy	Frozen pelvis	4	2*	
76	M	CA transverse colon	Ext. R hemicolectomy	A	4	6	Malignant polyp
68	M	CA prostate	Laparoscopic colostomy	Frozen pelvis	8	2	Died

CA, carcinoma; FAPC, familial adenomatous polyposis coli; PE, pulmonary embolism; FH, family history; CEA, carcino-embryonic antigen; Ext., extended; mets, metastases; LOS, length of stay.

Table 2. Summary of laparoscopic procedures undertaken
in 37 patients

	n
Right hemicolectomy	13
Left hemicolectomy	5
Sigmoid colectomy	3
Anterior resection	9
Subtotal colectomy + IRA	2
Reversal of Hartmann's operation	3
Defunctioning colostomy	2
(Full mobilisation of transverse colon	4)

Table 3. Histological diagnoses
of 37 patients undergoing
laparoscopic procedures

Colonic carcinoma (Dukes stage)	n
A	4
B	19
C	7
D	3
Familial polyposis	1
Lymphoma	2
Prostate carcinoma	1

involved laparoscopic manipulation in non-colonic malignant disease, and
to date there has not been a single port site recurrence or complication relating to the procedure despite often widely disseminated cancer. Table 3 lists the
histological diagnoses in the cases in which colonic procedures were performed.

The pathologists could not differentiate in terms of length of specimen or
nodal status between specimens obtained by open surgery and those obtained
in a laparoscopically assisted procedure.

Complications occurred in four cases: two of postoperative ileus due to
adhesions (postoperative lengths of stay were 14 and 26 day respectively), one
of urine retention (postoperative stay 7 days), and one of chest infection (postoperative stay 7 days). The average postoperative length of stay overall was 5.3
days (range 2–26); this was reduced to 4.5 days (range 2–6) if the cases with
complications were left out of the calculation.

The two cases of post-operative bowel obstruction were in elderly females
with bulky pelvic tumors that required extensive mobilisation of the rectum
leaving bare pelvic wall to which small bowel adhered. These patients both
initially did superbly, mobilising well and passing flatus on the 2nd day, but
then suffered obstruction on or about the 5th day. Conservative management
worked in one patient but open surgery was needed in the second, who subsequently developed a deep venous thrombosis and small pulmonary embolism,
accounting for her prolonged in-patient stay of 26 days.

Discussion

These cases represent the experience of a single surgeon and the results compare favourably with those of conventional surgery as well as with published reports of laparoscopic cases. They are neither selected nor randomized and do not form part of a trial. The reason for this is that the surgical approach is based on a pragmatic philosophy, so that in each case the advantages of a laparoscopic approach are utilised as far as individual circumstances allow. At the very least, laparoscopy permits staging of the disease and siting of an optimal incision. If, in addition, mobilisation of relevant quadrants of the colon is achieved, then further gains are made as regards siting the incision to facilitate the resection and anastomosis. In the case of the synchronous tumors at splenic flexure and distal sigmoid, it was possible to perform all the upper abdominal mobilisation laparoscopically and complete the more difficult pelvic procedure through a small Pfannenstiel incision. For this reason the length of the incision should carry little emphasis per se; the point is, it should always be big enough to complete the task. Abraham Lincoln was once asked by a heckler eager to ridicule his tall stature, "How long should a man's legs be?" "Long enough to reach the ground!" was the reply. This philosophy seems equally pertinent to the incision in laparoscopically assisted surgery. The pressure on the surgeon to perform is huge and, as in laparoscopic cholecystectomy, conversion must not be equated with failure. The obsessive and headlong rush to try to perform all surgical procedures through a keyhole should be resisted and a period of consolidation introduced to allow surgical skills to catch up witch modern technology. It is absurd to try to perform a totally intracorporeal procedure when one still has to make a hole big enough to safely retrieve the specimen, and until the pathologists allow the surgeon to morcellate the colon, it seem logical to concentrate on the physiological approach and utilize this incision to good advantage.

Conclusion

As surgical experience grows, the day will come when total intracorporeal laparoscopic colonic resections for cancer will be achieved in most cases. That day has yet to arrive, and the surgical fraternity must not be tempted to forget the lessons of the past in the pursuit of raw technological advance. The demands of the lay public and hospital administrators for success with the latest technologies (often supplemented with the word "laser") must be resisted and our enthusiasm tempered with common sense. Carcinoma of the colon is the second commonest cancer in the western world, and the majority of conventionally operable cases are amenable to sensible laparoscopically assited surgery. In time, technology will solve many of our immediate problems, but until then I would plead for a period of consolidation and reevaluation if we are truly to serve our patients.

References

1. Geis WP, Coletta AV, Jacobs M, Placensia G, Charles K (1994) Benefits of complexity scales in laparoscopic colectomy. Int Surg 79:230–232
2. Rouffet F, Hay J-M, Vacher B et al. (1994) Curative resection for left colonic carcinoma: hemicolectomy vs. segmental colectomy – a prospective, controlled, multicentre trial. Dis Colon Rectum 37:651–659
3. Turnbull RB, Kyle K, Watson FR et al. (1967) Cancer of the sigmoid colon. The influence of the no-touch isolation technique on survival rates. Ann Surg 166:420–425

Laparoscopic Operations in Colorectal Cancer

A. Kuthe, K. Reichel, and H. Faust

Introduction

While laparoscopic cholecystectomy and enterolysis have been introduced as standard procedures in almost all clinics, and while laparoscopic inguinal hernioplasty and appendectomy are becoming increasingly important, laparoscopic surgery of the colorectum has hitherto been performed in a very small number of centers. This seems prudent as there are still a considerable number of questions to be answered; in particular, there is still disagreement about the appropriate indication. A very low complication rate has been shown in the papers reporting on laparoscopic colorectal surgery [3, 4, 8, 12, 16, 21], but then the patient populations involved were selected. Moreover even though all laparoscopic colon surgeons repeatedly see a better postoperative course than after conventional procedures [2, 3, 13, 16, 20, 21], so far no factual evidence of benefit to the patients by laparoscopic techniques has been produced [20].

Although nearly all operations in the colon are now carried out laparoscopically, most surgeons do not accept colorectal cancer as a good indication for performing these procedures. First, there are doubts about the transferability of the proven oncological standards of conventional operations to the laparoscopic technique, and, secondly, the lack of long-term follow-up studies is cited as an objection to operations in colorectal cancer [10]. Exploratory and staging procedures, palliative resections of metastasized tumors, and colostomies are to some extent accepted, but curative resections are rejected outside controlled studies in specialized centers [10].

Over the years, colorectal surgeons have established conventional surgical procedures adapted to tumor location which take into account not only local tumor spread but also lymphatic dissemination [9, 11]. These procedures include the lymphatic drainage areas along the named vessels adjoining the tumor back to their origin on the superior mesenteric artery or the abdominal aorta [6]. Well-documented long-term follow-up studies of these techniques exist [6, 11], so the surgeon becomes the most important factor in the long-term prognosis [6, 11, 19]. To ensure equally good results laparoscopically, it is essential for these procedures to be transferred in toto from conventional to laparoscopic surgery. For that reason, and due to local anatomic conditions, some sites of colorectal tumors seem to be more suitable for laparoscopic procedures than others. Thus, tumors of the middle and distal third of the sigmoid colon and of the proximal third of the rectum appear to be very well suited to laparoscopic treatment, since lateral dissection of the descending colon and sigmoid, radicular removal of the inferior mesenteric artery, and mobilization of the left colic flexure can be carried out quite easily [12]. Abdominoperineal excision in cases of distal rectal tumors may be regarded as equally well siuted, as dissection of the mesorectum along the posterior and anterior sheat of the pelvic connective tissue membrane is easy and there is no problem with specimen recovery [12, 13, 14].

Resection of tumors of the middle third of the rectum, however, is technically more demanding, and the transection of the lower rectum using available staplers is difficult, so this tumor location seems to be less suitable. Tumors of the proximal third of the sigmoid and the descending colon require left hemicolectomy, which in turn requires dissection of the gastrocolic ligament and in some cases radicular removal of the medial colic artery. Tumors of the transverse colon need extended hemicolectomies, and tumors of the right colon need central removal of the right colic artery [9]. Because, of the difficulty of identifying the superior mesenteric artery and its branches, and because of the awkwardness of laparoscopic dissection of the gastrocolic ligament [8], tumors in these locations seem poorly suited to laparoscopic resection at present, although laparoscopic procedures have already been carried out for tumors in these locations [4, 8, 12, 16, 20, 21].

Case Experience

Patients

Between July 1, 1992, and September 15, 1995, we started 109 colorectal operations laparoscopically. Among these were 58 rectosigmoid resections including 33 for cancer (there were 4 conversions to open surgery: severe adhesions in 2 cases, obesity in 1, and stapler failure in 1) 36 abdominoperineal rectal excisions for cancer (3 conversions, due to bleeding during perineal dissection in 2 cases and the inferior mesenteric artery in 1), 1 right hemicolectomy for cancer of the cecum, and 7 palliative colostomies. We ended 63 resective operations laparoscopically (Table 1). The mean age of these 63 patients (35 female and 28 male) was 68 years (range 40–84 years).

Operative Technique

For the reasons given above, we confined ourselves to tumors in the following locations: the middle and distal third of the sigmoid colon and the proximal

Table 1. Number of laparoscopic resective procedures performed in cases of colorectal cancer

	Rectosigmoid resection	Abdomin-operineal excision	Right hemi-colectomy	Total
Conversions to open surgery	4	3	0	7
Laparoscopic operations begun	29	33	1	63
Operations completed laparoscopically	33	36	1	70

third of the rectum (operated on with extended sigmoid resection) and the distal rectum (operated on with abdominoperineal rectal excision). There was one right hemicolectomy in our series, in a patient with a big cecal polyp which turned out to be a carcinoma.

Our operative technique for rectosigmoid cancer is as follows. The surgeon and the cameraman stand on patient's right, the assistant on the left, using two monitors. The trocar site for the camera is located in the midline two finger widths above the umbilicus, and there are two 10-mm trocars in the right lower abdomen (for the surgeon) and in the left (for the assistant).

After lateral mobilization of the lower descending colon, including exposure of the left ureter, the serosa is incised to the right of the sigmoid mesocolon in the region of the promontory, followed by tunneling of the mesosigmoid. Dissection of this avascular space up to the inferior mesenteric artery, cutting its origin on the aorta, is followed by dissecting the inferior mesenteric vein and the left colic artery. After dissection of the avascular zone between the left colic artery and the first sigmoid artery, the arcade vessels are cut and further lateral mobilization of the descending colon carried out as far as the left flexure, with mobilization of the latter as well if necessary. The lower descending colon is then cut by stapler and the mesorectum is mobilized dorsal, by almost as far as the peritoneal reflection.

Rectosigmoid Resection. After tunneling the rectum and cutting it by stapler, a maximum length of 10 – 12 cm remaining, the mesorectum is cut 2 cm lower by stapler as well. The specimen is packed into a bag and recovered through a 4 – 5 cm laparotomy that includes the lower left trocar site. Delivering the descending colon through this laparotomy, the anvil is fixed by a purse-string suture, and after repositioning of the descending colon the laparotomy is closed. Transanal circular stapling of the anastomosis is followed by a leakage test, irrigation, and drainage.

Abdomionperineal Excision. After cutting the peritoneal reflection, the mesorectum is dissected totally to the levator muscles, with clipping or cauterization of the medial rectal arteries. At the same time the perineal procedure is performed, and after opening the levator dorsally the specimen is passed through, ending the operation from the perineal approach. The colostomy is performed starting at the site of the upper left trocar, and the descending colon is fixed to the left lateral abdominal wall by suturing, followed by irrigation and drainage after perineal closure.

TNM Staging

Table 2 classifies the 63 patients with laparoscopically completed procedures according to TNM stage. The pTN stages were determined as were the number of involved lymph nodes: 13 (6 – 36) among the patients with rectosigmoid resections, 12 (6 – 9) among those undergoing abdominoperineal rectal excision, and 32 in the patient with the right hemicolectomy. The M stages were all determined preoperatively.

Table 2. TNM tumor stages in the 63 patients with colorectal cancer in whom surgery was completed laparoscopically

Stage	Rectosigmoid resection (n)	Abdominoperineal excision (n)	Right hemicolectomy (n)
pT1N0M0	7	0	0
pT2N0M0	3	5	1
PT3N0M0	7	9	0
pT4N0M0	0	1	0
pT2N1M0	1	0	0
pT3N1M0	6	7	0
pT4N1M0	1	0	0
pT2N3M0	1	0	0
pT3N3M0	1	4	0
pT2N1M1	0	1	0
pT3N1M1	0	2	0
pT3N2M1	0	1	0
pT3N3M1	2	2	0
pT4NxM1	0	1	0
Total	29	33	1
Lymph nodes	13 (6–36)	12 (6–39)	32

Perioperative Complications

Intraoperative Complications

In the rectosigmoid resection group, one lesion of the small bowel caused by enterolysis was oversewn laparoscopically. One lesion to the colon caused by a Babcock clamp was treated in the same way. In one case stapler failure (cutting without stapling) necessitated conversion to open surgery.

In the abdominoperineal excision group, one case of bleeding from the inferior mesenteric artery necessitated conversion to an open procedure, as did two cases of bleeding from the perineal dissection. One lesion to the urethra in the perineal part of the procedure was oversewn.

Postoperative Complications

In the rectosigmoid group, leaking of the anastomosis on day 6 after surgery, due to a tube placement, required an open revision and colostomy in one case. In one case obstruction due to adhesions caused, by the drainage tube was treated by laparoscopic enterolysis (day 10 after surgery). In one case bleeding from the spleen (on day 7 after surgery) necessitated open splenectomy. One case of hematoma in the area of a trocar site and four cases of infection after specimen-recovery laparotomy were treated conservatively.

In the abdominoperineal excision group, bleeding from the medial rectal artery in one case was stopped laparoscopically (on day 1 after surgery), as was a case of epigastric vessel bleeding (day 3 after surgery). One case of obstruction due to Richter's hernia (day 7 after surgery) in the peritoneal closure of pelvic floor (which we performed until this case) required open enterolysis, as did one case of obstruction due to a loop of small bowel adherent to the lesser pelvis (10 months after surgery). One patient died without operation in another hospital due to obstruction caused by adhesions misinterpreted as cancer recurrence (4 months after surgery). One colostomy had to be enlarged (2 months after surgery), Sixteen cases of perineal wound infection were treated conservatively and seven others operatively.

Follow-up

Of the 63 patients with laparoscopically completed operations, 1 has been lost to follow-up (Table 3). Another 6 patients were operated on recently and have not yet attended their first follow-up examination. So far 9 patients have died (Table 4). Thus, we have 47 patients in follow-up at present, with a mean follow-up time of 15 months (range 3 – 37 months).

Table 4 gives details about the patients who died. In the rectosigmoid group, one died of infarction of the bowel due to embolism, one of progression of liver metastasis, and one (stage pT3N3M0) of liver and abdominal metastasis. In the abdominoperineal group one patient died of acute heart failure and one of obstruction due to small bowel loop fixed behind the colostomy (since then we fix the descending colon laterally) misinterpretated elsewhere as tumor recurrence (autopsy showed no recurrence). Two patients of hepatic failure caused by progression of liver metastase. One patient operated on for stage pT4NxM1 recurrent anal cancer died of diffuse metastatic disease, as did another operated on for stage pT3N3M0 rectal cancer.

Table 5 shows all patients currently in follow-up. Half of them are periodically examined by us and half of them elsewhere. In the rectosogmoid group one patient operated on in stage pT3N1M0 developed a solitary liver meta-

Table 3. Follow-up of patients with laparoscopically completed operations

	Rectosigmoid resection ($n = 29$)	Abdominoperineal excision ($n = 33$)	Right Hemi-colectomy ($n = 1$)	Total ($n = 63$)
No. of patients lost to follow-up	0	1	0	1
No. of patients with < 3 months follow-up	4	2	0	6
No. of deaths	3	6	0	9
No. of patients with > 3 months follow-up	22	24	1	47
Average follow-up time in months (range)	14.9 (3 – 32)	14.6 (3 – 37)	27	15.0

Table 4. Tumor stage and cause of death in the nine patients who died

Patient age (years)	TNM stage	Cause of death	Time from surgery to death
Rectosigmoid resection			
89	pT3N1M0	Bowel infarction	4 months
71	pT3N3M1	Progression	13 months
79	pT3N3M0	Metastasis	12 months
Abdominoperineal excision			
81	pT3N0M0	Acute heart failure	4 weeks
62	pT3N3M0	Bowel obstruction by adhesions	4 months
73	pT3N3M1	Progression	2 months
65	pT3N3M1	Progression	1 month
69	pT4NxM1	Metastasis	8 months
66	pT3N3M0	Metastasis	20 months

Table 5. Tumor stages of the patients still in follow up

TNM stage	n
Rectosigmoid resection ($n = 27$)	
pT1N0M0	7
pT2N0M0	3
pT3N0M0	6
pT3N1M0	4[a]
pT4N1M0	1
pT2N3M0	1
Abdominoperineal excision ($n = 24$)	
pT2N0M0	5
pT3N0M0	8
pT3N1M0	5
pT3N3M0	2
pT2N1M1	1
pT3N1M1	2[b]
pT3N2M1	1[b]
Right hemicolectomy	
pT2N0M0	1

[a] 16 months after surgery: right hemihepatectomy for solitary metastasis.
[b] Progression of liver metastasis.

stasis 14 months after surgery and underwent a left hemihepatectomy; so far no recurrence has been seen in any other patient. In the abdominoperineal group all three patients with liver metastasis have progression without local recurrence 6, 7, and 9 months after surgery respectively. All other patients are recurrence-free so far. We have not seen any metastases in trocar sites to date.

Discussion

Due to the considerable technical difficulties involved, the practice of laparoscopic colorectal surgery is not spreading as fast as that of other laparoscopic procedures. Furthermore, in cases of malignancy there are not only technical problems to be solved: it must be shown that laparoscopic surgery can produce results that equal or even surpass those of conventional techniques. So the main point in this patient population is the long-term follow up of as many patients as possible. A more favorable perioperative course would be a pyrrhic victory if it were to be paid for by a higher rate of recurrence.

We think that standardized conventional procedures are totally convertible to laparoscopy for tumors in certain locations. These locations are the middle and distal thirds of the sigmoid colon the proximal and third of the rectum, operated on by extended sigmoid resection, and the distal third of the rectum, operated on by abdominoperineal rectal excision. En bloc resection of the associated lymphatic drainage areas is easy since the oncological approach is mainly through avascular areas and mobilization of the left colic flexure is possible. The middle third of the rectum is now more difficult to handle in the absence of flexible staplers, but complete mobilization of the mesorectum down to the pelvic floor is possible, as we learned doing abdominoperineal rectal excisions.

In regard to all other tumor sites there are some doubts about fulfillment of the principles of cancer surgery, especially because of difficulties in locating the origin of the branches of the mesenteric superior artery and the high technical demands of dissecting the gastrocolic ligament. That is why we think it is wiser to limit laparoscopic procedures with curative intent to colorectal tumors in the sites mentioned, until curative laparoscopic procedures have become established. In any case, these are the sites where most colorectal tumors are found. There is no doubt about the necessity of a recovery bag impermeable to fluids and cells.

We think that our experience as well as that of others shows that even during the learning curve laparoscopic colorectal surgery is a safe procedure with a low complication rate [2, 8, 12, 16–18, 21, 22]. We want to emphasize that in our patients there were no cases of postoperative pneumonia, thrombosis, embolism, sepsis, and or death. Our mean operation time is close to 200 min, which is becoming acceptable.

Not only the longer operation times but also the instruments required of course make laparoscopic operations more expensive than conventional procedures [2, 8, 21]. This may turn out to be compensated by the low perioperative complication rate [21] and possibly better long-term results. However, discussing the costs seems premature at a time when the medical or curative value of this procedure has yet to be proved.

Of course we cannot make definitive statements about long-term results at present, but our results to date seem to be comparable to those of conventional procedures [4, 6, 11]. We have not hitherto discovered any cases of metastasis at trocar sites, which have recently been more and more under discussion [1, 5, 7, 15], It is possible that these unfavorable events may be unusual occurrences in small series, but we must be very attentive to this problem.

In conclusion, we think that we may take the experiences so far as a basis to continue along the path we have started; i. e., curative laparoscopic procedures for colorectal cancer are permissible in appropriate centers carefully monitoring the long-term results.

References

1. Alexander R, Jaques B, Mitchell K (1993) Laparoscopic assisted colectomy and wound recurrence. Lancet 341:249–250
2. Alexander S, Keriakian G, Kasper G, Hearn A (1995) Laparoscopic assisted colectomies versus open colectomy. J Laparoendosc Surg 5:1–6
3. Chindasub S, Charntaracharmong C, Nimitvanit C, Akkaranurukul P, Santitarmmanon B (1994) Laparoscopic abdominoperineal resection. J Laparoendosc Surg 4:17–21
4. Franklin M, Rosenthal D, Norem R (1995) Prospective evaluation of laparoscopic colon resection versus open colon resection. Surg Endosc 9:811–816
5. Fusco M, Paluzzi M (1993) Abdominal wall recurrence after laparoscopic assisted colectomy for adenocarcinoma. Dis Colon Rectum 36:858–861
6. Gall F, Hermanek P (1992) Wandel und derzeitiger Stand der chirurgischen Behandlung des colorectalen Carcinoms. Chirurg 63:227–234
7. Guillou P, Darzi A, Manson J (1993) Experience with laparoscopic colorectal surgery for malignant desease. Surg Oncol 2 [Suppl 1]:43–50
8. Guillou P (1994) Laparoscopic surgery for diseases of colon and rectum – quo vadis? Surg Endosc 8:669–671
9. Herfarth C, Runkel N (1994) Chirurgische Standards beim primären Coloncarcinom Chirurg 65:514–523
10. Hermanek P, Wittekind C (1994) In wieweit sind laparoskopische Verfahren in der onkologischen Chirurgie vertretbar? Chirurg 65:23–28
11. Hermanek P Jr, Wiebelt H, Riedl S, Staimmer D, Hermanek P (1994) Langzeitergebnisse der chirurgischen Therapie des Coloncarcinoms. Chirurg 65:287–297
12. Jacobs M, Verdeja J, Goldstein H (1991) Minimally invasive colon resection. Surg Laparosc Endosc 1:144–150
13. Köckerling F, Gastinger I, Schneider B, Krause W, Gall F (1992) Laparoskopische abdomino-perineale Rektumexstirpation. Laparoendosk Chir 1:99–113
14. Köckerling F, Gastinger I, Schneider B, Krause W, Gall F (1992) Laparoskopische abdomino-perineale Rektumexstirpation mit hoher Durchtrennung der Arteria mesenterica inferior. Chirurg 63:345–348
15. O'Rourke N, Price P, Kelly S, Sikora K (1993) Tumor inoculation during laparoscopy. Lancet 342:368
16. Puente J, Soza J, Sleeman D, Desai U, Tranakas N, Hartmann R (1994) Laparoscopic assisted colorectal surgery. J Laparoendosc Surg 4:1–7
17. Riedel S, Wiebelt H, Bergmann H, Hermanek P Jr (1995) Postoperative Komplikationen und Letalität in der chirurgischen Therapie des Coloncarcinoms. Chirurg 66:597–606
18. Safi F, Beger H (1994) Morbidität und Letalität der operativen Therapie des colorectalen Carcinoms. Chirurg 65:127–131
19. Schwenk W, Hucke H, Graupe F, Stock W (1995) Ist der Chirurg ein prognostischer relevanter Faktor nach RO-Resektion colorectaler Carcinome? Chirurg 66:334–343
20. Slim K, Pezet D, Stencl J, Lagha K, le Roux S, Lechner C, Chipponi J (1994) Prospective analysis or 40 initial laparoscopic colorectal resections: a plea for a randomized trial. J Laparoendosc Surg 4:241–245
21. Tucker J, Ambroze W, Orangio G, Duncan T, Mason E, Lucas G (1995) Laparoscopically assisted bowel surgery. Surg Endosc 9:297–300
22. Zucker K, Pitcher R, Martin D, Ford R (1994) Laparoscopic-assisted colon resection. Surg Endosc 8:12–18

Laparoscopic Resection of the Colon:
Indications, Patients Selection, Results to date

U. Hildebrandt

Introduction

Laparoscopic surgery combines traditional operative techniques with the new minimal-access technology. The term "laparoscopically assisted" is appropriate, since an incision is usually made for removal of the resected specimen.

Laparoscopic colon resection to treat benign disease has not encountered opposition [1], laparoscopic excision of the rectum in cases of cancer is accepted [2], but laparoscopic resection of the colon is controversial [3]. The leading argument against it is the fear that oncological standards will be sacrificed. The question raised is whether the required extent of resection, central ligature of the vessels and complete resection of the lymphatic drainage area can be achieved laparoscopically. Peritoneal spreading of tumor cells and the implantation of abdominal wall metastases are feared [4]. Leaving subjective opinions to one side, the goal of laparoscopic surgery is to benefit the patient. The measurement of this benefit is derived from the results of laparoscopic cholecystectomy: less trauma, less pain, early convalescence, short hospitalization. These were the goals that prompted us to use laparoscopic resection in cancer of the colon.

Indication for Laparoscopic Surgery

Cancers of the caecum and ascending colon close to the caecum, sigmoid carcinomas and rectal carcinomas in which excision was indicated were included. Cancers which could be seen laparoscopically to extend beyond the bowel wall were excluded.

Patients

Nine patients had a tumor in the region of the caecum and proximal ascending colon, 17 patients a tumor in the area of the sigmoid colon and three patients a low rectal carcinoma. Patient age was from 30 to 75 years, with an average of 61 years.

Operative Technique

Our operative technique changed over time, with increasing experience and under the influence of ongoing discussion. The current procedure is described below. We never operate laparoscopically on visibly extramural and infiltrating tumors. Whether a tumor is extramural or infiltrating is decided after inserting the optic through the first trocar.

Right Hemicolectomy

The operation begins with division of lateral adhesions and mobilisation of the caecum. After mobilisation, the colon lumen is closed distal to the tumor with a ligature tied extracorporeally. The retroperitoneum is incised in the medial direction in an arc beginning at the caecal pole. In this way, the terminal ileum is mobilised sufficiently. The spermatic or ovarian vessels are dissected with the dissecting swab. The ureter becomes visible in the retroperitoneum during the blunt dissection in the medial direction. The ileocolic transition area is skeletonised and the ileum is divided from the caecum with the linear cutter. Holding the caecum taut with Babcock forceps, the end artery of the superior mesenteric artery, the ileocolic artery, becomes visible. It is divided after making an opening in the mesentery where a main branch goes to the terminal ileum. The hepatic flexure is then mobilised. By pulling the ascending colon medially, the band-like attachment of the hepatic flexure can be divided with scissors. Small bleeding points are coagulated, and larger visible vessels are clipped. When the hepatic flexure is pulled medially, the duodenum comes into view and is pushed laterally with the dissecting swab. The linear stapler is inserted through the right upper trocar and the gastrocolic ligament is divided as far as the falciform ligament. The hepatic flexure is held taut and the right colic artery is dissected at its origin from the superior mesenteric artery and divided. The same applies to right-sided branches of the middle colic artery and their accompanying veins. The ascending colon is divided with the linear cutter distal to the tumor. The tumor-bearing segment of the ascending colon is placed in a specimen bag. The terminal ileum and the remainder of the ascending colon are each grasped with a Babcock forceps. The gas is released and a gridiron incision is made under the right costal margin. The specimen bag is removed through this incision and the Babcock forceps are used to bring the two bowel ends outside the abdomen. If necessary, the hepatic flexure is now resected also. The ileotransverse colostomy is made with an all-layer continuous suture. After replacing the bowel, the abdomen is irrigated through the mini-incision. The incision is closed in layers and the remaining trocars are removed.

Sigmoid Resection

For laparoscopic sigmoid resection, the operating table is head-down and tilted 30° to the right side. This displaces the small bowel to the right upper abdomen. The operation begins with division of the lateral adhesions of the descending colon and sigmoid colon. The descending mesocolon is stretched taut and the peritoneum is incised along the line of the aorta. The origin of the inferior mesenteric artery is sought and the artery is closed and divided with Ethicon PDS clips. The retroperitoneum is incised further along the lower margin of the duodenum and the pancreas to expose the inferior mesenteric vein, which is clipped. The descending colon is held medially and the spermatic or ovarian vessels are pushed laterally with the swab. The ureter is always exposed in its course. The bowel lumen is closed distal to the tumor with an extraperitoneally tied ligature. The splenic flexure is mobilised fully. This is followed by skeletonisation of the descending colon and interruption of bowel continuity. The sigmoid colon is held taut with the Babcock forceps distal to the tumor and the retroperitoneal incision is continued distally over the sacral promontory. The level of resection is just above the peritoneal reflection, and the reflection is occasionally incised. The tissue plane between the parietal and visceral pelvic fascia is opened in front of the sacral promontory. After complete mobilisation of the proximal third of the rectum, the mesorectum is divided with the linear cutter. The segment of bowel distal to the ligature is irrigated transanally with saline before division of the rectum. The rectum is divided with the linear cutter. The descending colon is grasped with Babcock forceps and the gas is released. The gridiron incision is made in the left lower abdomen. The dissected specimen is removed in a bag through this incision and the descending colon is pulled through to the outside of the abdomen using the Babcock forceps and, if necessary, more is resected outside the abdomen. The press-on disc is sutured in and the descending colon is replaced in the abdomen. It is irrigated liberally through the incision. The gridiron incision is closed and the anastomosis is made under laparoscopic vision. A drain is placed in the pouch of Douglas, the incision is closed and the trocars are removed.

Results

In four more patients with a colon carcinoma, the operation had to be continued in the conventional way. In one case, the colon was opened with the grasping forceps, with leakage of bowel contents. Obesity was the reason for conversion in one patient, and in two cases there was a colon carcinoma which extended visibly beyond the bowel wall.

Complications

An anastomotic leak occurred in one patient on the 4th day after right hemicolectomy. Despite immediate dissolving of the anastomosis and daily peritoenal lavage, the patient died of irreversible sepsis. He had underlying Waldenström's disease and was receiving immunosuppressive treatment.

One patient had delayed wound healing after laparoscopic rectal excision. All of the other patients were complication-free.

Tumor Stages

The distribution of tumors according to TNM stage was as follows:

To No	1	T3 N1 M1	2
T1 N2	2	T3 N2	2
T2 No	4	T3 N3	4
T3 No	10	T4 No	1
T3 N1	3	T4 N1 M1	1

Postoperative Course

The postoperative inpatient hospital stay was 9 – 18 days for patients with colon carcinoma (average 12.6 days). The patients only required at the most four injections for piritramide for pain relief. Compared to conventionally operated patients, there was no significant difference in analgesic consumption and no significant difference in experience of pain, which was measured on an analogue scale. Laparoscopically operated patients were fully mobilised significantly earlier, i. e. they could leave the ward unassisted.

Follow-Up of Colon Carcinoma Patients

Three patients who had evidence of distant metastases at the time of the primary operation (two in the liver, one in the lung) have died. Liver metastases have since been diagnosed in three more patients. In one patient, a sigmoid stenosis required dilatation. No patient had a local recurrence or recurrence at the trocar sites or in the mini-incision site.

Discussion

Laparoscopic resection of colon tumors was introduced because it appeared possible to extend the potential advantages of laparoscopic cholocystectomy – less pain, early mobilisation and short hospitalization – to colon resection. The technical feasibility was quickly demonstrated [5].

The laparoscopic operative techniques are not uniform. The concept of "laparoscopic resection" means that mobilisation, skletonisation, resection and anastomosis are performed entirely within the abdomen. The size of the resected specimen determines the size of the incision. "Laparoscopically assisted" implies that the operation is performed partly intracorporeally and partly outside the abdomen. The proportion of operative stages that are performed laparoscopically varies greatly in the literature [6–8], and often laparoscopic technique is limited to mobilisation of the colon. The mobilised segment of bowel is drawn outside the abdomen through an incision and the further steps – skeletonisation, resection and anastomosis – are continued conventionally. This procedure is particularly suitable for colon adenomas and is simple to perform.

As used for carcinoma [9], laparoscopic colon resection has rightly been called into question [10]. The conventional technique of colorectal surgery is clearly defined [11] and is regarded as the oncological standard. Laparoscopic operating technique is a variant which has the same oncological goal, namely Ro resection through minimal access routes. It cannot fully imitate the course of the conventional resection technique. A cardinal point of laparoscopic operating on the large bowel is the principle of traction and countertraction. The mesocolon must be stretched in order to identify the origin of the main vessels so that they can be divided there. The first operative step therefore is mobilisation and stretching of the mesocolon. Ligature of the colon lumen, likewise a component of the Turnball principle [12], can be performed simply and efficiently by means of the extracorporeal ligation technique in an early phase of mobilization. The no-touch principle during laparoscopic surgery means grasping the bowel with Babcock forceps as far as possible from the tumor and meticulously avoiding opening the bowel.

The number of lymph nodes resected is often regarded as one of the yardsticks of the quality of oncological resection. The minimum requirements for the N category of the TNM classification have been defined [13].

The extreme variation from one institution to another in the number of lymph nodes removed is well-known. Previous investigations therefore compared the number of lymph nodes removed in laparoscopically resected specimens with the number of lymph nodes removed in conventional operations and arrived at comparable results [14].

There are no reports of selection criteria for laparoscopic resection of colon carcinoma apart from the exclusion of bulky tumors. We have hitherto excluded tumors in the border region of two lymphatic drainage areas, in the proximal transverse colon and the splenic flexure, because of the necessity of extended hemicolectomy, and also tumors which could be seen laparoscopically to be extending through the wall on the antimesenteric border (T4). In two cases, we saw a contraction of the serosa at operation without visible tumor. Microscopic infiltration of the serosa was recognised on histological examination. This does mean stage T4 by definition, but intraperitoneal spread of tumor cells is not inevitable when infiltration of the serosa is visible only microscopically.

Twenty-one colon carcinomas were stage T3 on histology, i.e. the tumor was penetrating the mesocolon. Stage T3 is reached when the tumor can be seen microscopically to penetrate the tunica muscularis propria. It therefore seems very dubious to accept T2 carcinomas for laparoscopic resection while excluding T3 carcinomas. At present, there is no diagnostic procedure which can distinguish between stage T2 and T3 preoperatively. The distinction is barely possible even during operation. In an ongoing prospective study, we are investigating the accuracy of colon endosonography in establishing tumor stage [15]. Low-grade transmural spread into adjacent fat tissue does not in our opinion represent a risk of peritoneal tumor spread during laparoscopic operative procedures when performed by experienced surgeons. This has also been confirmed by our follow-up results. We have no evidence of local recurrence, peritoneal tumor seeding or metastases in the abdominal incision and trocar sites. Despite this, the following are the currently accepted exclusion criteria for laparoscopic colon resection: tumor in the border zone of two lymphatic drainage areas, carcinomas of the transverse colon and visible extramural tumor growth.

If the benefit for the patient of laparoscopic procedures is assessed, the main benefit is the early full mobilisation after surgery.

Conclusion

Laparoscopic colon resection can be performed with the same safety as conventional operations. The minimal access results in significantly earlier full mobilisation of the patient. With strict patient selection [16] and an experienced surgeon colon carcinomas can be resected laparoscopically with the same degree of oncological safety. Minimally invasive does not mean minimally effective.

References

1. Brune IB, Schönleben K (1992) Laparoskopische Sigmaresektion. Chirurg 63:342–344
2. Köckerling F, Gastinger I, Schneider B, Krause W, Gall FP (1992) Laparoskopische abdominoperineale Rektumexstirpation mit hoher Durchtrennung der A. mesenterica inferior. Chirurg 63:345–348
3. O'Rourke NA, Heald RJ (1993) Laparoscopic surgery for colorectal cancer. Br J Surg 80: 1229–1230
4. Nduka CC, Monson JRT, Menzies-Gow N, Darzi A (1994) Abdominal wall metastases following laparoscopy. Br J Surg 81:648–652
5. Phillips EH, Franklin M, Carroll BJ, Fallas MJ, Ramos R, Rosenthal D (1992) Laparoscopic colectomy. Ann Surg 216:703–707
6. Zucker KA, Pitcher DE, Martin DT, Ford RS (1994) Laparoscopic assisted colon resection. Surg Endosc 8:12–18
7. Monson JRT, Darzi A, Carey PD, Guillou PJ (1992) Prospective evaluation of laparoscopic assisted colectomy in an unselected group of patients. Lancet 340: 831–833
8. Monson JRT, Hill ADK, Darzi A (1995) Laparoscopic colonic surgery. Br J Surg 82:150–157
9. Sackier JM, Slutzki S, Wood C, Negri M, Moor EV, Halevy A (1993) Laparoscopic endocorporeal mobilisation followed by extra-corporeal sutureless anastomosis for the treatment of carcinoma of the left colon. Dis Colon Rectum 36:610–612
10. Fine AR, Lanasa S, Gannon MP, Cline CW, James R (1995) Laparoscopic colon surgery: report of a series. Am Surg 61:412–416
11. Herfarth C, Runkel N (1994) Chirurgische Standards beim primären Coloncarcinom. Chirurg 65:514–523
12. Wiggers T, Jeekel J et al. (1988) No-touch isolation technique in colon cancer: a controlled prospective trial. Br J Surg 75:409–415
13. Hermanek P, Wittekind C (1994) Inwieweit sind laparoskopische Verfahren in der onkologischen Chirurgie vertretbar? Chirurg 65:23–28
14. Franklin ME, Ramos R, Rosenthal D, Schuessler W (1993) Laparoscopic colonic procedures. World J Surg 17:51–56
15. Hildebrandt U, Schüder G, Feifel G (1994) Preoperative staging of rectal and colonic cancer. Endoscopy 26:810–812
16. Hildebrandt U, Feifel G (1995) Laparoskopische viszerale Chirurgie (editorial). Zentralbl Chir 120:345

Surgery for Rectal Cancer: Is It a Laparoscopic Procedure?

Lars Påhlman

Introduction

Almost all colorectal procedures can be performed laparoscopically [1, 2]. The main question is of course whether every procedure *should* be performed laparoscopically, and, especially, whether colorectal cancer should be [3–5]. Port-site metastasis is an important problem, which seems to be less important in rectal cancer surgery [6]. In rectal cancer, laparoscopic surgery has been performed with good preliminary results [7, 8]. However, several aspects have to be thought about, such as low or high ligation of the inferior mesenteric artery, lateral clearance, total mesorectal excision, nerve-sparing surgery and sphincter preservation.

Ligation of the Inferior Mesenteric Artery

Ligation of the inferior mesenteric artery flush to the aorta does not influence survival. However, it facilitates surgery, and it is necessary if a low anterior resection is planned [9, 10]. Therefore it is essential to learn this technique as well as how to ligate the inferior mesenteric vein high up under the pancreas. Both these particular technical feats are no more difficult to perform in a laparoscopic procedure than in open surgery [8]. If an abdominal-perineal excision is planned, however, it is not necessary to ligate these two vessels, as proximally as when a low anterior resection is performed.

Lateral Clearance

This is the most important part of rectal cancer surgery. Total mesorectal excision following the embryological plane will end up automatically with a good lateral dissection [11, 12, 13]. It is actually as easy to do this laparoscopically as in open surgery. If the procedure is started dorsally from or just in between the pelvic nerves and the rectal fascia, it is no problem to find the right plane dorsally and then do the total mesorectal excision. When the dissection turns laterally, the right plane will be found and easily followed. A well-known risk is damage to the left ureter. If the procedure starts with division of the inferior mesenteric artery, it is often easy to find the left ureter if the dissection proceeds form the right side and under the sigmoid colon [14]. When the ureter has been identified in this way, the peritoneal adhesions to the left part of the abdomen can be cut and the ureter will easily be visualized and not damaged. Lateral clearance is no more difficult with a laparoscopic procedure either.

Total Mesorectal Excision

This technique has become popular during the last 10 years and is probably one of the reasons why the incidence of local recurrence has been reduced [11, 12]. The main question is of course when total mesorectal excision should be carried our. In higher tumors, i. e. tumors situated 15 cm form the anal verge, total mesorectal excision is probably unnecessary. However, even in these cases the technique of following the embryological plane is important, and when the rectum has been mobilized totally it can be decided how to cut into the mesorectum at a proper distance from the tumor, while avoiding a cone effect. In lower tumors, however, it is often very difficult to create an anastomosis 5 cm distally to the tumor without having a cone effect [15, 16]. In these cases it is probably easier to do a total mesorectal excision, ending up with a more a less coloanal anastomosis. Due to the lack of good laparoscopic suturing instruments, it is in my opinion still too early to recommend low anterior resection as a laparoscopic procedure. The anastomosis cannot safety be done as a coloanal anastomosis. If the bowel is simply cut without any clamps, it is necessary to perform a purse-string suture. Of course this purse-string suture can be placed from below, but the rectal tube has to be everted through the anus, which has been recommended by some surgeons. The risk of damaging the sphincter during such a procedure is high, and patients with a very low anastomosis often need a good sphincter because they suffer from urgency and slight incontinence.

Another important question when a low anterior resection is performed is the distance from the tumor to the end of the bowel which has been argued about. It is not necessary to have a 5-cm margin since tumor cells rarely spread intramurally more than a few millimeters. A distal margin of 1 cm can be enough [12, 16]. With this knowledge, it is now very common in high specialized centres that 85–90 % low anterior resections are performed. This means that with tumors situated 4 or even 3 cm from the anal verge continence can sometimes be savaged with good sphincter function. It is almost impossible to do such operations laparoscopically [12], and there is an obvious risk if too many rectal cancers are approached laparoscopically that the operation will end up as an abdominoperineal excision due to difficulties in finding the exact plane for division of the bowel.

Summary

In my own experience, high division of the inferior mesenteric artery, good lateral clearance and total mesorectal excision without damaging the nerves are all possible in a laparoscopic procedure. The view is excellent, and my feeling is that when a rectal tumor is excised laparoscopically it is done even better than when it is done by open surgery. Therefore, an abdominoperineal excision is a superb operation when it is done laparoscopically. There is no problem with specimen retrieval, which can be done from below, and the operation does not jeopardize oncological principles. However, a low anterior resection is extremely difficult to do laparoscopically and should be avoided. A high anterior resection can be justified, but it is mandatory that the 5-cm rule is applied in this group of patients. It is especially important that the mesorectum be divided 5 cm below the tumor. This can be a tricky part of the laparoscopic procedure, indicated that even a high anterior resection may jeopardize oncological principles.

Reference

1. Falk PM, Beart RW, Wexner SD et al. (1993) Laparoscopic colectomy: a critical appraisal. Dis Colon Rectum 36:28–34
2. Monson JRT, Hill ADK, Darzi A (1995) Laparoscopic colonic surgery. Br J Surg 82:150–157
3. Guillon PJ, Crazi A, Monson JRT (1993) Experience with laparoscopic colorectal surgery for malignant disease. Surg Oncol 2 [Suppl 1]:43–49
4. Cohen SM, Wexner SD (1993) Laparoscopic colorectal surgery for cancer: the Cliveland Clinic Florida experience. Surg Oncol 2[Suppl 1]:35–42
5. Wexner SD, Cohen SM (1994) Laparoscopic colectomy for malignancy – advantages and limitations. Surg Oncol Clin N Am 3:637–643
6. Wexner SD, Cohen SM (1995) Port site metastases after laparoscopic colorectal surgery for cure of malignancy. Br J Surg 82:295–294
7. Dodson RW, Cullado MJ, Tangen LE, Bonello JC (1993) Laparoscopic-assisted abdominoperineal resection. Count Surg 42(1):42–44
8. Koeckerling F (1994) Laparoscopic abdominoperineal excision with high transection of the inferior mesenteric artery. Surg Oncol Clin N Am 3:731–743
9. Pezim ME, Nicholls RJ (1984) Survival after high or low ligation of the inferior mesenteric artery during curative surgery for rectal cancer. Ann Surg 27:729–733
10. Grinell R (1965) Results of ligation of inferior mesenteric artery at the aorta in resections of carcinoma of the descending colon and sigmoid colon and rectum. Surg Gynecol Obstet 120:1031–1036
11. MacFarlane JK, Ryall RD, Heald RJ (1993) Mesorectal excision for rectal cancer. Lancet 341:457–460
12. Kranjia ND, Schache DJ, North WR, Heald RJ (1990) "Close shave" in anterior resection. Br J Surg 63:673–677
13. Adam IJ, Mohamdee MO, Martin EG et al. (1994) Role of cirucmferential margin involvement in the local recurrence of rectal cancer. Lancet 344:707–711
14. Påhlman L, Arvidsson D (1994) Anterior resection. Surg Oncol Clin N Am 3:711–716
15. Williams NS (1984) The rationale for preservation of the anal sphincter in patients with low rectal cancer. Br J Surg 71:575–581
16. Williams NS, Dixon MF, Johnston D (1983) Reappraisal of the 5 centimeter rule of distal excision for carcinoma of the rectum: a study of distal intramural spread and patients' survival. Br J Surg 70:150–154

Complications of Minimally Invasive Colon Surgery: An Error Analysis

A. Franke, K. Lebrecht, H. A. Richter and S. Zeyfang

Introduction

While laparoscopic surgery already represents the "gold standard" for cholecystectomy, the same cannot (yet) be said of the minimally invasive approach to colorectal resection. However, with the enormous progress in the field of minimally invasive surgery, laparoscopic colorectal surgery is being employed increasingly widely [2, 3, 5 – 11]. After performing more than 2000 laparoscopic procedures, we began carrying out laparoscopic resections of the sigmoid colon in May 1993.

We were interested in questions of technical feasibility as well as the quality control which we always pursue, including a critical error analysis (Table 1).

Patients and Results

The error analysis discussed here covers laparoscopically assisted sigmoid and rectal resections and one colectomy for familial polyposis coli. We operated on 42 patients with benign and 19 patients with malignant diseases of the distal colon during the period from May 1993 to August 1995 using this method (Table 2).

The preoperative work-up consisted of colonoscopy carried out by ourselves, if necessary with biopsy, colon contrast studies (in acute diverticulitis

Table 1. Minimally invasive colorectal resection: factors investigated

Technical feasibility	Clip applicator
	Linear stapler
	Mini laparotomy
	Waterproof and cell-proof bag
	Circular stapler
Prompt early postoperative recovery	Gentle operation
	Low analgesic consumption
	Shorter postop. gastrointestinal atony
	Early mobilization
Safety of laparoscopic vs conventional large bowel surgery	Ligation of inferior mesenteric artery near its origin
	Duration of operation
	Minimization of complications
	Quality control/error analysis

Table 2. Indications for minimally invasive colorectal resection in 61 patients

	Male	Female
Benign disease (n = 42)		
Sigmoid diverticulitis	8	21
Sigmoid diverticulitis, sealed perforation	1	1
Sigmoid diverticulitis, perforated	1	–
Sigmoid diverticulitis with vesical fistula	1	2
Sigmoid endometriosis with stenosis	–	1
Redundant sigmoid with symptoms of volvulus	–	1
Sigmoid adenoma	2	1
Rectal adenoma	–	1
Familial polyposis coli	1	–
Total	14	28
Malignant disease (n = 19)		
Sigmoid carcinoma T2/T3	2	10
Sigmoid carcinoma with liver metastases	–	1
Rectal carcinoma T2/T3	2	3
Rectal carcinoma with liver metastases	1	–
Total	5	14

only), an intravenous urogram to show the course of the ureters, measurement of tumor markers in the cases of malignancy, upper abdominal and endo-sonography and computer tomography. Colon contrast studies were done on the seventh to tenth day after surgery to assess the anastomosis.

The statistical data are shown in Table 3. Tables 4 and 5 give a precise listing of *all* complications in accordance with our quality control, whatever their clinical relevance.

Table 3. Statistical data on 61 patients undergoing minimally invasive colorectal resection between May 1993 and August 1995 (means and ranges)

	Patient sex		Patient age (years)		Operation time (h:min)		Hospital stay (days)	
	M	F	M	F	M	F	M	F
Benign	14	28	51 (31–70)	63 (33–84)	3:10 (1:55–5:15)	2:50 (1:30–5:30)	19 (10–86)	17 (5–53)
Malignant	5	14	69 (54–80)	69 (54–83)	2:35 (1:35–3:50)	2:50 (1:40–3:45)	14 (12–16)	18 (11–36)
Subtotal	19	42	56 (31–80)	65 (33–84)	3:00 (1:35–5:15)	2:50 (1:30–5:30)	17 (10–86)	17 (5–53)
Total	61		62 (31–84)		2:55 (1:30–5:30)		17 (5–86)	

Table 4. Intraoperative complications ($n = 11$) during minimally invasive colorectal resection in 61 patients: error analysis/quality control

	n	Treatment
Bleeding from superficial epigastric artery (trocar puncture site)	1	Local ligation
Minor bowel-wall injury due to stapler	5	Laparoscopic oversewing
Major bowel-wall injury during insertion of circular stapler	2	Laparoscopic resection
Negative from the patient's/surgeon's point of view:		
Problem with extraction due to tumor size	1	Somewhat extended mini-laparotomy, extracorporal anastomosis
Insufficient anastomosis	1	Conversion
Colovesical fistula	1	Conversion

Table 5. Postoperative complications ($n = 20$) after minimally invasive colorectal surgery in 61 patients: error analysis/quality control

	n	Treatment	Hospital stay (days)
Clinically silent anastomotic leak	3	None	17[a]
Negative from the patient's point of view:			
Wound infection (trocar puncture site, mini-laparotomy)	7	Wound cleansing	19[a]
Acute cholecystitis	1	Laparoscopic cholecystectomy	18
Aspiration pneumonia	1	Intensive care	38
Negative form patient's/surgeon's point of view:			
Caecal perforation	1	R hemicolectomy, repeated lavage	86
Infected haematoma in pouch of Douglas	1	Aspiration of pouch of Douglas	36
Secondary haemorrhage (mesocolon/pelvirectal) (1 death)	4	1 × Relaparoscopy 3 × relaparotomy (1st or 2nd day)	17[a]
Anastomotic failure with sepsis (2 deaths)	2	Relaparotomy, ileostomy, repeated lavage	32[a]

[a] Average.

Discussion

The average patient age of 62 years is typical of large bowel disease, but 80-year-old patients also tolerated the procedure well. The average operation time was 2 h 55 min, while the benign inflammatory illnesses naturally took on average 20–30 min longer. We found only a small difference between this and conventional large bowel surgery.

Due to the billing and financing system for hospital charges which was still in force during the assessment period, the postoperative hospital stay was deliberately prolonged for financial reasons in many cases.

We had initially operated only for benign disease (diverticulitis), and turned to rectosigmoid malignancies later after becoming familiar with critical opinions [4] which persuaded us of the technique of ligation of the inferior mesenteric artery near its origin [8], extraction of the prepared specimen using a waterproof and cell-proof bag, and the comparable number of lymph nodes removed in laparoscopically resected sigmoid diverticulitis and conventionally surgery on sigmoid carcinomas. We limited ourselves to T2 and small T3 tumors and two palliative operations in the presence of advanced distant metastases.

For error analysis and quality control, we worked out a list of possible complications which could occur in minimally invasive colon surgery (Table 6). We assessed the results of our laparoscopic rectosigmoid resections according to this list.

At first, *all* complications were included, including those which were not noted as such by the patient at all. These include, for example, intraoperative findings such as bleeding or injury to the bowel wall. These situations can be

Table 6. Minimally invasive colorectal resection: list of *possible* complications, for use in quality control

---

Complications from the patient's point of view

Without technical surgical problems
☐ Wound: haematoma, seroma, abscess
☐ General: thrombosis, pneumonia, myocardial infarct, cerebrovascular accident, etc.

Due to technical surgical problems
☐ Conversion of the operative procedure for anatomical reasons
☐ Conversion of the operative procedure because of intraoperative complications

Complications from the technical surgical point of view:

Without significant disadvantages for the patient
☐ Lesions of the small bowel or bladder due to inflammation: laparoscopic oversewing possible
☐ Clinically silent anastomotic leaks

With disadvantages for the patient
☐ Insufficient anastomosis: conversion
☐ Ureteric injury: conversion
☐ Secondary haemorrhage: reoperation
☐ Anastomotic breakdown with septic complications: reoperation

---

rectified intraoperatively laparoscopically without sequelae [2]. They cannot be blamed on the method and so are no different from those of conventional methods and are of no clinical relevance for the patients.

In one case, we had to extend our usual 4-cm mini-laparotomy incision as the tumor was too big. A hand-sutured anastomosis in our first laparoscopic colon procedure appeared so unsafe to us that we concluded the operation conventionally. Another conversion had to be performed subsequently on one occasion only in a case of a very extensive colovesical fistula.

Our intraoperativ "errors" identified in 11 patients and the 3 clinically silent anastomotic leaks would not have been listed at all for the conventional procedure, but they are not typical of minimally invasive surgery and do represent a certain loss of comfort in the context of a laparoscopic operation.

Despite similar bowel preparation and antibiotic prophylaxis, wound infections ($n = 7$) are – as in conventional surgery – probably impossible to avoid totally; in laparoscopic surgery they occur at the trocar puncture sites or the extraction incision, even when the specimen bag is used to prevent contact between the bowel and the abdominal wall. They are locally limited, however, and are much less serious than after laparotomy.

Acute postoperative cholecystitis and aspiration pneumonia, which occurred in one patient on the 3rd postoperative day, can likewise not be blamed on the minimally invasive method.

The postoperative hospital stay is at any rate increased by all complications, even those of slight clinical relevance. This must be taken into account from the economic point of view in the future.

Eight cases deserve particular attention. Death occurred in 3 cases; as a result of anastomotic breakdown with sepsis and multi-organ failure in 2 patients and multi-organ failure in an 80-year-old patient despite relaparotomy and control of haemorrhage. Of the two patients who died after anastomotic breakdown, one, who was also being treated with cytostatic drugs for non-Hodgkin's lymphoma, had diverticulitis and a vesical fistula. This patient died of sepsis despite laparotomy, ileostomy and repeated lavage. A second, 70-year-old patient had a similar postoperative course. It remains a matter for discussion whether suture dehiscence of stapled anastomoses can be linked to a laparoscopic operation [1], as this can also occur after conventionally performed stapled operations.

In addition, five cases of secondary haemorrhage in the pelvis were recorded. Treatment was in one case by aspiration through the pouch of Douglas and in one case by relaparoscopy; relaparotomy was necessary in three cases. Despite this, on 80-year-old patient died of multi-organ failure.

We are particularly concerned about the occurrence of secondary haemorrhage, which has also been observed by other authors [2, 6, 7, 10]. In each case, the laparoscopic operation had been completed without a conspicuous source of bleeding or bleeding tendency. Linear staples and clip applicators cause visually secure control of bleeding. This raises the question of whether the increased intra-abdominal pressure temporarily prevents bleeding that would otherwise be apparent. This is suspected by Herold et al. [5] also. More meticulous control of bleeding and a longer pelvic inspection at the end of operation with the intra-abdominal pressure greatly reduced should help to clarify this matter.

Conclusion

The critical assessment of our error analysis permits the conclusion that clinically relevant complications such as breakdown of stapled anastomoses occur in only small numbers and are comparable to those in large series of conventional procedures. The accepted improvement in patient comfort brought by laparoscopic procedures outweighs them. Quality control is essential and must also take into account the patient's psychological condition and his or her assessment of the procedure. It is important to rectify any exaggerated expectations patients may have of laparoscopic procedures.

References

1. Christen D, Buchmann P, Klinger K (1994) Probleme beim Einstieg in die laparoskopische Colonchirurgie. Langenbecks Arch Chir Suppl II (Kongressbericht): 231–233
2. Faust H, Reichel K (1995) Laparoskopische Kolonresektion – Ist eine onkologische Resektion auf laparoskopischem Wege möglich? Zentralbl Chir 120:392–395
3. Fowler DL, White SA (1991) Laparoscopy-assisted sigmoid resection. Surg Laparosc Endosc 1:183–188
4. Hermanek P, Wittekind C (1994) Inwieweit sind laparoskopische Verfahren in der onkologischen Chirurgie vertretbar? Chirurg 65:23–28
5. Herold A, Schiedeck T, Müller G, Bruch HP (1994) Minimal invasive Colonchirurgie. Coloproctology 16:338–394
6. Kleine U, Kraas E (1995) Indikation zur laparoskopischen Dickdarmchirurgie. Zentralbl Chir 120:400–404
7. Kleine U, Kraas E (1995) Laparoskopische Hemikolektomie rechts. Minim Invasive Chir 4: 24–28
8. Köckerling F, Gastinger I, Schneider B, Krause W, Gall FP (1992) Laparoskopische abdominale Rectumexstirpation mit hoher Durchtrennung der Arteria mesenterica inferior. Chirurg 63:345–348
9. Marema RT (1993) Die laparoskopische Kolonresektion. Eine Übersicht über 50 Fälle. Chir Gastroenterol Interdiszipl Gespr 9:20–23
10. Müller G, Herold A, Schiedeck T, Bruch HP (1995) Laparoskopische Rektumchirurgie. Minim Invasive Chir 4:33–40
11. Woisetschläger R, Sulzbacher H, Rieger R, Schrenk P, Wayand W (1994) Laparoskopisch-assistierte Kolonchirurgie. Coloproctology 16:335–340

III Principles

General Principles of Laparoscopic Colorectal Surgery

H.M. Schardey and G. Meyer

General Preparation for Surgery

Before laparoscopic colorectal surgery, the patient's large bowel is prepared with an antegrade lavage the day before the intervention. All patients ought to wear antiembolism stockings and receive low-molecular-weight heparin as thromboembolism prophylaxis, perioperative single-shot antibiotic prohylaxis on the day of surgery and have a urethral catheter placed. Adhesion ultrasonography on the day before laparoscopy helps to identify the safest port of entry if previous abdominal operations have been carried out in the patient. If extensive adhesions are expected, a blunt Hasson trocar combined with Minilaparotomy should be available as primary access. Alternatively, a special blunt, translucent trocar with bilateral cutting edges, the Optiview trocar (Ethicon Co.) in combination with a 0° laparoscope may ensure a safe abdominal entry. For operations on the sigmoid rectum, especially reoperations, preoperative transurethral placement of ureteral catheters may facilitate the identification of the ureter and therefore improve the speed and safety of the procedure.

Positioning of the Patient

The modified dorsolithotomy position has proven ideal for laparoscopic colorectal operations. Positioning the stirrups at a 45° angle allows adequate access to the abdomen during the laparoscopic portion of the procedure, while good perineal access for resection, stapling, or endoscopy may be attained by bringing the stirrups to a straight-up position. The patient is in the supine position on a foam rubber sheet, which prevents slippage and allows good weight distribution. Between the foam rubber and the operating table is a heating mattress. The best position for the arms is in bilateral adduction, which allows unimpaired movement of the surgeon and assistants. If one of the arms needs to be abducted for monitoring purposes, it shoud be the one on the other side from the operator. The arms are wrapped in cloth or foam padding for safety. Since gravity and not retraction is the primary force by which the bowel is moved out of the field of vision, the patient is secured with supporters on the shoulders and both sides, which prevents slippage during extreme repositioning from side to side or from Trendelenburg to anti-Trendelenburg.

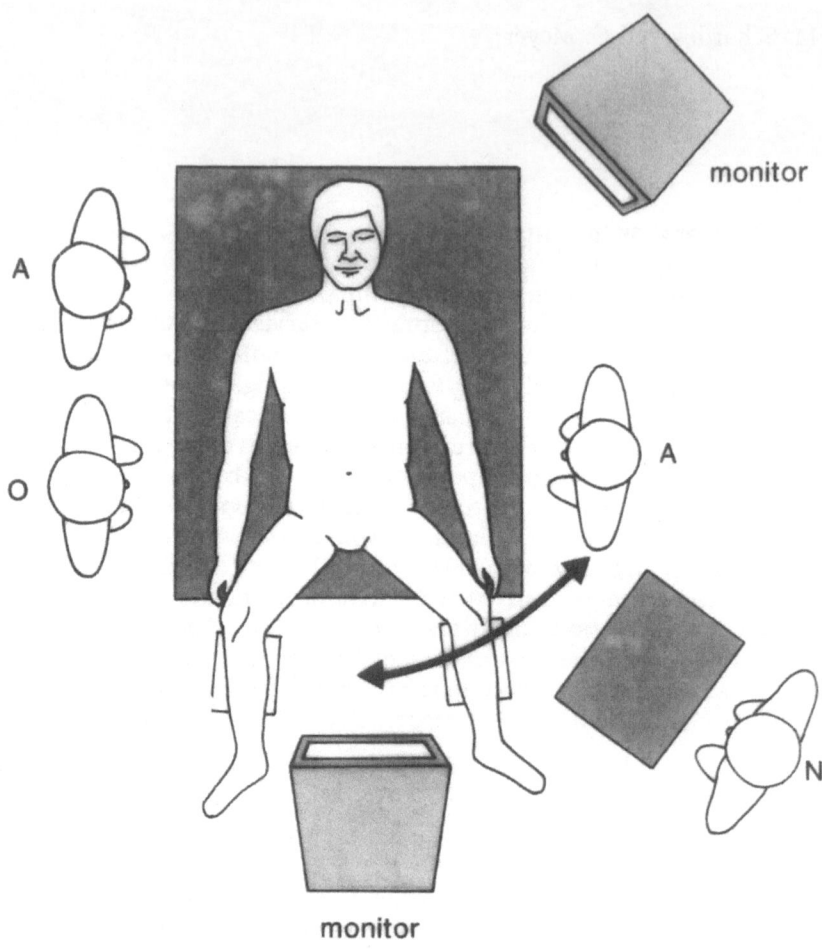

monitor

monitor

Fig. 1. Position of the patient and the surgical team in surgery of the left colon or rectum. *O*, operator, *A*, assistants, *N*, cameraman

For operations on the sigmoid and rectum the surgeon stands on the right and the first assistant on the left side of the patient (Fig. 1). The main monitor is located between the patient's legs and the additional monitor to the left of the patient's left shoulder. The cameraman may stand near either shoulder of the patient, although he is usually positioned on the patient's left. However, especially during mobilization of the splenic flexure the second assistant may stand on the right of the patient. During operations on the right or transverse colon the surgeon stands between the patient's legs, the second assistant on the left side of the patient, and the first assistant cephalad to the latter. The main

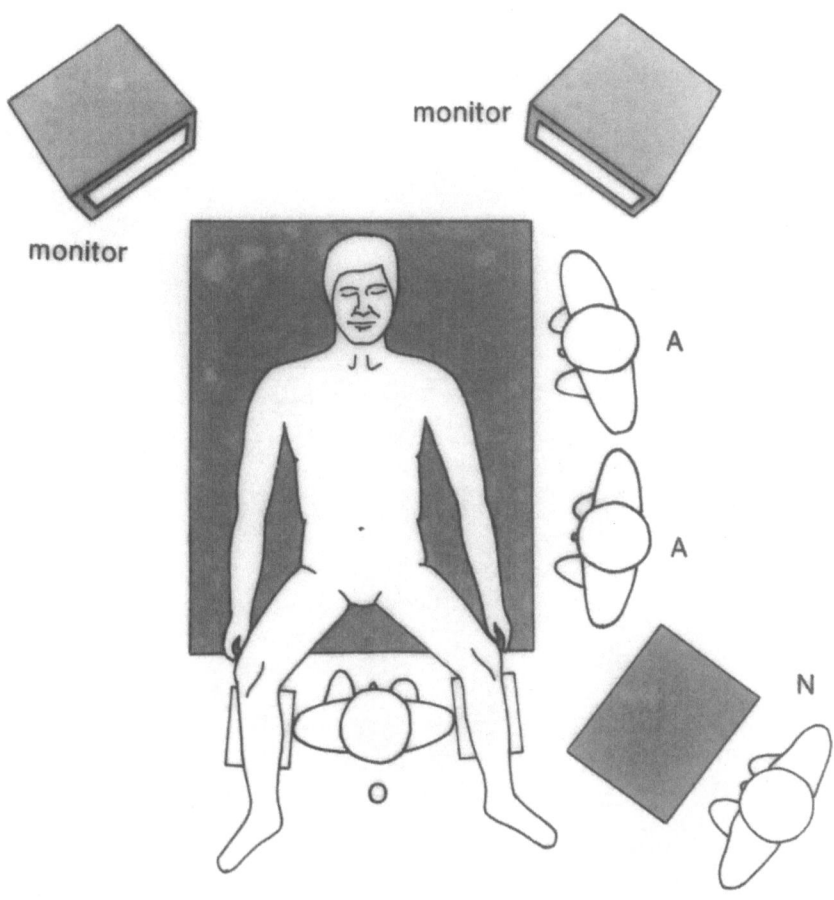

Fig. 2. Position of the patient and the surgical team in surgery of the right or transverse colon

monitor stands near the right shoulder and the second monitor either near the left shoulder or the right hip of the patient, depending on whether the anastomosis is to be constructed more to the right or the left side of the patient (Fig. 2).

Trocar Placement

For laparoscopic colorectal operations, which are usually complex, four or five trocars are required. The best access is gained if the trocars are placed in a

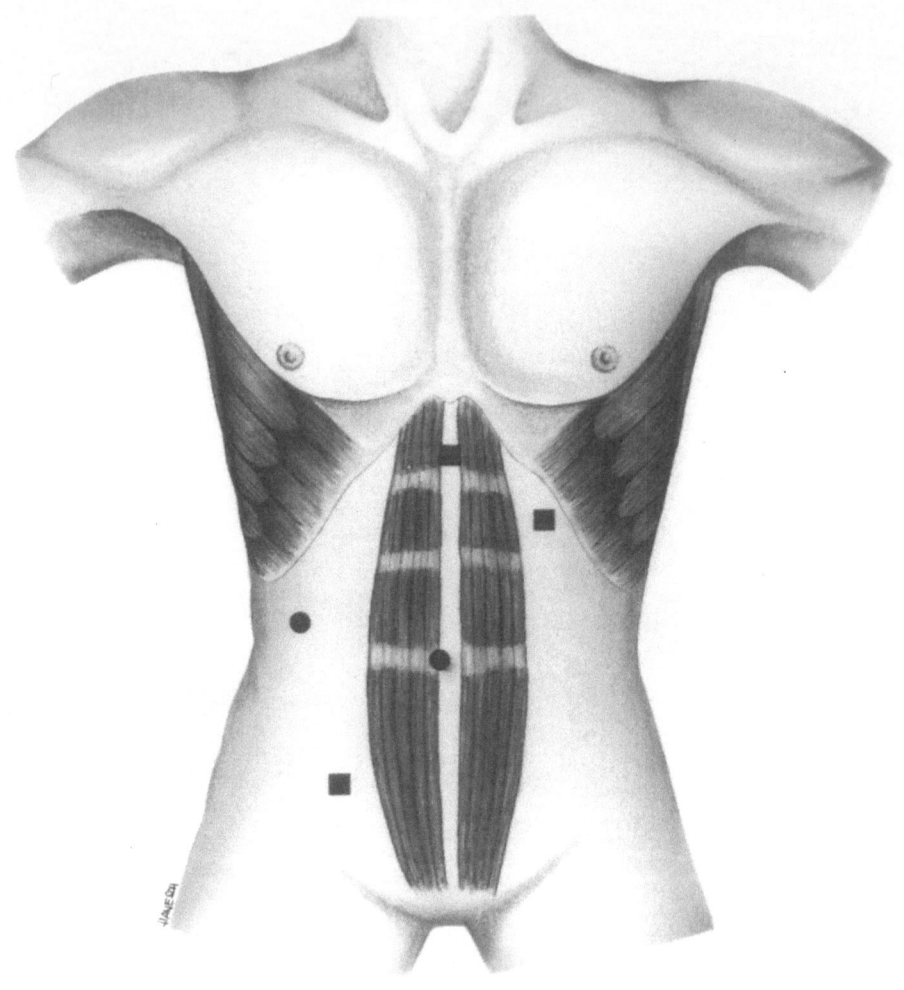

Fig. 3. Position of the trocars in surgery of the left colon or rectum

semicircular fashion so as to surround the surgical site as much as possible
(Figs. 3, 4). The initial trocar is usually introduced at the inferior or superior
crease of the umbilicus, because the abdominal wall is thinnest at this level.
However, an adequate distance to the surgical site should be maintained, and a
higher or lower port site may be chosen. Each trocar should be introduced in a
direct alignment towards the planned surgical field, so that after introduction,
even when the sheath is not being held, it will naturally point to the surgical
site. This reduces the pressure on the sheath which would otherwise interfere

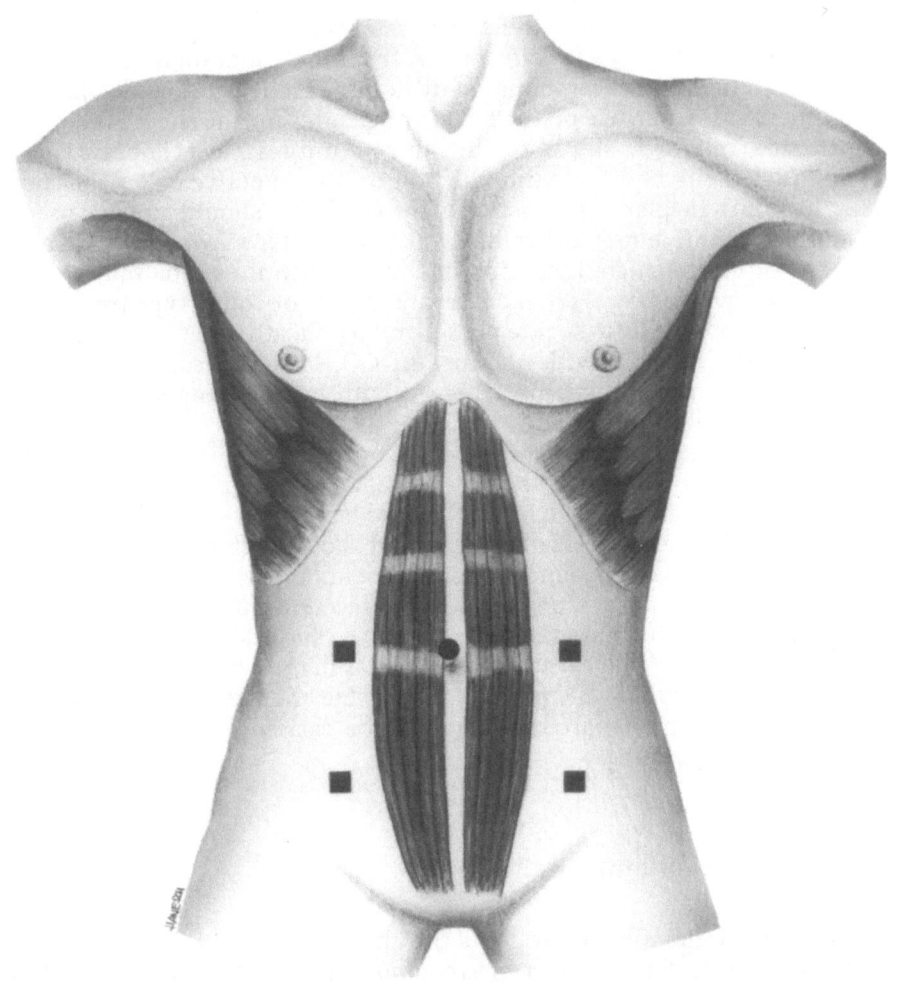

Fig. 4. Position of the trocars in surgery of the right or transverse colon

with the senitivity of touch and feeling necessary to palpate tissue. This is especially helpful in obese patients. Skin incisions for the secondary trocars should in any case be made avoiding the transilluminated vessels of the abdominal wall. It is also essential when choosing the secondary trocar sites that sufficient distance is kept between trocars to prevent scissoring. The introduction of these ports is carried out under visual control only.

With the exception of Hartmann procedures or simple loop colostomies, most laparoscopic colorectal operations are relatively long procedures, which are associated with an increasing tendency of trocar sheaths to dislocate over time and an attendant loss of the peritoneal seal against the sheath, with continuous leakage of CO_2 from the abdominal cavity. With a little forethought however, hours of difficulty can be prevented. One of the main measures is the use of a self-retaining collar for the sheath (grip). The detachable retentive sleeve is introduced until it just appears in the abdominal cavity. By tightening the bolt on the retentive collar the sheath may be fixed in place. A plastic retentive sleeve should not be used in combination with a metal sheath, because the latter may act as a capacitor and any electrical current coming in contact with the metal may spark to adjacent organs or bowel [1]. If a retentive sleeve or collar-type trocar is not available, another way to secure the secondary sheath is to tie the sidearm of the sheath to the skin with a suture. If CO_2 leakage occurs despite precautions, good results may be achieved with purse-string sutures around the fasciotomy and/or the skin.

We recommend the use of large trocars only, measuring 10–12 mm in diameter, right from the start of the procedure, and the employment of reducers for smaller instruments. The most ideal are large trocars with automatic reducers. Large trocars increase flexibility and allow the choice of the best angle of approach with any instrument in use. Depending on the particular circumstances, even the laparoscope may be introduced through other trocars than the umbilical one to obtain the best view of the surgical site. If 60-mm linear staplers are to be employed, at least one trocar in the contralateral abdominal wall needs to measure 15–18 mm. If at all possible, the specimen extraction and if necessary the minilaparotomy ought to be carried out at the site of this largest incision.

Locating the Lesion Intraoperatively

Because it is impossible to evaluate the characteristics of the pathology by palpation, we prefer intraoperative colonoscopic location of the lesion and of the resection margins. Prior to intraoperative colonoscopy the proximal bowel need to be occluded with a clamp to prevent inflation of the entire intestine. Once the lesion has been located, it is identified laparoscopically and marked with a suture (Fig. 5), which is better than using a clip, dye or electrocoagulation, because it is much easier to recognize and can also be used to manipulate the bowel during preparation. The proximal and distal resection margins are marked as well. With continuous suction to remove all the air, the colonoscope is extracted before the operation starts. During the procedure, manipulation of the intestines may be facilitated by using a bowel suspender, which is a rubber hose or plastic tape-like string introduced through one of the trocars, placed around the colon, and closed with a suture or a clip. A suspender is especially helpful when a loop colostomy is planned, because the bowel can be pulled through the abdominal wall by traction on the suspender [1].

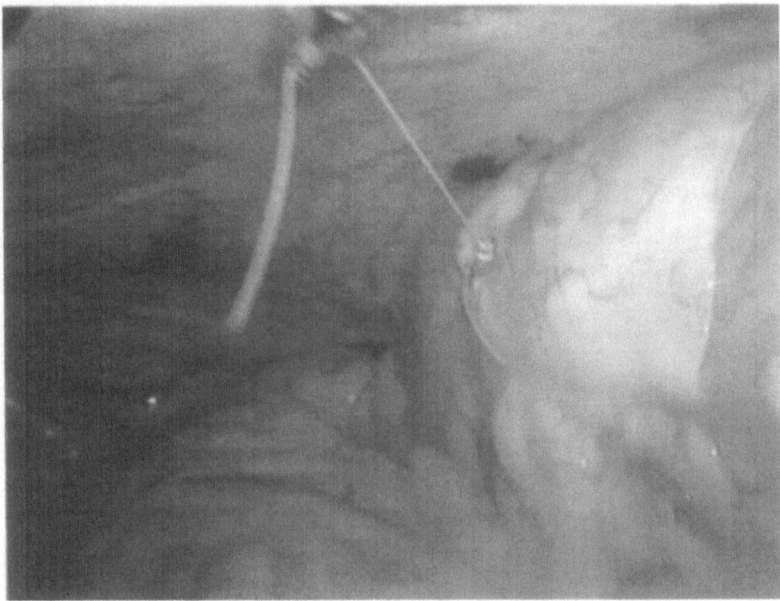

Fig. 5. Suture marking of the lesion and the resection margins during intraoperative colonoscopy at the beginning of the procedure

Surgical Strategy

Laparoscopic operations on the colon or rectum should only be carried out by at least two surgeons experienced in laparoscopic surgery. Effectiveness as a first assistance requires special knowledge, and during the course of the operation there are many preparatory steps that are easier to carry out from the position of the first assitant. While the technique of laparoscopy is very different from the technique of the conventional open operation, the tactical approach to the lesion, the surgical strategies, and the final goals are identical. The well-known standards of conventional surgery therefore also apply to laparoscopic surgery and must be met. These are an identical extent of resection for potentially curatively resectable malignant tumors, preliminary central ligation of vessels, ligation of the bowel lumen, and regional lymphadenectomy.

The surgeon works bimanually. Sharp or blunt tissue dissection is carried out under traction and countertraction using electrical scissors, grapsers, dissectors, or swabs. As an alternative a monopolar electric hook or ultrasound dissector may be employed. For the manipulation of the bowel, special swab-bearing forceps have proven to be ideal; fan retractors seem less suitable. Preparation of the rectum may be aided by moving it to and from with a transanally introduced rectoscope. The uterus may be kept out of the way with stay sutures, lifting it up against the ventral abdominal wall. These sutures are

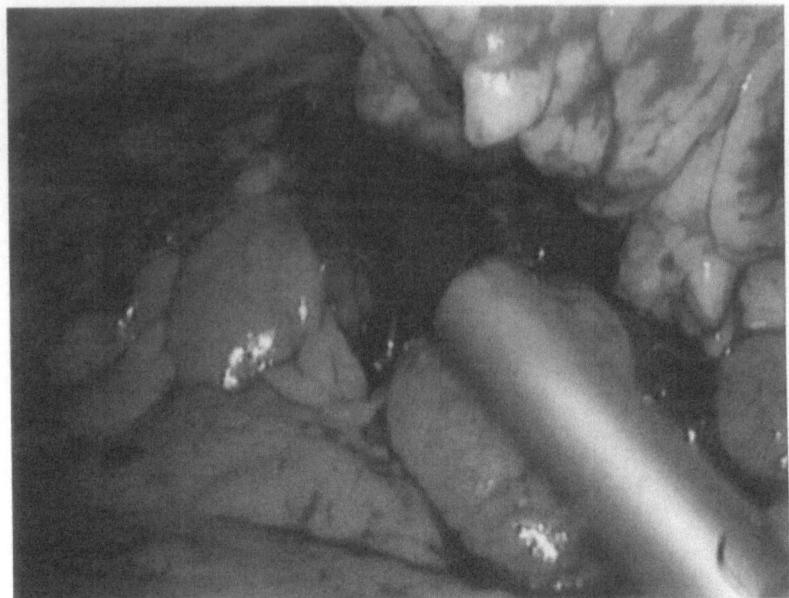

Fig. 6. Placement of resorbable clips during dissection

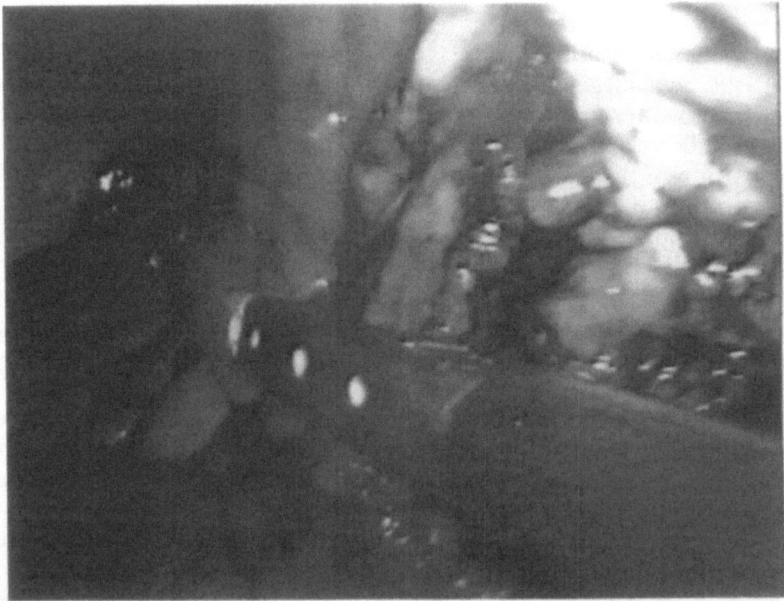

Fig. 7. Transection of the inferior mesenteric artery (A) and vein (V) with the linear cutter

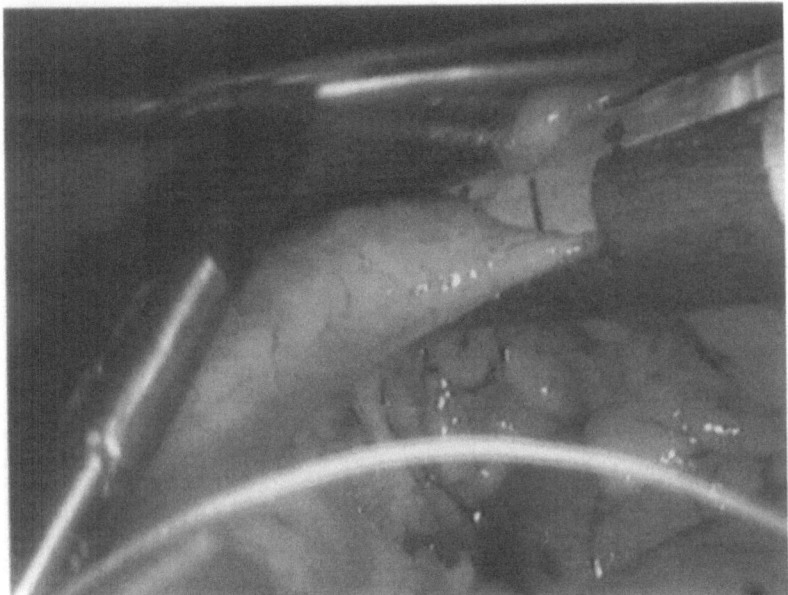

Fig. 8. Transection of the colon with the 60-mm linear cutter

placed transcutaneously and run beneath the latum ligament and back to the outside, where they are tied ventrally to the skin.

Any vessel may be clipped and then transected with scissors. We prefer resorbable clips (Fig. 6), because they have the additional advantage of resisting dislocation. Major vessels (Fig. 7) and the mesentery may be transected with the linear staplers employing a white or gray magazine, a technique which we favor because of the speed and unsurpassed degree of safety. The bowels are also transected with linear staplers using a blue or green magazine (Fig. 8); here we chose the 60-mm linear staplers in order to transect the colon with one bite. For determination of the magazine type and staple size, special measuring instruments are available. The colon should remain closed as long as possible to avoid bacterial contamination of the abdomen.

Mobilization of the colon begins with transection of the right or left paracolic gutter. The splenic flexure (Fig. 9) is always mobilized in larger resections of the left colon or rectum. The same holds true for visualization of the ureter (Fig. 10). A lens cleaner and a gas recirculating pump, which clears the intraabdominal smoke developing during electrocoagulation, greatly speed up the procedure.

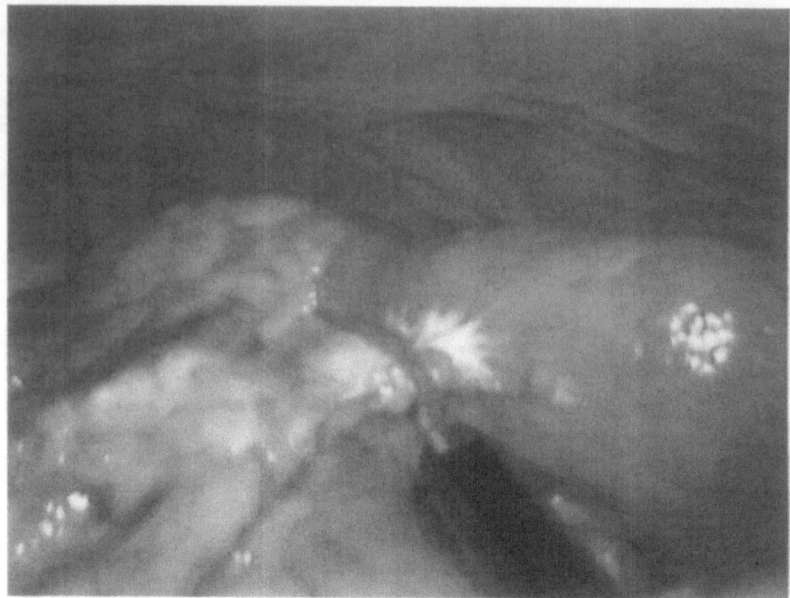

Fig. 9. Mobilization of the splenic flexure during resection of the left colon or rectum

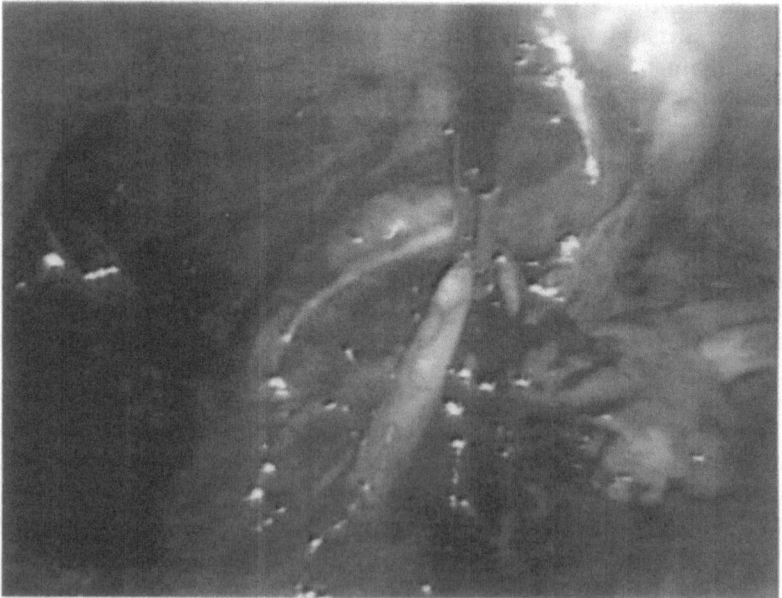

Fig. 10. Preparation and visualization of the ureter during resection of the left colon or rectum

Retrieval of the Specimen

We use large retrieval bags in laparoscopic colorectal surgery to isolate the resected specimen from the peritoneal cavity and abdominal wall (Fig. 11). This is especially important when laparoscopic bowel surgery is performed for cancer. If completely intracorporeal procedures with end-to-end anastomoses are carried out [2, 4], the specimen remains in the air-, water- and celltight

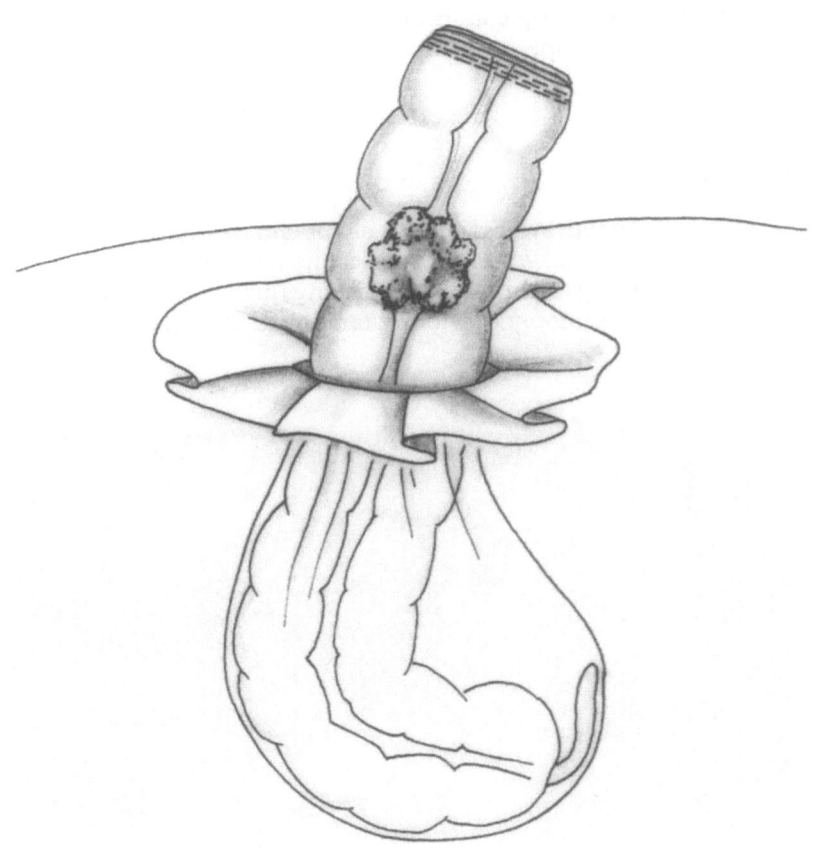

Fig. 11. The resected specimen is always placed intracorporeally in a large water- and celltight retrieval bag and then extracted through a trocar incision or minilaparotomy

retrieval bag until the end of the operation. The bag is then removed through incision for the largest trocar, which is usually 15 mm [4] or 33 mm [2]. Specimens containing only benign lesions or metastasized tumors may undergo morcellation within the retrieval bag before being extracted, and in those cases enlargement of the incision is never required. During laparoscopically assisted procedures in our department only the anastomosis or part of the fashioning of the anastomosis is carried out after evisceration of the colon end. The entire preparation, resection, and placement of the specimen into the retrieval bag are done intracorporeally. Once that point in the operation has been reached the site of the anastomosis determines which trocar incision will be converted to a minilaparotomy for extraction of the specimen followed by performance of the anastomosis. If the anastomosis is to be carried out with laparoscopic assistance, the minilaparotomy is closed with sutures and the pneumoperitoneum reestablished before the final steps are carried out [5].

End of the Operation

Final inspection should be carried out at the end of the laparoscopic procedure, with a detailed survey of the surgical field to look for visceral injuries and bleeding. Lowering the intra-abdominal pressure to below 5 mmHg allows recognition of any venotomy previously tamponaded by the 15 mmHg pneu-

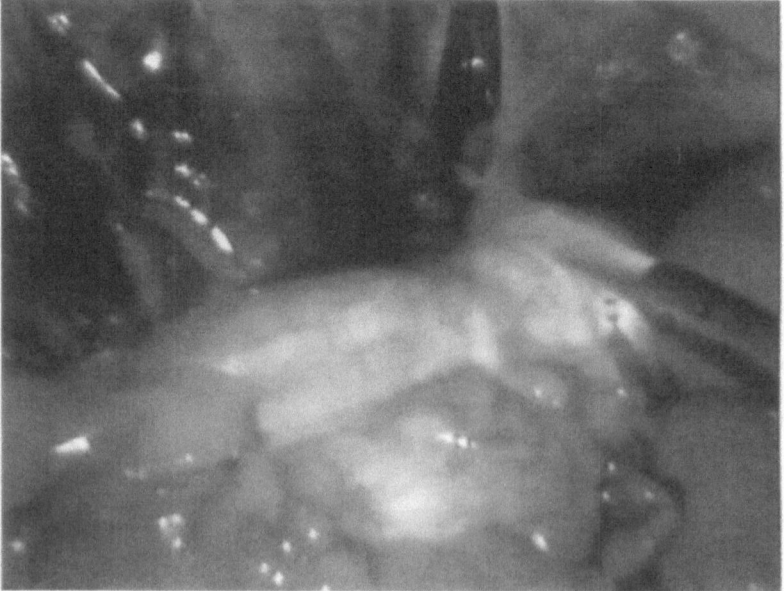

Fig. 12. Underwater test of the suture line during the final colonoscopic check

moperitoneum. This pressure reduction, however, may lead to a complete obstruction of vision in the majority of patients. The problem may be solved by intermittent pressure reduction with reinsufflation for inspection. At this point, 500–2000 ml warm saline solution may be introduced into the abdominal cavity. As the irrigant fills the abdomen, examination of the abdomen and surgical sites continues. The anastomosis is always checked endoscopically for hemorrhage, patency, and leakage. Again the colon is clamped proximal to the anastomosis to prevent obstruction of vision by the inflated intestines. With irrigation of the anastomosis, the underwater test confirms that the suture line is airtight (Fig. 12). Final intraoperative colonoscopy also allows the surgeon to check that the lesion has been completely removed, something which can occasionally be a problem, e. g., in polyposis.

After suctioning of the irrigant, a drainage (20 Charr Robinson) is placed near the anastomosis or at the lowest point in the abdomen. Prior to removal of the ports fibrin sealant may be applied to the anastomosis. This step is of course optional, because the benefit of fibrin sealant for anastomotic healing is debated [6]. The placement of Endo-Close sutures before removal of the sheaths, if correctly executed, ensures closure of the fascial and peritoneal defects. As an alternative, direct suturing with the needleholder or the Deschamps instrument may be adequate. The fascia of all port entries larger than 5 mm should be closed with sutures.

References

1. Soper NJ, Odem RR, Clayman RV, McDougall EM (1994) Essentials of laparoscopy. Quality Medial Publishing, St Louis
2. Köckerling F, Schneider I, Gastinger I, Schneider B, Gall FP (1993) Laparoskopische Tabaksbeutelnahtklemme für die minimal invasive kolorektale Chirurgie. Minim Invasive Chir 2 : 68–75
3. Lange V, Meyer G, Schardey HM, Schildberg FW (1991) Laparoscopic creation of a loop colostomy. J Laparoendosc Surg 1 : 307–312
4. Meyer G, Lange V, Rau HG, Schardey HM, Schildberg FW (1994) Laparoskopische Einzelklammernaht – erste klinische Erfahrung. Chirurg 65 : 361–366
5. Ravo B, Bagnato J (1994) Surgery of the left colon. In: Meinero M, Melotti J, Maouret PH (eds) Laparoscopic surgery in the nineties. Masson, Milano pp 306–313
6. Van der Ham AC, Kort WJ, Weijma IM, Jeekel H (1993) The transient protection of incomplete colonic anastomoses with fibrin sealant: an experimental study in the rat. J Surg Res 55 : 256–260

Anesthetic and Monitoring Considerations in Patients Undergoing Laparoscopic Colectomy

F. L. Greene

Although standard anesthetic techniques and methods of monitoring patients are similar for both open celiotomy and minimal access procedures, there are concepts which need to be highlighted regarding the issues of safety for patients undergoing surgical procedures with associated pneumoperitoneum. This paper will deal with the physiological consequences incurred during laparoscopic colectomy which may also be seen in other forms of minimal access surgical procedures utilizing pneumoperitoneum. In addition, discussion of appropiate monitoring techniques is included which will inform both the anesthesiologist and the surgeon of the importance of these concepts.

Anesthesia During Laparoscopic Colectomy

The bulk of anesthetic techniques which are provided for both diagnostic laparoscopy and laparoscopic colectomy fall under the heading of "general anesthesia." This allows overall airway control, muscle relaxation, and the adequate development of pneumoperitoneum which will allow for both laparoscopic-assisted and intra-corporeal techniques of laparoscopic colectomy [1]. These procedures will generally necessitate anesthesia for operations 1–4 h, and anesthesia needs to be controlled to insure adequate airway and ventilation during these procedures. Increased intra-abdominal pressure may require an increase in ventilation pressures during the procedure [2]. In addition, the change of position required during laparoscopic colectomy may affect ventilatory pressure. This applies to both steep Trendelenburg positioning to perform lower abdominal and pelvic laparoscopic procedures and reversed Trendelenburg for dissection in the upper abdomen [3]. Use of a nasogastric tube is mandatory to assure a reduction of the anatomical problems related to a full stomach as well as the potential for aspiration. Placement of a urethral Foley catheter is always important because of the need to monitor urine output carefully during lengthy operations.

Basic monitoring during general anesthesia includes continuous monitoring of heart rate with electrocardiography, blood pressure monitoring, precordial or esophageal monitoring, and pulse oximetry. Since the advent of carbon dioxide pneumoperitoneum it has been advised that end-tidal carbon dioxide be routinely monitored using capnography. Carbon dioxide is rapidly absorbed because its solubility is 35 times that of nitrogen and 20 times that of oxygen [1]. In cases of hypoventilation, hypercarbia may develop and have adverse effects on cardiac function. It is especially important to monitor end-tidal carbon dioxide in patients with chronic obstructive pulmonary disease, although it is important to realize that this technique may underestimate serum carbon dioxide levels. In these situations, it may be important to perform arterial blood gas analysis during the procedure.

Anesthetic techniques are varied and may be applied according to the experience of the anesthesiologist. Common agents include halothane, isoflurane, and enflurane, which are given along with nitrous oxide. It is important to remember that the addition of nitrous oxide may lead to bowel distention, which may have an adverse effect on an attempt to perform laparoscopic colectomy [4]. It is important to mention this point to the anesthesiologist and to discuss this at the initiation of the case. An additional side effect of nitrous oxide may be increased nausea and vomiting for the patient after laparoscopic procedures, which indicates that this gas may have a direct effect on intestinal motility and distention. In addition to the usual inhalational anesthetics, intravenous drugs such as propofol, etomidate, and midazolam have become common agents during laparoscopic procedures [5]. One of the great benefits of propofol is the rapid recovery following anesthesia, which is especially helpful in diagnostic laparoscopic procedures. Propofol also causes less postoperative nausea and vomiting.

Neuromuscular blockers may be used routinely during laparoscopic colectomy and other forms of minimal access surgery and are, in fact, important to assure relaxation of the abdominal and diaphragmatic musculature. It is virtually impossible to establish an adequate pneumoperitoneum of 12–14 mmHg in a patient who is not relaxed on the operating table. Neuromuscular blocking agents may be reversed at the conclusion of the procedure and, in fact, have been used in the outpatient setting. At present, there is virtually no indication for regional or local anesthesia during the performance of laparoscopic colectomy. The sympathectomy effect of spinal anesthesia my be beneficial, however, in producing sympathetic blockade with a resultant reduction in bowel distention.

Physiologic Monitoring During Laparoscopic Colectomy

Most physiologic changes that occur during laparoscopic colectomy are the result of the effects of anesthetics as well as the changes associated with the establishment of pneumoperitoneum and the positioning of the patient. Although abdominal wall lift devices have been recommended by some [6], laparoscopic colectomy is currently performed using intra-abdominal distention created by carbon dioxide pneumoperitoneum. For patients who may not be good candidates for carbon dioxide pneumoperitoneum (e.g. those with chronic obstructive pulmonary disease) it may be appropriate to use lift devices to reduce the physiologic changes mentioned.

The major changes during pneumoperitoneum are hemodynamic and pulmonary in nature. Several excellent studies, using both animal models and the human, have shown the hemodynamic effects caused by pneumoperitoneum at pressures of 12–20 mmHg in the abdomen [7]. Pressure in the inferior vena cava and portal venous system has been observed to increase and is associated with decreased flow in the superior mesenteric artery and portal vein. These events are important in patients with underlying cardiac disease or hepatic dysfunction. The effects on liver flow and splenic blood flow may be minimized by reducing insufflation pressure to 8–12 mmHg.

Cardiac function is directly affected in that cardiac output and stroke volume may decrease during pneumoperitoneum. Underlying cardiac disease in patients undergoing laparoscopic colectomy must be fully evaluated in order to monitor the patient properly and minimize these effects. We have shown that the use of transesophageal echocardiography may be important to discern subtle changes in cardiac chamber size prior to the development of arrhytmias which are associated with pneumoperitoneum [8]. Cardiac dysfunction may be worsened by respiratory acidosis secondary to carbon dioxide pneumoperitoneum. Although other agents such as nitrous oxide have been advocated for development of pneumoperitoneum, carbon dioxide remains the agent of choice because of its noncombustible characteristics. As operative intervention, especially during laparoscopic colectomy, is associated with prolonged exposure to pneumoperitoneum, hypercapnia and acidosis may result. This calls for increased awareness of physiologic changes and the use of standard monitoring devices as well as invasive techniques such as arterial monitoring to allow routine blood gas analysis.

Alternative gases, such as helium, have been studied in both animals and humans [9]. The major drawback of helium is that it is much less soluble than carbon dioxide in blood and serum and thus may carry an increased risk of gas embolism. Future utilization of both alternative gases and lift devices may reduce the physiologic consequences of laparoscopic colectomy.

Because of the increased pressure in the vena cava created by pneumoperitoneum, stasis of blood occurs in the venous system of the legs and may increase the risk of deep vein thrombophlebitis or postoperative embolic phenomena following laparoscopic colectomy. It is important to use compression devices from the beginning of the operation, and we have found that compression pumps on the legs are quite effective in reducing the possibility of thrombosis. Enhanced coagulation has also been noted in patients with malignancies. This association is particularly important when laparoscopic colectomy is utilized for carcinoma of the colon and rectum, which increases the possibility of thrombotic episodes. In addition, the creation of pneumoperitoneum has been shown to cause an endogenous rise in arginine vasopressin, which is associated with a rise in hypercoagulation parameters in some patients. [10]. Thus, the technique of pneumoperitoneum will increase the potential risk of hypercoagulation in patients with malignancies. Although frequent and repetitive measurement of coagulation parameters is not thought to be helpful in this setting, the use of compression devices on the lower extremities is once again extremely important to reduce the stasis associated with the hypercoagulable state.

Conclusion

The surgeon who is undertaking laparoscopic colectomy must be aware of the physiologic changes created by the operative technique and should work closely with his or her anesthesia colleagues in providing appropriate monitoring for hemodynamic and pulmonary evaluation. It is important to remember that although many of the physiologic consequences noted in laparoscopic colectomy are similar to those associated with traditional open celiotomy, the addition of pneumoperitoneum and the change in patient position over a prolonged period of time may create an environment of additional hazard to the patient.

References

1. Andrus CH, Wittgen CM, Naunhaim KS (1994) Anesthetic and physiologic changes during laparoscopy and thoracoscopy: the surgeon's view. Semin Laparosc Surg 1: 228–240
2. Alexander GD, Noe FE, Brown EM (1969) Anesthesia for pelvic laparoscopy. Anesth Analg 48: 4–18
3. Marco AP, Yeo CJ, Rock P (1990) Anesthesia for a patient undergoing laparoscopic cholecystectomy. Anesthesiology 73: 1268–1270
4. Taylor E, Feinstein R, Soper N, White PF (1991) Effect of nitrous oxide on surgical conditions during laparoscopic cholecystectomy. Anesthesiology 75: 541–543
5. Bailie R, Craig G, Restall J (1989) Total intravenous anesthesia for laparoscopy. Anaesthesia 44: 60–63
6. Tsoi E, Organ CH Jr (1995) Abdominal wall lifting devices as alternatives to pneumoperitoneum, Semin Laparosc Surg 2: 205–208
7. Ishizaki Y, Bandai Y, Shimomura K et al. (1994) Safe intraabdominal pressure of carbon dioxide pneumoperitoneum during laparoscopic surgery. Surgery 114: 549–554
8. Dorsay DA, Greene FL, Baysinger CL (1995) Hemodynamic changes during laparoscopic cholecystectomy monitored with transesophageal echocardiography (TEE) Surg Endosc 9: 28–134
9. Leighton TA, Liu SY, Bongard FS (1993) Comparative cardiopulmonary effects of carbon dioxide versus helium pneumoperitoneum. Surgery 113: 527–531
10. Nussey SS, Bevan DH, Ang V, Jenkins JS (1986) Effects of arginine vasopressin infusions on circulating concentrations of platelet AVP, factor VIII C and Von Willebrand factor. Thromb Haemost 55: 34–36

Assessment of Operative Difficulty and Postoperative Recovery in Laparoscopic Surgery of the Colon

P. O. Nyström and S. Skullman

Introduction

Laparoscopic bowel surgery is more difficult than cholecystectomy, hernia repair or appendectomy. Neither the training of surgeons nor the development of instruments or methods has yet reached the stage of routine. Much less is reported about laparoscopic colorectal operations than was ever reported about the previous achievements in laparoscopic surgery [1]; indeed, there is reason to believe that many thousands of bowel procedures are attempted or completed as laparoscopic operations without any protocol or organised follow-up of results. One reason is probably that it is not clear how laparoscopic bowel surgery should be described when it is so often a combination of closed and open techniques. The dubious terms "assisted" and "converted" have been used to get round this uncertainty. It is also likely that many surgeons have been disappointed with the technical difficulties of this method of surgery. Moreover, it is not at all clear that the postoperative course is any better than after expert open operation [2, 3]. A programme was designed in our institution to address these problems of laparoscopic bowel surgery.

Patients and Methods

Patients

Ninety-eight patients have been operated on laparoscopically for colorectal disease in the course of 3 years (1993–1995). The operations were performed for a variety of conditions and indications encompassing both malignant (31 patients) and benign disease (67 patients), as shown in Table 1. No particular selection criteria were used. Patients age and body mass index were the same as for similar open operation. Many of the patients had had a previous abdominal operation. The decision to operate laparoscopically was made mainly on logistic grounds (availability of surgeons and time). Most operations were performed by at least two out of a pool of six colorectal surgeons with varying previous experience of laparoscopic technique. This therefore represents our early experience.

For several years a data base of colorectal operations has been kept in the institution for reasons of quality assurance. The information relates to age,

Table 1. Numbers of laparoscopic colorectal operations performed in Linköping 1993–1995

Operation	
Resections	37
Right colon	7
Left colon	20
Low anterior resection	5
Abdominoperineal resection	3
Total colectomy	2
Non-resections	61
Ileostomy/colostomy	16
Ileorectal anastomosis	9
Colorectal anastomosis	7
Rectopexy	14
Mobilisation without resection	6
Other	9

sex, diagnosis, procedure, operation time and blood loss, complications and postoperative stay. In addition, an index score defining the technical content of the operation and another index score defining the postoperative recovery are entered prospectively, as described below. From this data base, information on groups of similar patients with open operations was retrieved for comparison with those undergoing the closed operation. Owing to the great variety of the laparoscopic operations, it was impossible to obtain perfectly matched controls for the comparisons.

Completeness of Laparoscopic Operations

All laparoscopic operations are reported according to the principle of "intention to treat", meaning that if the laparoscope was introduced into the abdomen with the intention of completing one or more steps of the operation with laparoscopic assistance, the operation is deemed laparoscopic. The terms "assistance" and "conversion" have not been used because they are open to various interpretations. The completeness of the laparoscopic operations was therefore determined from the number of steps that were performed with the laparoscope. In resections of the colon and rectum the steps were as follows:

Step 0 Laparoscopy only or interrupted dissection
Step 1 Completed mobilisation of peritoneal reflections
Step 2 Division of the segmental artery and vein
Step 3 Division of the bowel on one or both sides of the lesion
Step 4 Completion of an anastomosis or a stoma

A predetermined scheme for a complete laparoscopic bowel resection allowed extracorporeal resection and anastomosis in right-sided colon lesions, while on the left side the complete operation required all of steps 1–4 to have

Table 2. Steps completed with laparoscopy in colorectal operations

Surgical steps completed	Resections (n = 37)		Non-resections (n = 61)	
	n	%	n	%
Laparoscopy only	1	3	12	20
Mobilisation	10	27	5	8
Division of segmental artery	9	·24	–	–
Division of bowel	3	8	–	–
Completed laparoscopic reconstruction	14	38	44	72

been performed with the closed technique. The specimen was removed through a coeliotomy that was large enough for convenient delivery of the bowel. The proximal resection of the bowel was usually done extracorporeally. Anastomose on the right side were done with a linear stapler, while those on the left side were performed with circular stapler introduced transanally. In two complete abdominoperineal resections the specimen was removed through the perineal wound and the stoma was fashioned laparoscopically.

In non-resections no segment of bowel was removed, but often a stoma was fashioned or an ileo-rectal or colo-rectal anastomosis was performed for restoration of bowel continuity (Table 1). Completeness of the laparoscopic operation then required that the anastomosis or stoma was performed without a coeliotomy. The same criterion was used for completeness of other non-resections, e. g. rectopexy. The degree of completeness by the above criteria for all 98 operations is shown in Table 2.

Technical Content of the Operations

All our open and closed operations are scored by the principal surgeon upon completion of the operation. Scores are given on an analogue scale as follows:

0: technical content at most up to an imaginary median difficulty in the surgeon's own experience (0 – 50th percentile);
1: technical content between the 51st and 75th percentile;
2: technical content among the worst 25 % in the surgeon's experience (76th – 100th percentile).

The surgeon assigns a score to each of seven variables: visibility (exposure), disturbing bleeding (oozing), dissection, reconstruction, demand on own technical skill, demand on own judgement, and psychological stress experienced. The scores for all variables are totalled to give a maximum score of 14, but scores above 5 are unusual in open surgery and half of open operations are scored zero. The score is related to the operation time, blood loss, postoperative recovery and stay, as well as complications in open surgery.

Postoperative Recovery

A recovery score was constructed from the following information: the post-operative day when the patient had a normal acute physiology score with the APACHE II system (maximum 2 points); the day when body temperature was 37.8 °C or less for a full 24 h; the day when stools were passed or stoma content was in excess of 100 ml; the day when more than 1000 ml nutrition was tolerated by the oral route. The days were totalled and 4 was detracted from the sum to achieve a scale with a zero starting point for the patient who had fully recovered on the 1st postoperative day. Typical scores are 3–6 for non-resections (minor intra-abdominal operations) and 7–10 for colonic resections.

In open surgery this recovery score is a sensitive measure of the postoperative course, which is related to the operation index above as well as the diagnosis and procedure. It is almost independent of patient age and sex. The recovery score is a better measure of the immediate postoperative course than length of hospital stay, which varies greatly between hospitals.

Results

The diagnosis was cancer in 31 patients and non-malignant previous or current disease in 61 patients. A bowel resection with anastomosis or stoma was performed in 37 patients. An anastomosis with or without bowel resection was performed in 50 patients. The types of operations are shown in Table 1. To give a fuller understanding of the variety of these procedures, the operation time and blood loss in patients with malignant and benign diagnoses are shown in Fig. 1 and 2.

The median postoperative stay was 7 days after an operation for cancer and 6 days after operation for non-malignancy. Five patients were reoperated on for complications. Three had postoperative bleeding, but in each instance the bleeding had ceased at reoperation and no cause could be indentified. One patient was reoperated on for anastomotic dehiscence and another for dehiscence of the incision wound. One patient died postoperatively. This patient suffered postoperative bleeding (reoperated) and subsequent anastomotic dehiscence (reoperated) caused by necrosis due to thrombosis of the middle colic artery.

Fig. 1. Operation times in laparoscopic operations. Each mark represents one patient

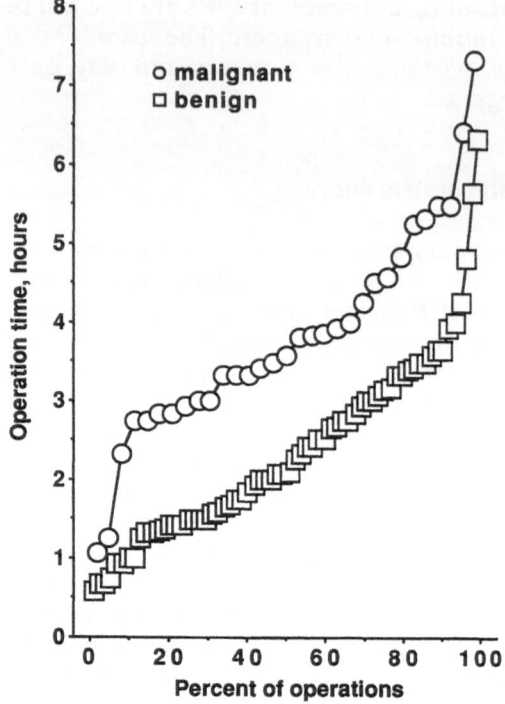

Fig. 2. Operative blood loss in patients undergoing laparoscopic operation

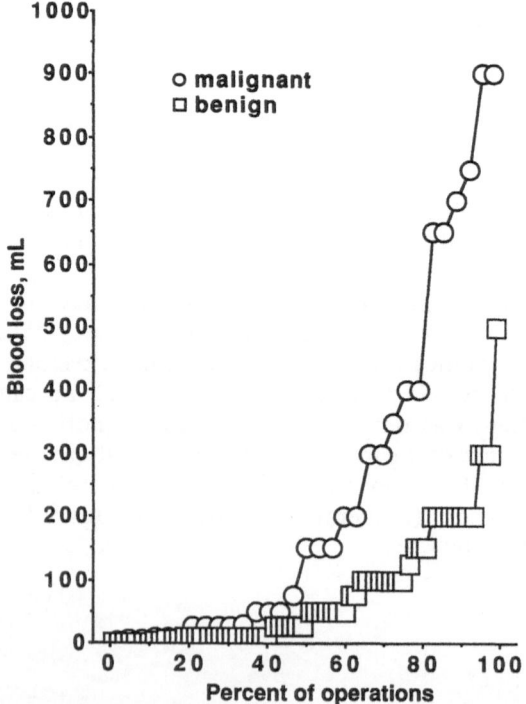

Technical Content of the Operation

The analysis of the technical scores assigned to the operation showed scores consistently about one point higher in closed than in open operations (Tables 3, 4). Laparoscopic resections scored higher than laparoscopic non-resections (Fig. 3, 4). A further comparison of the relative distribution of points showed that points were assigned especially for difficulty of dissection,

Table 3. Postoperative patient recovery and operation technical score in laparoscopic non-resections compared with similar open operations[a]

	Laparoscopic non-resection[b] ($n = 61$)		Open non-resection[c] ($n = 112$)		Open ileo-rectal anastomosis ($n = 27$)		Open colo-rectal anastomosis ($n = 24$)	
	Mean	SD	Mean	SD	Mean	SD	Mean	SD
Recovery score	4.6	4.0	5.0	3.5	6.1	2.5	9.3	3.3*
Temperature	2.2	1.7	2.2	1.6	2.4	1.0	2.8	1.6
Gut motility	2.8	1.7	2.6	1.3	2.7	0.7	4.4	1.2*
Enteral feeding	2.4	1.6	3.2	2.1	3.8	1.5	4.8	1.6*
Operation score	1.5	2.1	0.7	1.4	0.7	1.3	1.3	2.1

* Statistical difference from laparoscopic operation, $p < 0.05$.
[a] Recovery score is the global assessment of recovery (arbitrary units.) Temperature, gut motility and enteral tolerance are given as the postoperative day on which the patient satisfied the defined criteria see Patients and Methods.
[b] See Table 1 for case mix.
[c] No anastomoses, 68 % ileostomy/colostomy formation.

Table 4. Postoperative recovery and operation technical score in laparoscopic colon resections compared with similar open operations

	Laparoscopic resection[a] ($n = 37$)		Laparoscopic anastomosis[a] ($n = 50$)		Open resection[b] ($n = 263$)		Open anastomosis[c] ($n = 623$)	
	Mean	SD	Mean	SD	Mean	SD	Mean	SD
Recovery score	9.0	5.2	7.8	5.0	8.1	3.7	8.1	4.4
Temperature	2.7	1.7	2.5	1.6	2.6	2.2	2.7	2.4
Gut motility	3.9	1.4	3.5	1.5	3.8	1.4	3.4	1.4
Enteral feeding	4.7	2.2	4.2	2.2	4.6	1.8	4.8	2.2
Operation score	2.2	2.0	2.2	1.9	1.0	1.7	1.3	2.0

[a] See Table 1 for case mix.
[b] Right and left colon resections only, no stomas.
[c] Anastomosis of small bowel, ileocolic, colon, colorectal, coloanal, ileorectal, and ileoanal, some with protective ileostomy.

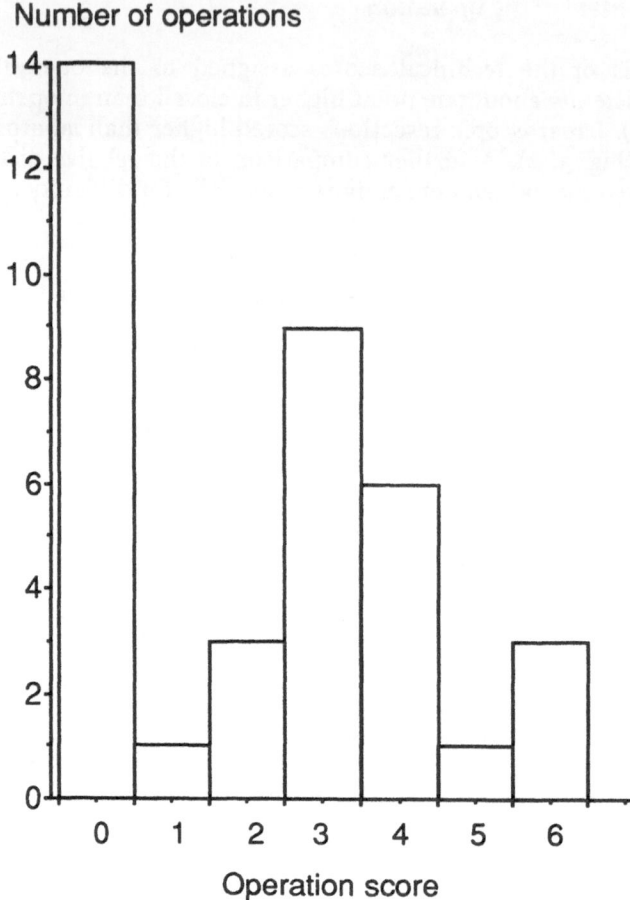

Fig. 3. Distribution of operation technical scores in laparoscopic bowel resections

demands on technical ability and demands on judgement. Exposure was good and disturbing bleeding was not a major problem, judging from the scores. Few points were assigned for the anastomosis or stoma after resections, but in non-resective operations rather more points were assigned for the reconstructive phase of the operation (Fig. 5).

Postoperative Recovery

Recovery varied considerably between patients and reflected among other things the diagnosis and the procedure performed. Recovery was clearly longer after resections than after non-resections, and after procedures including an anastomosis versus those without an anastomosis ($p < 0.001$) in

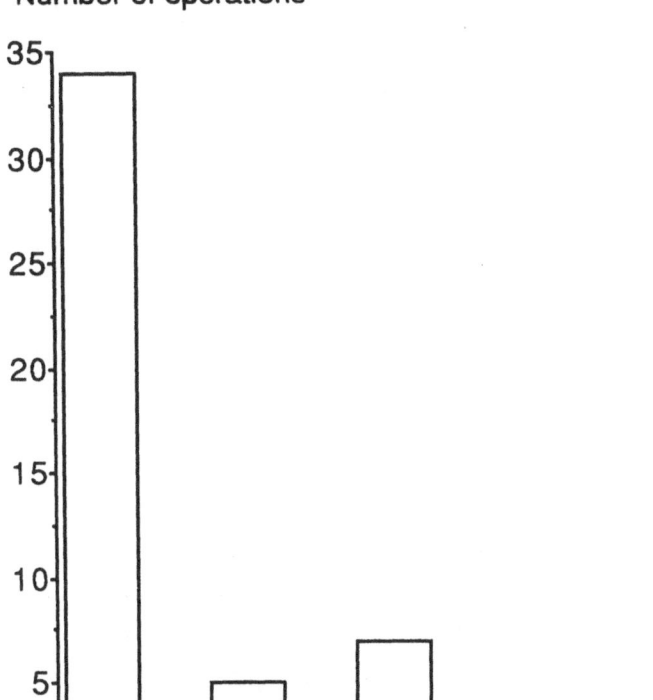

Fig. 4. Distribution of operation technical scores in laparoscopic non-resections

both comparisons; Figs. 6, 7). While these differences were obvious, the comparison between laparoscopic and open operations was more problematic and showed less difference.

Table 3 shows the comparisons between laparoscopic and open non-resective operations, including ileo- and colostomy, reconstructive colorectal or ileorectal anastomosis, as well as procedures where the bowel had not been entered. Except for open colorectal anastomosis, no statistical differences were found between closed and open operations.

Table 4 also compares laparoscopic and open operations, with the laparoscopic procedures subdivided into those with resection (irrespecitve of anastomosis) and those with an anastomosis (irrespective of resection). There was remarkable agreement in all comparisons, both for the global recovery score and for the individual components of the index.

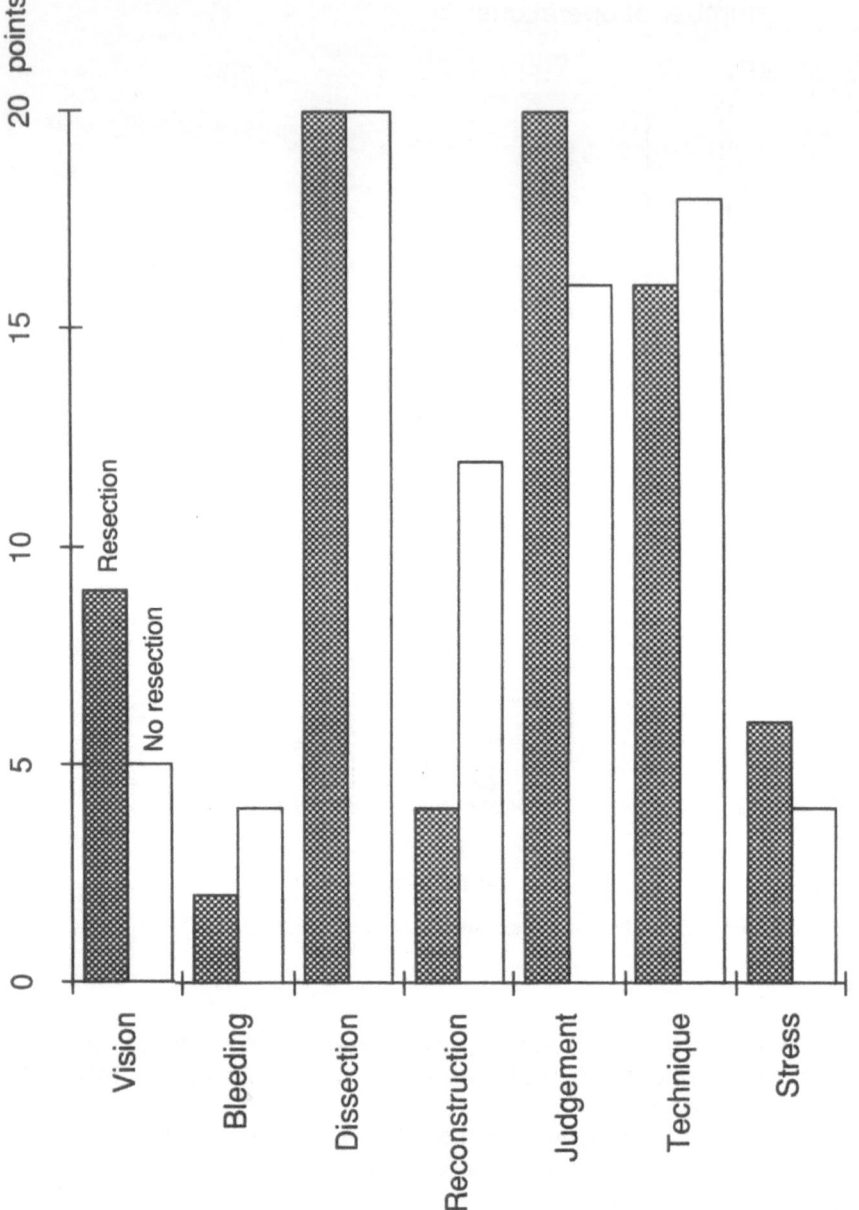

Fig. 5. Total number of score points assigned for each element in the operation technical score for resections ($n = 37$) and non-resections ($n = 61$)

Fig. 6. Postoperative recovery after laparoscopic resections and non-resections. Arbitrary units, $p < 0.001$

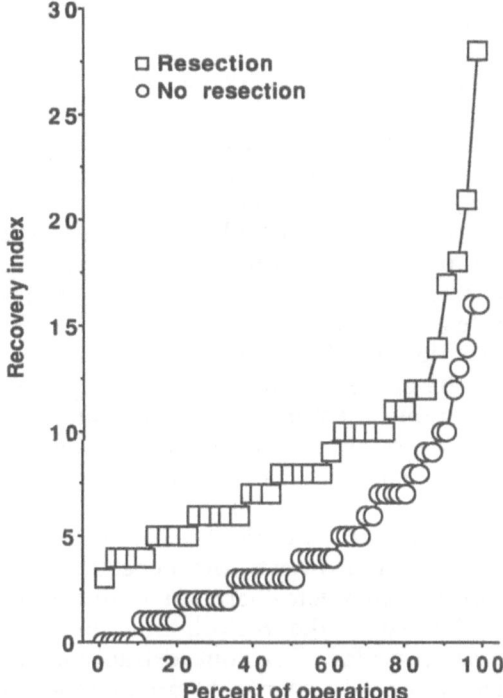

Fig. 7. Postoperative recovery in laparoscopic procedures with and without an anastomosis. Arbitrary units, $p < 0,001$

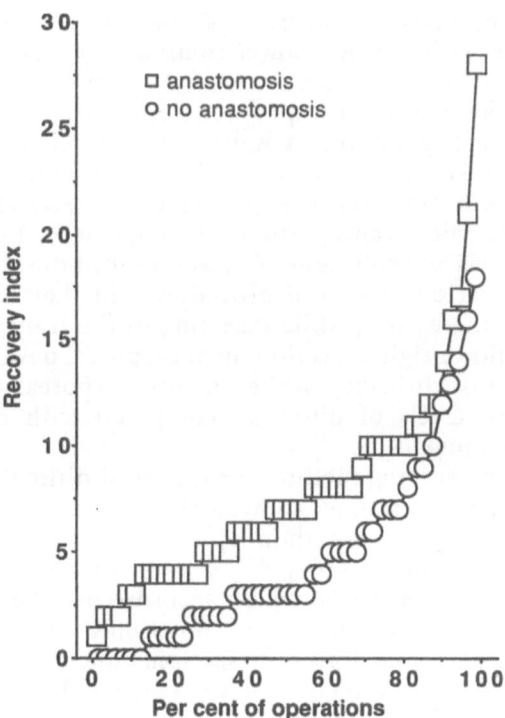

Discussion

It is expected that laparoscopic surgery will come to be as common for colorectal diseases as it is for upper gastrointestinal diseases. However, before it can be the preferred operative method for a large proportion of the procedures now done with an open technique a tremendous educational effort will be needed, because colorectal surgeons have less experience with laparoscopic techniques. It is not known how long the learning period is but some 20 operations are needed before operation time approximates that of open surgery [4]. Our approach has been to train our whole group of colorectal surgeons, with the ultimate goal of turning laparoscopic operations into routine. Consequently, the operations we report represent those performed while still in training.

We were able to perform complete laparoscopic resection in only 38% of the resections attempted, whereas as many as 72% of non-resections were completed laparoscopically. For a complete operation, each of four steps had to be performed laparoscopically according to a predetermined schema for each procedure. It recognized, however, that it is permissible, because it is easier, to resect and anastomose the bowel extracorporeally in right hemicolectomy. However, the ileocolic artery must be divided intracorporeally for a complete operation. In resections on the left side the bowel had to be divided at the rectosigmoid junction intracorporeally, while the proximal resection was done extracorporeally. The anvil of the circular stapler was introduced into the proximal segment, which was returned to the abdomen, and the coeliotomy was closed to allow a renewed pneumoperitoneum for the intracorporeal anastomosis. In operations where a stoma is fashioned or when bowel continuity is restored by ileorectal or colorectal anastomosis, completeness of the operation required there to have been no coeliotomy at all except at the stoma site.

We suggest that counting the number of steps actually performed laparoscopically describes the potential of the laparoscopic method and the current level of expertise more precisely than using the conversion rate, which is always subject to judgement. A similar approach was assumed by Geis and colleagues [5], who ranked the skill that is required to perform the various standard procedures. In their opinion right colon resection was the easiest, while resection of the transverse colon was the most difficult. In right resection, intracorporeal devascularisation added one more level of difficulty, while an intracorporeal anastomosis added a further three levels of difficulty compared with extracorporeal resection and anastomosis.

The scoring method for technical difficulty that we have long used for all our operations showed that surgeons rated laparoscopic operations as more difficult than open operations – no surprise. However, 37% of resections and 57% of non-resections were scored as of median difficulty or easier, which accords with the general experience that laparoscopic operations are sometimes remarkably simple with excellent exposure and quick dissection. Since less than half of the resections could be completed as an entirely laparoscopic procedure, the conclusion must be that the degree of difficulty increases very steeply. The instruments occasionally seem desperately inadequte for the handling of a bulky bowel.

It is believed that laparoscopic operation can allow a reduction of operative trauma and therefore of systemic inflammation, with quicker recovery after the operation [6]. We attempted to match our closed operative series with historical and contemporary open operative controls from the same registry to investigate this question. Admittedly these comparisons were deficient in several respects. It must also be borne in mind that many of the laparoscopic operations were incomplete procedures, and quicker recovery is not to be expected when a significant part of the operation was performed with an open technique. Judging from our results, there was no indication that laparoscopic operations were associated with less inflammation (fever), earlier restoration of bowel motility, or earlier tolerance of enteral feeding. Other have reported similar recovery after laparoscopic colonic operations [7], or have found marginally better recovery in comparison with historical controls or in comparison with patients whose operations were converted [8]. One study reported exceptional recovery and discharge within 2–3 days postoperatively after a combination of laparoscopy, epidural analgesia, and early mobilisation and enteral feeding [9].

Only a proper randomised design will be able to provide better answers about the presumed benefits of laparoscopic bowel surgery. In all likelihood it will take more than laparoscopy alone to significantly improve outcome after colorectal surgery. We remain confident, however, that laparoscopy will change many old surgical concepts.

References

1. Monson JRT, Hill ADK, Darzi A (1995) Laparoscopic colonic surgery, review. Br J Surg 82:150–157
2. Falk PM, Beart RW, Wexner SD et al. (1993) Laparoscopic colectomy: a critical appraisal. Dis Colon Rectum 36:28–34
3. Kmiot WA, Wexner SD (1995) Laparoscopy in colorectal surgery: a call for careful appraisal. Br J Surg 82:21–25
4. Simons AJ, Anthone GJ, Ortega AE, Franklin M, Fleshman J, Geis WP (1995) Laparoscopic-assisted colectomy learning curve. Dis Colon Rectum 38:600–603
5. Geis WP, Coletta AV, Verdeja J-C, Plasencia G, Ojogho O, Jacobs M (1994) Sequential psychomotor skills development in laparoscopic colon surgery. Arch Surg 129:206–212
6. Senagore AJ, Kilbride MJ, Luchtefeld MA, MacKeigan JM, Davis AT, Moore JD (1995) Superior nitrogen balance after laparoscopic-assisted colectomy. Ann Surg 221:171–175
7. Milsom JW, Lavery IC, Church JM, Stolfi VM, Fazio VW (1994) Use of laparoscopic techniques in colorectal surgery: preliminary study. Dis Colon Rectum 37:215–218
8. Senagore AJ, Luchtefeld MA, Mackeigan JM, Mazier WP (1993) Open colectomy versus laparoscopic colectomy: are there differences? Am Surg 59:549–554
9. Bardram L, Funch-Jensen P, Jensen P, Crawford ME, Kehlet H (1995) Recovery after laparoscopic colonic surgery with epidural analgesia, and early oral nutrition and mobilisation. Lancet 345:763–764

Cytological Examinations After Intraoperative Lavage in Colon Carcinoma Patients Undergoing Conventional and Laparoscopic Surgery

U. Bonk, P. Hanisch, B. M. Helmke, K. Lebrecht, H. A. Richter, and A. Franke

At present we have had relevant experience in minimally invasive surgery for about 6 years – even less for the majority of minimally invasive procedures. We are in an ongoing stage of learning and studying trying to make sure that we draw tight conclusions to that we can compare the results of conventional and minimally invasive surgery. One question we asked was whether there are any differences between cytological slides after Intraoperative lavage in conventional and laparoscopic surgery for cancer of the colon.

Method

In the first weeks of 1995 peritoneal lavage was carried out before surgery (A), during surgery (B), and after surgery (C). About 1000 ml of the fluid from each of the three lavages was immediately delivered without further preparation to the Institute of Pathology.

The pathologists had no information as to which method of operation had been chosen in each case. The fluid specimens were centrifuged. The cytological slides were produced using the cytocentrifuge and were subjected to standard staining techniques.

Results

Tables 1 and 2 show the results for the total of 26 patients undergoing surgery. Cancer cells were only detected in the first lavage fluid, (A) from two patients. Both patients had advanced-stage cancer and underwent conventional

Table 1. Clinical data of patients undergoing conventional surgery

Code	Age	Gender	Tumor	Stage				Grade	Positive findings in lavage fluid
				T	N	M	R		
8	46	f	Sigmoid	3	0	x		2	–
3	51	f	Rectum	2	0	x		2	–
7	51	f	Rectum	2	0	x		2	–
2	52	f	Rectum	3	0	x		1	–
22	60	m	Coecum	is					–

Table 1 (Fortsetzung)

Code	Age	Gender	Tumor	Stage				Grade	Positive findings in lavage fluid
				T	N	M	R		
23	61	m	Ascending colon	3	1	x		2	–
1	65	m	Sigmoid	3	1	x		2	–
13	69	f	Coecum	4	3	x		2	+(A)
9	70	f	Rectum	4	2	x		2	–
25	71	f	Coecum	3	2	x		3	–
6	73	f	Sigmoid	3	1	1		2	–
5	74	m	Rectum	3	0	x	2	2	–
12	75	f	Descending colon	3	1	x		2	–
16	77	m	Ascending colon	3	0	x		2	–
19	79	f	Sigmoid	3	2	x		2	–
11	82	f	Coecum	2	0	x		2	–
24	82	f	Rectum	4	1	1		3	–
18	83	m	Descending colon	is					–
20	83	f	Sigmoid	3	0	x		2	–
14	85	f	Sigmoid	4					+(A)

is, in situ.

Table 2. Clinical data of patients undergoing laparoscopic surgery

Code	Age	Gender	Tumor	Stage				Grade	Positive findings in lavage fluid
				T	N	M	R		
15	57	f	Rectum	is					–
17	66	f	Sigmoid	3	1	x		2	–
26	70	m	Sigmoid	3	2	x		2	–
4	80	m	Sigmoid	3	1	x		3	–
10	80	f	Sigmoid	2	0	x		2	–
29	83	f	Rectum	is					–

surgery. In none of the patients undergoing minimally invasive surgery were tumor cells detected in the peritoneal lavage. All other peritoneal lavage fluids were free of tumor cells but showed the presence of mesothelial and blood cells.

Discussion

Peritoneal lavage is an accepted technique in both the staging and the treatment of gynaecological tumors, e.g. in stage Ic of ovarian carcinoma.

Mesothelial cells in peritoneal lavages contain some morphological characteristics which differ from those of spontaneously shed cells [1, 2]. These include:

- Large, even honeycomb-like formations
- Round to oval cores with a soft core membrane
- Frequently, noticeable small round nucleoli
- Granular chromatin

In addition there are also massively degenerated cells.

Although adenocarcinoma of the colon was the main cancern in our series, cytologists must always be familiar with the multitude of possible differential diagnoses of benign or malignant lesions which are detected using the lavage technique.

A synopsis of typical cytological patterns which may be found in a peritoneal lavage fluid is given below [3 – 8]:

Malignant Tumors

Lung: Epidermoid carcinoma

- Usually single cells
- Nuclei irregular, frequently indented or lobulated, rim interrupted
- Nucleoli prominent, multiple and deformed
- Cytoplasm thick, distinct border degenerative vacuolation
- Cell clusters flat, "Cobblestone" appearance

Lung: Cylindrocellular Adenocarcinoma

- Large, highly differentiated single cells, cuboid or cylindrical typically double-nucleated (like the soles of two feet)
- Nucleus round or oval, hyperchromatic, eccentrically located, giant nuclei possible
- Nucleoli prominent, roundish, occasionally absent
- Secretory vacuoles in single cells
- Cell cluster: lobular, acinar or rosettes, usually without mucus vacuoles

Lung: Large Cell Carcinoma

- Large single cells
- Nuclei polymorphous, varying in shape and size
- Nucleoli prominent, occasionally multiple and deformed
- Cytoplasm ill-defined, scanty or abundant

Lung: Small Cell Carcinoma

- Cell groups with nuclear moulding: "Indian file" or "vertebra-like"
- Nuclei polymorphous, chromatin dense
- Nucleoli usually absent
- Cytoplasm scanty, poorly preserved

Breast: Ductal Carcinoma

- Cell Balls
- Cells unimorphous, relatively small
- Nucleus round to oval, hyperchromatic
- Nucleus small or absent
- Cytoplasm dense, sharp-bordered
- Vacuoles usually absent

Breast: Undifferentiated Carcinoma

- Dissociated single cells (free cell type) or "indian files"
- Distinct anisocytosis, double or multinucleation
- Nucleoli multiple
- Vacuoles facultative, mucus rare

Ovarian Carcinoma

- Polymorphism
- Mucus, occasional psammoma bodies, conspicuous
- Anisocytosis in papillomatous clusters
- Solid groups of small cells besides large cell clusters with vacuolation
- Nuclei varying in shape and size
- Chromatin coarse, hyperchromatic
- Nucleoli large, frequently multiple
- Giant secretory vacuoles ("signet ring" cells, "soap-bubble-like")

Colon Carcinoma

- Polymorphic formations
- Clusters of tall, columnar cells with nuclear palisading
- Nuclei large, round, lobated or kidney-like, eccentrically located
- Nucleoli distinct, occasionally multiple
- Cytoplasm abundant, vacuolated, mucus production in all cases

Stomach Carcinoma

- Frequently large cellulated
- Single layered "histiocytic" cells, large tubular and/or poorly differentiated clusters
- Nuclei large, hyperchromatic, granular chromatin, multinucleation
- Nucleoi large, frequently multiple
- Cytoplasm abundant, vacuolated ("signet ring" cells)
- Mucus production

Gallbladder Carcinoma

- Cylindrical or cuboidal single cells and morula-like papillary clusters
- Nuclei roundish, relatively large, hyperchromatic, chromatin coarse
- Nucleoli round, centrally located
- Cytoplasm intensely basophile, occasional secretory vacuoles (mucus)

Pancreas and Bile Duct Carcinoma

- Two cell types
- Papillary clusters of small, cuboid, uniform cells, occasional nuclear palisading, nuclei hyperchromatic, cytoplasm granular
- Abundant polymorphous cells, layering in groups or clusters, nuclei notably clear, round or oval, chromatin fine, granular nucleoli small and round
- Cytoplasm occasionally vacuolated (usually empty)

Hypernephroma

- Large histiocyte-like cells
- Nuclei round or oval
- Nucleoli single, prominent, roundish
- Cytoplasm abundant, foamy PAS + (diastase instable)
- Symplasm inside cell clusters

Melanoma

- Polymorphous, immature, single cells with and without pigment
- Nuclei ovoid, occasionally lobulated, chromatin fine, densely reticular
- Nucleoli single, roundish
- Double or multinucleation
- Cytoplasm fine, granular with grey to black pigment (DOPA +, Schmorl +)
- Melanophages

Mesothelioma (Epithelial Type)

- Single cells and morula-like clusters, large cells with only one nucleus
- Nuclei hyperchromatic, chromatin coarse
- Nucleoli prominent (non-obligate)
- Cytoplasm cuboidal, varying in shape, size and staining, occasionally fine or large vacuolated
- Hyaluronic acid increased

Fibrosarcoma

- Single cells and formations with fibrous intercellar substance
- Nucleus ovoid, spindle-shaped, chromatin irregular, coarse
- Nucleoli non-obligate
- Cytoplasm scanty or moderately abundant, ill-defined

Non-malignant Conditions

Indications of Tuberculosis

- Richness of cells
- Preponderance of mature lymphocytes
- Lymphocyte aggregates (detritus)

- Reactive lymphatic cells
- Occasional epitheloid cells
- No local reaction (rare mesothelial cells)

Rheumatoid Arthritis

- Hypersegmentation of granulocytes
- Phagocytes
- Multinucleated, frequently tailed giant cells (comet cells)
- Detritus in the background

Lupus Erythematosis

- Neutrophils and lymphocytes
- Plasma-like cells
- Detritus
- Rare mesothelial cells
- LE cells, rosettes, globules

Pancreatitis

- Colour beer-brown
- Degenerative and reactive mesothelial cells
- Erythrocytes, sometimes eosinophils
- Amylase increased

To sum up, none of the peritoneal lavage fluids from patients undergoing laparoscopic surgery for cancer of the colon yidded any tumor cells. So far, the postoperative course of all patients has been unremarkable. We are of the opinion that patients treated using this operative technique have no higher risks of tumor recurrence than patients who underwent conventional surgery.

References

1. Covell JL, Carry JB, Feldmann PS (1985) Peritoneal washings in ovarian tumors. Potential sources of error in cytologic diagnosis. Acta Cytol 29 : 310 – 316
2. Johnson TL, Kumar NB, Hopkins M, Hughes JD (1988) Cytologic features of ovarian tumors of low malignant potential in peritoneal fluids. Acta Cytol 32 : 513 – 518
3. Luesley DM, Williams DR, Ward K, Redmann CR, Lawton FG (1990) Prospective comparative cytologic study of direct peritoneal smears and lavage fluids in patients with epithelial ovarian cancer and benign gynecologic disease. Acta Cytol 34 : 539 – 544
4. Sneige N, Fernandez T, Copeland LJ, Katz RL (1986) Mullerian inclusions in peritoneal washings: potential source of error in peritoneal washings. Acta Cytol 30 : 271 – 276
5. Zuna RE, Mitchell ML, Mulick KA, Weijchert WM (1989) Cytohistoligic correlation of peritoneal washing: cytology in gynecologic disease. Acta Cytol 33 : 327 – 336
6. Greenebaum E (1993) Fine needle aspiration of cystic ovarian lesions and peritoneal washing cytology. Course material, Houston
7. Ehya H (1993) Diagnostic problems in effusion cytology Course material, Hahnemann University School of Medicine, Philadelphia
8. Lin F (1993) Cytopathology of serous effusions. Course material, University of California Irvine Medical Center, Orange

Complexity of Laparoscopic Colon Procedures and Program Development

W.P. Geis, E.J. Brennan, and H.C. Kim

Introduction

In contrast to laparoscopic cholecystectomy, laparoscopic colectomy represents a category of procedures of varying complexity and varying risks. It is assumed that surgeons who undertake to perform laparoscopic colon procedures are experienced surgeons, and therefore the varying complexities attributed to laparoscopic colectomy center entirely upon the new skills which are necessary to perform the laparoscopic components of the procedures. The key to success, therefore, is to be aware of the laparoscopic skills required for each procedure and to choose cases judiciously, based on knowledge of their individual complexities. The three laparoscopic skills required to perform the spectrum of laparoscopic colectomy procedures are laparoscopic mobilization, laparoscopic devascularization, and laparoscopic anastomosis [1].

It is not necessary that all three laparoscopic skills be utilized in all colectomy procedures. Knowledge and understanding of which skills are required for each procedure allows the surgeon to choose colectomy cases which require fewer skills early in his or her learning experience, thus allowing successful performance of safe and efficient laparoscopic surgery during the learning process for the surgeon. This allows the surgeon to acquire dexterity in the three laparoscopic colectomy skills in a sequential fashion [2]. Moreover, the use of a Complexity Scale provides the surgeon with an instrument to quickly determine the complexity of, and the skills required for, various laparoscopic colectomy procedures [1].

Three factors which strongly influence the development of a successful laparoscopic colectomy program are the use of a Preceptor to guide the surgeon educatee, operating room team development to support the surgeon educatee, and the frequent performance of laparoscopic colectomy procedures to reinforce the educational process for the surgeon and team members. Lastly, the laparoscopic operating room team is exposed to varying case complexities independent of the technical complexities for the surgeon. The awareness of these complexities influences the successful development of a laparoscopic team. Each of these factors represent an important contribution to successful vs unsuccessful program development in laparoscopic colon resection. Each will be discussed here.

Complexities of Laparoscopic Colon Procedures

Strategy

The important factors which provide an environment to comfortably learn and accomplish the three laparoscopic colectomy skills and procedures are

1. positioning of the patient,
2. strategic placement of laparoscopic ports, and
3. room layout and positioning of the surgeon.

We place all patients supine, followed by elevation and separation of the lower extremities to a modified lithotomy position using Allen stirrups. The thighs are parallel to the anterior abdominal wall to avoid their obstructing the use of instruments through laparoscopic ports. Both upper extremities are placed at the patient's sides to accommodate the surgeon and team member positions, the robotic arm, and the appropriate placement of monitors.

Strategic placement of laparoscopic ports minimizes the complexity of procedures by establishing an excellent visual field, and facilitates traction and countertraction laparoscopically. In most colon resections, four 10 to 12-mm ports are used. Two ports are placed in the quadrant of the abdomen most distant from the expected work in order to maximize versatility of atraumatic instrumentation when performing retraction, traction, and countertraction. The camera port is located to facilitate the normal hand-eye axis for the surgeon and is usually at the umbilicus. The fourth port is a working port which accommodates mobilization and devascularization utilizing the endoshears or harmonic scalpel [3].

The surgeon and assistant stand at locations which face the work and maintain a normal hand-eye axis. For sigmoid and left colon resection, the monitors are on the left side of the patient and the surgeon is on the right side of the patient. During right colon resection, the monitors are along the right side of the patient and the surgeon is on the left side of the patient or between the legs. The position of the patient also minimizes complexity, the patient is placed in a "right side up" position, during left colon resection in a "left side up" position, and in the reverse Trendelenburg position during transverse colon resection. Similarly, the rectum is mobilized using steep Trendelenburg position, and the hepatic flexure mobilized using reverse Trendelenburg and "right side up" position.

Psychomotor Skills

There are three laparoscopic psychomotor or manual skills which may be used by the surgeon during laparoscopic colectomy procedures. These are laparoscopic mobilization of the bowel, regional devascularization laparoscopically, and intracorporeal anastomosis. Not all three skills are required in every colectomy procedure. During the performance of right colon resection for benign disease, for example, the right colon including hepatic flexure and right transverse colon are mobilized and generously freed from the retroperitoneal structures. This intestinal segment may be removed through a mini-incision in the right hemiabdomen or the midline along with the intact segment of mesentery and adjacent proximal and distal bowel. The specimen is then devascularized and resected at the skin level, followed by performance of an extracorporeal anastomosis. The anastomotic segment is then placed carefully in the abdominal cavity and the procedure is essentially complete. In contrast, performance of laparoscopic right colon resection for malignant disease requires intracorporeal devascularization of the regional blood supply in order to accomplish a wide regional resection for cancer.

The use of one laparoscopic skill during certain procedures vs the use of two skills in others suggests how the surgeon may acquire these laparoscopic skills sequentially if he or she chooses cases judiciously during the learning phase [2]. Further, the third laparoscopic skill, intracorporeal anastomosis, is only required when the proximal and distal ends of the transected intestinal segments do not reach the skin level of the mini-incision. This circumstance occurs most commonly during laparoscopic sigmoid colectomy or low anterior resection. It is most often performed utilizing a circular stapler in the performance of a transrectal anastomosis. The skill of laparoscopic colonic anastomosis is most easily developed by laparoscopic closure of a Hartmann and colostomy. This third skill may also be learned sequentially by the laparoscopic surgeon.

Complexity Ratings and Scale

Each of the three laparoscopic skills adds complexity to the laparoscopic colectomy procedure. Further, we have documented that each of the skills is itself of variable complexity depending on which colectomy procedure is being performed (right colectomy vs left colectomy, etc.). We have assigned a numeric value to the complexity level of each skill required during each of the seven basic laparoscopic colectomy procedures [2]. The conversion of the complexity level of each of the skills to a numeric value allows the construction of a complexity rating for each of the colectomy procedures depending on whether one, two, or three skills are utilized. These ratings have been converted to a Laparoscopic Colectomy Complexity Scale.

Note that the complexity of each procedure is the sum of the complexities of each of the three laparoscopic skills utilized [1]. When two skills are utilized in a procedure, the total complexity is the sum of the complexity of the two skills; when one skill is utilized, the procedure complexity is equal to the laparoscopic complexity of the single skill used. The use of the Laparoscopic Colectomy Complexity Scale provides a unique was for the surgeon to develop his or her skills in a sequential fashion while simultaneously allowing the laparoscopic operating room team to develop its experience and skills by delineating the appropriate types of laparoscopic colectomy procedures to the performed early in the experienced laparoscopic surgeon and laparoscopic operating room team should choose their first cases from the least complex third of the Complexity Scale, while a more experienced surgeon and team may choose colectomy cases from the middle third of the Scale, and the advanced and experienced laparoscopic colectomy team and surgeon may choose even the cases which are in the most complex third of the Colectomy Scale. As a results, the team and surgeon continue to develop their skills and experience while simultaneously avoiding risk to the patient and unduly long operating times. This margin of safety and efficiency is reinforced during laparoscopic colectomy program development by the use of a Preceptor to modulate the educational experiences of the surgeon educatee and the operating room team.

Laparoscopic Colectomy Program Development

The successful development of a laparoscopic colectomy program involves a combination of structured and organized educational experiences for the surgeon, similar experiences for the operating room team, the use of surgeon Preceptor to help guide all members of the operating room team during early cases, and the judicious choice of appropriate laparoscopic colectomy cases from the Laparoscopic Colectomy Complexity Scale during the learning experiences in the operating room.

Preceptor Concepts and Case Efficiency

The use of a Preceptor as the experienced surgeon/teacher during laparoscopic colectomy procedures allows the Preceptor to provide guidance for the surgeon preceptee and instruction and help for the operating room team, and to aid the anesthesiologist and other operating room personnel in their early experiences. In 70 experiences as Preceptor for laparoscopic colectomy procedures, we observed that the operative times for surgeon preceptees were reasonably short, were not associated with technical mishaps, and provided a reference for the expected length of laparoscopic colectomy procedures [4]. These procedures were the first or second procedures of their complexity performed by the surgeon preceptees. Further, these operative times were comparable to open colectomy operative times. It is notable that the addition of laparoscopic skills in incremental complexity was not associated with a gradual increase in operative times. Right colon resection, sigmoid colon resection, and even abdominoperineal resection exhibited comparable operating times. In contrast, low anterior resection, and abdominal colectomy add longer operating times – due largely to the increase in the quantity of work necessary – as opposed to the gradual increase in complexity of each procedure. Thus, strategic use of the Laparoscopic Colectomy Complexity Scale to sequentially increase the complexity of procedures as laparoscopic colectomy experience increases, avoids the phenomenon of inordinately long operative times associated with increasing complexity [5].

Laparoscopic Operating Room Team Complexity Score

The successful implementation of an efficient and productive laparoscopic room team is influenced by many factors which are independent of the technical complexity of the procedure for the surgeon. These factors include the amount of equipment utilized, the choreography of equipment utilized, the positioning of the patient, the complexity of the technology used, and the complexity of the case for the scrub nurse. Importantly, the operating room team must recognize the complexity as it affects them. We have devised and implemented a Laparoscopic Complexity Score for the operating room team utilizing a numeric scale. Each of the members of the team has rated the factors by numeric complexity [6]. The Operating Room Team Complexity Score is used to assess the choice of team members. New members of the team are not utilized in highly complex cases, but rather initially gain experience by participation in the least complex cases. As experience increases, the team member are placed on gradually more complex cases as indicated by the Complexity Score [6].

Factors Influencing Successful Implementation of Laparoscopic Colectomy Programs

We have had the opportunity to preceptor surgeon preceptees in the performance of their first or second laparoscopic colectomy at their own hospital while performing a laparoscopic colectomy for the patient of the surgeon preceptee. In each of these circumstances, we took the opportunity to evaluate the local hospital environment and the factors which may influence the success or failure of a developing laparoscopic colectomy program. Further 6–9 months later, we reassessed each hospital to evaluate whether a program had been implemented successfully or had failed. Local factors were again re-evaluated. Factors which were evaluated included sponsorship and strong support from top administrative management, support and technical help from the peer surgeon group, the number of colectomy cases preceptored at the hospital, the number of visits by the preceptor to the hospital, and the number of colectomy cases available per month for potential laparoscopic colectomy. Many surgeons and their teams are self-motivated, intuitive, and creative in continuing to pursue a self-learning process during program development. Moreover, every program that developed successfully following one or a few preceptorship experiences had strong administrative support which filtered through the hospital organization.

However, the two factors which most obviously influenced success during program development were the number of cases available per month for laparoscopic colectomy and the number of peer surgeons who supported and provided technical help to the program. Clearly, program development was unsuccessful when the number of cases available was less than 3–4 cases per month. In contrast, programs were almost universally successful when the number of cases available to the surgeon preceptees were 5–9 cases per month. The increased number of cases available for laparoscopic colectomy per month reinforces the mastering of the technical and choreographic aspects of the educational process in the operating room by repetition. Further, when procedures are performed more frequently, new and innovative improvements are generated by the team as well as the surgeons.

The last and very important factor influencing success is peer surgeon support. In programs where peer surgeon support is absent, the programs were universally unsuccessful. Peer surgeon support added confidence, manpower, additional cases referred from the peer surgeon group, and strengthened the commitment of the team. Programs with peer surgeon support were universally successful with one single exception where the problem was an insufficiency of cases to reinforce education and pursue program development.

We conclude that two factors are absolutely necessary for program development. These are peer surgeon support and a minimum of three to four cases per month. Further, the presence of strong administrative and management support of the program converts program development from a difficult and cumbersome task to a streamlined plan with strategic goals and identifiable parameters.

References

1. Geis WP, Coletta AV, Jacobs M, Plasencia G, Kim HC (1994) Benefits of complexity scales in laparoscopic colectomy. Int Surg 79 : 230 – 232
2. Geis WP, Coletta AV, Verdeja JC, Plasencia G, Ojogho O, Jacobs M (1994) Sequential psychomotors skills development in laparoscopic colon surgery. Arch Surg 129 : 206 – 212
3. Brennan, EJ, Kim HC, Geis WP (1995) 110 consecutive laparoscopic colectomies performed using the harmonic scalpel (LCS). Society of Laparoendoscopic Surgeons (abstract)
4. Geis WP, Kim HC (1994) Adoption of laparoscopic colectomy procedures: relationship to local factors and preceptorships. Int Surg 79 : 228 – 229
5. Geis WP, Kim HC (1994) Preceptors, complexity scales and local factors influencing success in laparoscopic colectomy procedures. Surg Endosc 8 : 545
6. Geis WP (1995) Safe and efficient implementation of minimally invasive surgery program in innovations 95. Models for Medical Management, May 1995

IV Laparoscopic Surgical Techniques

Laparoscopic Surgery of the Colon Our Experience of 142 Cases

S. Bonilauri, E. Tamborrino, T. Berselli, I. Selmi, A. Lanzani, and G. Melotti

Introduction

The extraordinary and continuing evolution of operative laparoscopy has already made it possible to perform endoscopic bowel resections. Nowadays the indications can be extended to both benign and malignant pathology amenable to surgical treatment. This is the result of an emerging laparoscopic culture, supported by an ever-improving surgical technique and by the availability of specific instruments, in particular mechanical staplers. Performing these procedures by the laparoscopic route, it is possible to reproduce faithfully all the stages of the corresponding open techniques and follow all the basic principles upon which they are based. The laparoscope provides optimum visualization of the operative field, allowing the identification, ligature, and transection of the vascular pedicles, lysis of adhesions, mobilization of the affected bowel, and its transection without soilage of the operative field.

From a diagnostic point of view, laparoscopy can offer a significant advantage prior to making a specific and definite therapeutic decision. From the therapeutic point of view, laparoscopy can exclude the possibility of a curative procedure, the laparoscopic procedure can be sufficient as a matter of principle. From a technical point of view the many unexplored potentials of the abdominal lifter should also be considered.

As to contraindications to this method, we include all the general contraindications to laparoscopy: severe coagulopathy, cardiac failure with precarious hemodynamic stability, and respiratory failure. The latter problem should be evaluated very carefully in view of the fact that it is not an absolute contraindication for short laparoscopic procedures (cholecystectomy, hernioplasty), but may become so for colon surgery, which usually takes longer (another hope for the abdominal lifter).

Local contraindications to be considered are those relating to the portion of bowel to the treaded: distention due to complete or incomplete bowel obstruction, a significant amount of adhesions from complications related to the pathology to be treated or to previous laparotomies, and fecal contamination of the abdominal cavity.

Obesity and the thickness of the mesocolon may make this surgical method more difficult, even if they are not considered a contraindication.

The advantages are those common to all laparoscopic techniques used to date. The disadvantages, such as the high cost and the longer operative time, relate to the state of this surgery at the present time and will change as the technique becomes more widely practiced and instrumentation is improved.

Technique

The position of the patient and of the surgical team and the operating room instrumentation correspond to the specific requirements of the procedure to be performed. Several positions have been proposed in which the patient is placed either with his legs spread or not, but in which the surgeon can place her or himself in different positions. This allows the possibility of modifying according to the stage of the procedure: on the right, on the left, the position of the surgeon or between the legs of the patient. The position of the laparoscope can also be changed to obtain an optimal view during the different stags of the procedure, performed either in the right or in the left area. To these changes are added, lastly the changes in position of the operating table: Trendelenburg or anti-Trendelenburg, right and left decubitus and combinations of these.

Our preferred position can be described as follows: for operations on the right colon, the patient is in the lithotomy position, allowing the surgeon to be between the legs, particularly during the dissection along the paracolic gutter. The assistants are on the left side of the patient during the phase of the procedure in which the surgeon is not between the legs of the patient, a position which is usually assigned to the first assistant. The scrub nurse is on the right level of the patient's pelvis. These are used as reference points during maneuvers with an operative direction toward the right suphrenic area or the right iliac fossa respectively. For the left colon the patient is positioned as for the right colon and the surgeon and assistant both stands on the right side of the patient with the monitor on the left side. The patient always has an indwelling bladder catheter and a nasogastric tube.

The choice of the type of access to the abdominal cavity is conditioned by the location, dimension, and number of the trocars to be used. As to dimensions, we insert trocars of large diameter (10 mm to 12 mm) to be able to utilize instruments of different caliber merely by changing the type of reducer.

Normally four to five trocars are used for the right colon: one for the laparoscope at the umbilical level or at the level of the transverse umbilical line, areal to the rectus muscle; a subxiphoid trocar; and in the left subcostal area at the level of the anterior axillary line. The fourth, in the right subcostal area, at the same level as the contralateral trocar is placed as far laterally as possible, while the fifth trocar, if needed, is introduced in a location between the right iliac fossa and the suprapubic area. If an extracorporeal anastomosis is planned as we always do, an incision will be made. The choice of location for this incision has to obey two anatomical requirements:

1. external aesthetic need, which suggests connecting two skin incisions already utilized for the trocars, and
2. a parietal element, by which the choice of the incision location is based both on the mobility of the viscera to be anastomosed outside the abdominal cavity, and on facilitating the performance of the anastomosis.

Lastly, it is important to plan the proper place for introduction of the abdominal lifter, such that it does not interfere with either the endoscope or the trocar cannulas.

For the left colon, the first trocar is inserted at the level of the umbilical incision and the following ones in positions which take into account the need to be sufficiently distant form one another to allow easy maneuvering of the instruments. In general the position is the same for the right colon but inverted.

Laparoscopic colorectal surgery does not require any particular instruments: graspers, dissectors, scissors, hepatic retractor, staplers (laparoscopic with both cartridges, vascular and parenchymal). If the anastomosis is to be performed extracorporeally, all the instruments for open surgery should be available and they may be combined in different ways with the laparoscopic ones.

As the exploration of the abdominal cavity is completed, and when a decision has been made, as to the choice of surgical procedure, the first stage begins. For the right colon the procedure start with the dissection of the greater omentum along its colonic insertion, followed by the opening of the right paracolic gutter. Theoretically this maneuver may be performed from the hepatic flexure downward or from the ileocecal valve upwards, with particular attention paid to possible peculiar anatomic situations of adhesions between the transverse colon and the ascending colon, the shape of the hepatic flexure, or a particularly low transverse colon. In general, the maneuver is performed from the ileocecal valve upwards, after having placed a grasper on the cecum-ascending colon and mobilizing it upwards and towards the left, using Endo-Shears and progressing upward along the right paracolic gutter.

During this dissection, even if it is performed along an avascular plane, some elements of risk for the iliac vessels should be considered, particularly if the angle of vision is not optimal or the tumor may cause an obstacle to optimal vision, due to a large size or to adhesions with the parietal peritoneum. In the anatomical region where these vascular structures are located, obviously the use of electrocoagulation is to be avoided and if needed can be performed only under strict visual control, elevating the tissue to be coagulated. Another safety measure is the positive identification of the right ureter, which is certainly favored by laparoscopic vision. The spermatic vessels have to be identified, as well as the kidney and the third portion of the duodenum as well. As an alternative, the next stage can be transection of the terminal ileum and identification of the ileocolic artery. These two surgical phases, which complete the dissection of the specimen to be resected, are conducted both before and after the hepatic flexure.

The characteristics of laparoscopic surgery have led us not to detach the hepatic flexure completely, to maintain a fixed point of traction on which the ileocolic area can be mobilized upward or the right transverse colon downward. In this way there is maximum possibility of applying tension over the mesentery and mesocolon for vascular resection by the laparoscopic route.

After having transected the terminal ileum and the right transverse colon with the Endo GIA-30 if necessary to obtain sufficient mobilization, the specimen can be exteriorized. After performing a minilaparotomy (with the previously mentioned characteristics), the pneumoperitoneum can be evacuated and the abdominal lifter ca be released. In this particular case, all the vascular ligatures will be performed outside the abdominal cavity (ileocolic, right colic and middle colic artery), the anastomosis can be performed conventional by and the mesocolon can be closed. The bowel is then returned to the abdominalcavity and the laparoscopy is resumed, either with pneumoperitoneum or by utilizing the abdominal lifter, to complete the final task of checking the result of the procedure and possibly completing the suturing of the mesocolon if this has not been completed extra-abdominally.

If the procedure has to be continued laparoscopically the next step is transection of the terminal ileum and proper securing of the major blood vessels. Identification of the blood vessels can be made easier by transection of the terminal ileum, which allows the ileocolic mesocolon to be opened progressively towards the prechosen area at which the transverse colon is to be transected. At the end of this dissection, the colon is transected with the Endo GIA-30, if this has not already been done, thus completing the detachment of the specimen.

This procedure appears to be completely sterile in view of the fact that resection and suture of the bowel is done with the Endo GIA.

The last stage of the procedure is represented by the terminolateral ileocolic anastomosis performed through a small subcostal laparotomy used also for the extraction of the specimen. Once the patency of the anastomosis has been verified, the procedure is concluded with reconstruction of the meso aspect of the terminal ileum and colon, followed by the final laparoscopic check.

The technique for the left colon starts mobilizing the colon along the left paracolic gutter with scissors and electrocoagulation. The splenic flexure is also dissected and this dissection is extended to the distal transverse colon. During this phase, the operating room table is rotated towards the right to maintain the bowel away from the operative field. The left ureter is identified. At this point the colon is suspended with two graspers and the right mesenteric wall is opened. Through this window the ureter is again seen and the left iliac vessels are dissected. Following these vessels, the aorta is identified and an extended lymphadenectomy is performed. According to the resection chosen, the inferior mesenteric artery or the sigmoid arteries are transected with the vascular Endo GIA or between clips. If a left hemicolectomy is chosen, the inferior mesenteric vein is transected close the duodenum.

The distal margin of resection is done with the Endo GIA across the colon. The proximal stump of the specimen is exteriorized from an incision made in the left iliac fossa. The colon is exteriorized for a sufficient length to perform the proximal transection, where a purse-string suture is performed and the anvil of the EEA mechanical stapler is placed. The proximal colon with the anvil of the EEA in place is then returned to the abdominal cavity and the base of the EEA stapler is inserted by the transanal route. The base of the instrument and the anvil are then placed in contact under laparoscopic control and fired to perform the anastomosis. The procedure terminates with inspection of the anastomosis and positioning of a drain.

Abdominoperineal resection is performed in the same way but the transection of the colon is done at higher level where the colostomy will be performed. After the releasing pneumoperitoneum, the perineal phase is performed as usual.

A very smart application of laparoscopy is to perform a colorectal anastomosis after Hartmann procedure. The steps are the same as for the colorectal anastomosis described above.

Our Experience

During the period from October 1992 to September 1995 142 patients underwent laparoscopic colon surgery in our department. There were 87 males and 55 females with ages ranging from 42 to 81 years (average 62 years). In 127 cases the procedure was performed for malignant disease and in 15 cases for other reasons as shown in Table 1.

In 114 cases (81%; 101 cases of malignancy, 13 cases for other reasons), the procedure was completed laparoscopically; in 28 cases (19%; 26 malignancies, 2 other) the procedure was converted to open surgery (Table 2).

The procedures performed are shown in Table 3.

Table 1. Reasons for laparoscopic colon surgery other than for malignant disease

	n
Reversal of Hartmann procedure	2
Benign disease	3
Diverticulosis	10

Table 2. Reasons for conversion to open surgery

	n
Hemorrhage	3
Small bowel injury	1
Technical difficulties[a]	24

[a] Technical difficulties were due to obesity, a large amount of adhesions, or unclear anatomy.

Table 3. Procedures performed in 114 patients

	n
Right colectomy	32
Left colectomy	68
Miles operation	6
Total colectomy	3
Segmental resection	3
Colorectal anastomosis after Hartmann procedure	2

Table 4. Morbidity after the operations completed laparoscopically

	n
Hemorrhage	2
Anatomotic leak	3
Small bowel obstruction	1
Wound infection	6
Perineal infection	1
Anastomotic stenosis	1

Mean operating times was 230 min (range 60–360 min). Mean operating times for the procedures were: right colectomy 170 min, left colectomy 250 min Miles oparation 230 min, total colectomy 270 min, segmental resection 90 min, colorectal anastomosis after Hartmann procedure 100 min.

Postoperative morbidity in the operations completed laparoscopically was 12.2% (Table 4). One patient with hemorrhage (bleeding from a mesenteric vessel) was treated by renewed laparoscopy and the other (bleeding from a rectal ligament) by laparotomy. The patient with small bowel obstruction (trocar site hernia) was treated by laparoscopy with a Maciol needle suture of the trocar wound. No general complications (e.g. pulmonary, urinary) or deaths occurred in our series.

The mean time for passage of flatus was 2 days and the average postoperative hospital stay was 8.6 days.

Discussion

In the literature, conversion from laparoscopic to open surgery of the colon has been reported at rates of 18% to more than 50%, often because of poor exposure of the operative field due to bleeding or visceral injuries not recognized, particularly when the omentum is very large, or because of technical problems. Complications reported are: splenic or vascular laceration, dehiscence of anastomosis, ileal injuries, wound infection, myocardial infarction, and urinary and pulmonary infection. The cost of laparoscopic surgery has been higher than that of traditional surgery, and if laparoscopic surgery of the colon is converted to open surgery, the cost of the hospital stay will even be increased.

On the basis of our experience we think that laparoscopic surgery of the colon is possible and sometimes easier than the open approach (for example, dissection of the splenic flexure is easier) and the average rate of complications is similar to that after open surgery. We make a practice of timing the procedure, and after a first evaluation, and starting the dissection we decide if is useful to carry on by the laparoscopic route or convert to open surgery.

If this procedure is performed for benign disease, the earlier return to normal life, due to increased patient comfort, saves money for the patient and for society and balances the higher cost of the procedure.

Reconstruction After Low Anterior Resection

Lars Påhlman

Introduction

Sphincter preservation in rectal cancer surgery has been widely accepted over the last two decades, with a marked decline in abdominoperineal excisions [1]. The rationale of having a 5-cm distal margin of clearance from the cancer has been challenged. Intramural tumor invasion is hardly ever more than 5 mm, indicating that in patients with a tumor situated 4 – 5 cm from the anal verge an anterior resection is possible [2]. There is no increase in local recurrence rate if a low anterior resection is performed for low rectal cancers instead of an abdominoperineal excision, and recent knowledge shows that the most important element in rectal cancer surgery is the lateral margin of clearance, i.e. the circumferential margin, not the distant one [2, 3]. With a total mesorectal excision, where the dissection is performed in the anatomical plane outside the rectal fascia and Denovilliers' fascia surrounding the rectum, the local recurrence rate can be kept very low in experienced hands [4]. If the mesorectum is totally excised and it is possible to divide the rectum distal to the tumor, a low colorectal or just a coloanal anastomosis can be performed without jeopardizing a curative outcome [5].

As a consequence of lower anastomosis, bowel function will be impaired, mainly due to lack of compliance of the neorectum, but also to poor sphincter function in patients with a very low anastomosis. Symptoms such as urgency, frequent bowel movements and occasional incontinence can be linked to loss of rectal reservoir function. Moreover, a reduction in anal resting pressure has been seen – the "anterior resection syndrome" [6, 7].

Review of the Literature

Non-randomized Trials

The first reports on coloanal anastomosis and reconstruction with a pouch were presented by two French groups in 1986 [8, 9]. In the study presented by Parc et al. [8] the descending colon and splenic flexure were mobilized, and a J-shaped, 8-cm-long, hand-sewn reservoir was created from the upper part of the sigmoid colon. From below, a mucosectomy just above the dentate line was performed up to the end of the rectal tube (2 – 3 cm long). The pouch was anchored by four stay sutures to the upper end of the sphincter and the mucosa was stitched with interrupted resorbable sutures to the dentate line. In total, 31 patients were included, and all had a diverting transverse loop colostomy. In this series no anastomotic complications occurred and the functional results were good with patients fully continent, day and night, 1 month after closure of the colostomy. No patient needed to wear a protective pad. The mean number of daily bowel movements was 1.6 after 1 month and 1.1 after 3 months. This group now has experience of more than 200 patients. In a review of 162 patients, urgency and incontinence were satisfactory in almost all (96 %), and the mean number of bowel movements was two per 24 h with no problems with multiple repeated defecations [9]. In this large series only 6 patients (4 %) had an anastomotic complication such as dehiscence, rectovaginal fistula or pelvic sepsis.

In other French study, reported by Lazorthes et al. [10] 45 patients with straight anastomosis were compared with 20 patients given coloanal anastomosis and colonic pouches of varying sizes. All patients underwent an abdomino-trans-sphincteric resection with a simultaneous abdominal and posterior trans-sphincteric approach. The rectum was divided and transected at the level of the anorectal junction. The J pouch was created with a 6-cm GIA stapler. Fourteen pouches were 6 cm long (i.e. one application), while in six patients a 12-cm pouch (i.e. two applications) was performed. The coloanal anastomosis was performed by hand and all anastomosis, including straight ones, were covered with a temporary transvesostomy. All patients were prospectively followed up every 3rd month. Anal manometry was performed in 19 patients without reservoir and 7 patients with a pouch. Fistulas and anastomotic dehiscence occurred in 7 patients. As in the other French study, patients with pouches were found to be doing better in terms of incontinence, urgency and laxative requirements. There was an inverse relationship between frequency of defecation and maximum tolerable volume of the neorectum. The manometric differences between large and small reservoirs indicate a risk of faecal impaction and retention if the reservoir is too large.

In a British study 13 patients underwent rectal excision and reconstruction with a coloanal anastomosis and a 10-cm-long colonic J pouch [11]. This group was compared with 15 patients operated upon with a straight coloanal anastomosis. Most patients had a proximal defunctioning stoma which was closed within 6 months. The anastomosis was performed by hand in the majority of the patients and with a circular stapler in a few cases. There was no significant difference in mean evacuation frequency, although the variance of frequency was significantly less in the reservoir group. Furthermore, no difference in continence, urgency, or ability to difference flatus from faeces was found, nor any difference in the compliance of the neorectum. They found a significant increase in rectal sensitivity, volume, and capacity. No firm data have been shown in this trail to support a coloanal anastomosis with a reservoir. However, the patients given a straight anastomosis had a substantially longer flow-up which probably skewed the results.

In a recently published Italian study [12], 44 patients had a coloanal anastomosis with a 7-cm-long colonic reservoir made from the distal sigmoid colon. The endoanal coloanal anastomosis was performed by interrupted resorbable sutures from below after a mucosectomy from the dentate line. Two pelvic abscesses were noticed in this group and seven patients developed a mild anastomotic stricture. In this series six patients developed local recurrence and the authors discussed whether the anastomotic technique with a mucosectomy could have an impact on local cure or not, but no data support that hypothesis.

At least two American centres have reported small series where the functional results seem to be superior if a small J pouch is used. Again, bowel frequency is better if a pouch is constructed, although the data rest on comparison with historical controls [13, 14]. In the study from the Memorial Sloan-Kettering Cancer Center functional results were good, with no need for enema or antidiarrhoeic medication.

In a consecutive series comprising 23 patients with a coloanal anastomosis combined with a J pouch, functional outcome was studied prospectively [15]. Pouch size was 9 cm. All patients but one had a defunctioning loop ileostomy. Mean bowel movement frequency approximately 7 months after ileostomy closure was 2.1 (range 1–4) per day. Urgency was reported in five patients and four had mild seepage. Some degree of incomplete evacuation was found in seven patients.

Randomized Trials

Three randomized trials have been published so far in this field. However, all of them are very small and no firm conclusions can be drawn from them. In one trial in Japan [16] only eight patients were studied as, according to the authors, it was found unethical to continue recruiting patients to the trail because of superior results in the pouch group. In another trail conducted in Spain [17], 30 patients were randomly allotted to receive a straight coloanal anastomosis or a J pouch, with 15 in each group. Reduced stool frequency was found in the pouch group, but no difference in urgency. In a trial in Singapore [18], 20 patients received a stapled straight anastomosis and 20 patients a 10-cm-long stapled colonic pouch. All patients had a defunctioning stoma. The median distance of the tumor from the anal verge was similar in both groups: 6 cm (range 4–8 cm). There was significantly higher use of anti-diarrhoeal medication, faecal urgency, nocturnal soiling, and usage of pads in the straight anastomosis than in the pouch group. It was concluded that functional results were superior in the pouch group.

In a Swedish multicentre trail [19] 100 patients were studied. Three patients were withdrawn, two due to inadequate bowel length for pouch construction and one who refused participation after randomization, leaving 47 patients with a pouch and 52 with a straight anastomosis. Patients with a tumor less than 12 cm from the anal verge were eligible and the level of the anastomosis in this study was determined by the meosrectal excision rather than by the location of the tumor. The anastomosis was done with a double staple technique and the colonic pouch, 6–8 cm long, was done with a GIA or TLC stapler on the proximal sigmoid or descending colon. The use of a temporary stoma was left to the discretion of the surgeon, and 71% in the pouch group and 59%

in the straight group had a loop transversostomy or a loop ileostomy. One patient in the pouch group died postoperative due to haemorrhage and subsequent multiorgan failure. A significant decrease in anastomotic leakage was found in the pouch group (2%, $n = 1$) compared to the straight group (15%, $n = 8$, $p = 0.03$). A questionnaire regarding bowel function was used preoperatively and at 2 and 12 months postoperatively. A significant reduction in frequency of bowel movements, noturanal movements, urgency, and incontinence score was found in the pouch group. However, the ability to evacuate the bowel changed slightly for the worse within the pouch group between the 2- and the 12-month follow-ups.

Controversies

Which Part of the Colon for the Reservoir?

It is not obvious which part of the colon should be used for pouch construction. The sigmoid colon is not always a perfect substitute, due to diverticulosis and poor vascular supply after a "high-tie" resection. Moreover, the sigmoid colon can be bulky and fatty and often harbours adenomas. With high ligation of the inferior mesenteric artery and, especially, high ligation of the inferior mesenteric vein under the pancreas, the left colon can easily be taken down to the anal verge. In my own experience, it happened once that the circulation in Riolan's arch was almost nil and a stoma had to be performed. In Uppsala we have also found a higher postoperative complication rate in patients in whom the sigmoid colon has been used for the reservoir.

Type of Anastomosis

Two techniques have been proposed, mucosectomy and a handsewn anastomosis or a stapled (single or double) anastomosis with a circular stapler. There is no rationale for performing a mucosectomy and an anastomosis down to the dentate line, for oncological principles: if a tumor is growing so far distally that a mucosectomy is necessary to achieve local cure, an abdominoperineal excision is probably a more appropriate procedure. However, data from one of the French series may indicate that handsewn anastomosis is safer when performed to the dentate line than to the distal remnant of the rectum [8]. On the other hand, according to the Swedish trial [19], anastomotic integrity is merely a matter of performing an end-to-side rather than an end-to-end anastomosis. Another explanation of better anastomotic healing may be that the pouch is quite bulky and fills out the empty presacral space, reducing the risk of a pelvic haematoma.

Pouch Size

The initial studies by Lazorthes et al. [10] demonstrated that a pouch should not be too large. Exactly how long the two limbs of the J pouch should be is not known.

To achieve good reservoir function in regard to bowel movements and urgency, a pouch size of 6–8 cm is probably necessary. However, the ability to empty the pouch has not been properly studied. Manometric data from the French group [10] indicate that evacuation can be a problem if the pouch is too large. The other French group reported evacuation problems in as many as 25% of patients; some of them had to take enemas [9]. These results can possibly be explained by the pouch size, which was 9 cm, i.e. quite large. Similar findings, i.e. a tendency to evacuation problems after a longer follow-up, were noted in the Swedish multi-centre trial [19]. All trials presented have a very short follow-up and it is not known whether difficulties with evacuation will increase with time or not. It is therefore essential that patients be followed for a longer period to solve this question.

Diverting Stoma

The rational of covering the anastomosis with a diverting stoma is the risk of a fatal outcome due to pelvic sepsis. In all series deaths will occur, and this complication must be avoided by every means possible. However, a covering stoma must be closed, and that procedure carries a potential risk of new complications. Furthermore, in a small number of patients the stoma will be permanent. In the Swedish trial [19] no leaks occurred in the group not given a diverting stoma. In Uppsala 50 pouches have been performed, 40 without diverting stoma. Only in one patient was a clinical leak present, and in one woman a rectovaginal fistula. Both underwent an emergency loop transversostomy, Recovery was uneventful, although one of the patients still has the stoma. It is better to monitor patients carefully postoperatively and select those with an indication of leakage for early reoperation for placement of a stoma. At that procedure it is important, with antegrade on-table lavage of the distal bowel segment, to prevent faeces passing the hole in the anastomosis with the risk of continuous infection.

Other Indications than Cancer

Other than rectal cancer, one indication for a coloanal anastomosis where a J pouch may be useful is in patients with a radiation injury to the intestinal tract, where resection of badly injured rectum is necessary. In addition, in cases with rectovaginal fistula or very low strictures a coloanal anastomosis is often required. In such cases pouch reconstruction is probably worthwhile [20].

Conclusion

A colonic pouch is in my opinion the treatment of choice for low rectal cancer, especially in patients with known metastases in whom palliative resection is planned. This group of patients will never reap the benefits of the relatively good function after a straight anastomosis, since this only becomes obvious after 1–2 years. One concern is, of course, the evacuation problem. Young patients may have a straight anastomosis, but in the Uppsala experience the evacuation problem seems not to deteriorate with longer follow-up. Moreover, most patients in Uppsala have had short-term high-dose preoperative radiotherapy, and this treatment seems not to interfere with the functional results.

References

1. Williams NS (1984) The rationale for preservation of the anal sphincter in patients with low rectal cancer. Br J Surg 71: 575–581
2. Williams NS, Dixon MF, Johnston D (1983) Reappraisal of the 5 centimeter rule of distal excision for carcinoma of the rectum: a study of distal intramural spread and patients' survival. Br J Surg 70: 150–154
3. Adam IJ, Mohamdee MO, Martin EG et al. (1994) Role of circumferential margin involvement in the local recurrence of rectal cancer. Lancet 344: 707–711
4. MacFarlane JK, Ryall RD, Heald RJ (1993) Mesorectal excision for rectal cancer. Lancet 341: 457–460
5. Kranjia ND, Schache DJ, North WR, Heald RJ (1990) "Close shave" in anterior resection. Br J Surg 63: 673–677
6. Williams NS, Price R, Johnston D (1980) The long term effect of sphincter preserving operations for rectal carcinoma on function of the anal sphincter in man. Br J Surg 67: 203–208
7. Williamson MER, Lewis WG, Holdsworth PJ, Finan PJ, Johnston D (1994) Decrease in the anorectal pressure gradient after low anterior resection of the rectum: a study using continuous ambulatory manometry. Dis Colon Rectum 37: 1228–1231
8. Parc R, Tiret E, Frileux P, Moszkowoski E, Joygue J (1986) Resection and colo-anal anastomosis with colonic reservoir for rectal carcinoma. Br J Surg 73: 139–141
9. Berger A, Tiret E, Parc R et al. (1992) Excision of the rectum with colonic J pouch-anal anastomosis for adenocarcinoma of the low and mid rectum. World J Surg 16: 470–477
10. Lazorthes F, Fages P, Chiotasso P, Lemozy J, Bloom E (1986) Resection of the rectum with construction of a colonic reservoir and colo-anal anastomosis for carcinoma of the rectum. Br J Surg 73: 136–138
11. Nicholls RJ, Lubowski DZ, Donaldson DR (1988) Comparison of colonic reservoir and straight colo-anal reconstruction after rectal excision. Br J Surg 75: 318–320
12. Leo E, Belli F, Baldini MT, Vitellaro M, Mascheroni L, Andreola S, Belloni M, Rebuffoni G, Lombardi F, Audisio R, Filiberti A (1994) Total rectal resection and colo- and anastomosis with colonic reservoir for low rectal cancer. Int J Colorectal Dis 9: 82–86
13. Drake DB, Pemberton JH, Beart RW Jr et al. (1987) Colo-anal anastomosis in the management of benign and malignant rectal disease. Ann Surg 206: 600–605
14. Cohen AM (1993) Colon J pouch rectal reconstruction after total or subtotal proctectomy. World J Surg 17: 267–270
15. Mortensen NJM, Ramirez JM, Takeuchi N, Humphreys MMS (1995) Colonic J pouch anal anastomosis after rectal excision for carcinoma: functional outcome. Br J Surg 82: 611–613
16. Kusunoki M, Shoji Y, Yanagi (1991) Function after anoabdominal rectal resection and colonic J pouch-anal anastomosis. Br J Surg 78: 1434–1438
17. Ortiz H, De Miguel M, Armendáriz P (1995) Coloanal anastomosis: are functional results better with a pouch? Dis Colon Rectum 38: 375–377
18. Seow-Choen F, Goh HS (1995) Prospective randomized trial comparing J colonic pouch-anal anastomosis and straight coloanal reconstruction. Br J Surg 82: 608–610
19. Hallböök O, Påhlman L, Krog M, Wexner SD, Sjödahl R. Randomised comparison of straight and colonic J pouch anastomosis after low anterior resection. Ann Surg in press
20. Lucarotti ME, Mountford RA, Bartolo DCC (1991) Surgical management of intestinal radiation injury. Dis Colon Rectum 34: 865–869

Laparoscopic Abdominoperineal Excision of the Rectum

A. Herold, T. Schiedeck, and H.-P. Bruch

Introduction

Jacobs in the USA carried out the first laparoscopically assisted operation on the colon in 1991 [11]. In the same year, entirely laparoscopic resections of the colon were reported. The first laparoscopic abdominoperineal excision of the rectum was performed in January 1992. In November 1992, the rectum was excised from a patient by the minimally invasive method for the first time in the Department of Surgery of the Medical University of Lübeck [14].

Indication for Laparoscopic Surgery

In recent years, excision of the rectum has been increasingly superseded by sphincter-preserving procedures in the treatment of rectal carcinoma. Intersphincteric resection has joined low anterior resection with coloanal anastomosis. In addition, a colon pouch is fashioned in many clinics in cases of very low resections. There remain 10%–20% of rectal carcinomas which require abdominoperineal excision if oncological principles are to be observed. Selection of patients for laparoscopic abdominoperineal excision is essentially exactly the same previously for the conventional procedure. An exception is in the case of infiltration of neighboring organs by a T4 tumor, because of the present paucity of experience in the field of laparoscopic cancer surgery. In addition, a T1 carcinoma smaller than 3 cm of a low-risk type without lymphatic invasion should be treated as before by transanal tumor excision. In summary, the following rectal tumors are suitable for laparoscopic surgical treatment: high-risk T1 tumors and T2 and T3 tumors which cannot be resected with preservation of continence.

If radio- and chemotherapy were contraindicated in an anal carcinoma or have been ineffective, or there is a recurrence of an anal carcinoma, laparoscopic abdominoperineal excision would be possible in these cases also [8, 10, 18, 22, 25, 27].

Preoperative Investigations

The usual preoperative investigations are performed, the same as before a conventional operation: total colonoscopy with histological confirmation of diagnosis, anorectal endoscopic ultrasonography and computed topography or magnetic resonance topography, hepatic ultrasound, tumor marker estimations and general tests in preparation for general anesthesia.

Orthograde bowel lavage is performed preoperatively and obligatory perioperative antibiotic cover is given. For reasons of safety, both ureters were provided with a double-J ureter stent in the operations performed hitherto. With increasing laparoscopic experience, this can be omitted.

Operative Procedure

The patient is placed on the operating table in the lithotomy position with bilateral shoulder supports. Support of the right side of the body can also be useful; this ensures that sliding of the patient is avoided if the head of the table is lowered and the table is tilted to the right. The insufflation gas is warmed in order to avoid cooling of the patient during the operation. In all laparoscopic operations, dissection is done with the endoscissors, the endodissector and bipolar electrocoagulation forceps. The colon is moved and held with atraumatic dissection swabs and a finger-like endoretractor. Traumatic grasping instruments are avoided. Smaller vessels are dealt with using electrocoagulation, and larger vessels with absorbable clips and, in exceptional cases, with a 30-mm endostapler. Very adipose mesentery and the bowel are dissected with the 30- or 60-mm endostapler.

The camera trocar is positioned 2–3 cm above the umbilicus in the midline via an open pneumoperitoneum. The three or four working trocars (12 mm) are inserted in a semicircle in the lower abdomen. Dissection begins at the descending and sigmoid colon with division of the left lateral fetal adhesions and of the peritoneum. If necessary, the entire splenic flexure can be mobilised in this plane. Dissection proceeds dorsal to the colon along Gerota's fascia until the left colon can be moved completely freely. To support it, the colon is pushed to the right using the dissecting swabs and the left ureter is identified clearly behind Gerota's fascia. Mobilisation and direct exposure are not necessary. Dissection from the left is continued as far as to the inferior mesenteric vein. The incision is continued below the sacral promontory as far as the anterior incision of the pouch of Douglas. The colon is then displaced to the left and the peritoneum on the right of the colon is incised. This incision is continued as far as the inferior mesenteric vein above the inferior mesenteric artery. Incision of the pouch of Douglas is completed below. After incision of the peritoneum on the right, the fat layer beneath it can usually be dissected bluntly so that it is possible to tunnel under the colon with its neurovascular bundles including the mesorectum and sigmoid mesocolon, mobilising it anteriorly using the endoretractor. The presacral fascial tissue plane is opened easily by this elevating the colon and is then dissected on to the level of the muscles of the pelvic floor. Approaching from behind, the presacral space is exposed in the anteriolateral direction on both sides and the medial rectal artery is divided with electrocoagulation or clips. Distal to the peritoneum of the pouch of Douglas, Denonvillier's fascia is incised and the rectum is dissected from behind the bladder, prostate or posterior vaginal wall down to the level of the pelvic floor muscles. Magnification of the camera optic and use of a 30° optic facilitates the entire dissection in the pelvis compared to the conventional operation. Dissection in the cranial direction is anterior to the aorta as far as the inferior mesenteric artery, sparing the nerve fibres. After circular exposure, the vessel is divided high, with double clips above and a single clip distally. The inferior mesenteric vein is clipped and divided in the same way a few centimeters above the artery. A thin mesocolon can be dissected easily with the scissors, and a stapler is used when the mesentery is fat. The colon is divided with the stapler in the region of the junction of the descending and sigmoid colon. The end-colostomy is constructed only after completion of the perineal stage of the operation.

The anus is incised in a circle and mobilised from the pelvis en bloc with the rectum. This is done by the conventional operating technique. The resected specimen consisting of the anal canal, rectum, sigmoid colon including the entire mesentery is removed through the perineal incision. The pelvic floor muscles and skin are sutured closed in layers. Drainage is abdominal only and is placed later when using the laparoscopic method.

After closure of the perineal wound, the pneumoperitoneum is restored, the operative site is inspected for bleeding, irrigated copiously and one or two Easy-Flow drains are placed in the pelvis. If there is an adequate peritoneal margin, the pelvic floor peritoneum can be closed with a laparoscopic suture. After releasing the pneumoperitoneum, the descending colon is brought to the surface in the conventional manner at the upper left trocar incision site after adequate extension of the skin and fascia. Fixation of the intra-abdominal limb of colon is omitted [1, 3, 14, 16, 19, 24].

Results

Twelve patients have undergone laparoscopic abdominoperineal excision of the rectum by this technique so far. In the same period, 15 patients have been treated by open surgery. In these patients, the reasons why laparoscopic operation was not performed were the presence of a second tumor coexisting, cardiopulmonary disease, tumor growth beyond the colon and refusal by the patient to undergo laparoscopic treatment. The tumor stage extended from T2N0M0 to T3N3M1 (the last patient had palliative surgery in the presence of known liver metastases).

The average age of the patients was 63 years (range 51–82 years). The postoperative stay in the intensive care unit was 1.5 days on average (range 1–3 days). The duration of operation dropped from 7–8 h early on to 4–5 h as experience – also of other laparoscopic colon procedures – increased. The long duration of operation is also partly a result of the "one team" policy. On average, patients were able to leave hospital after 14 days (range 11–22 days) (Table 1).

Table 1. Operative data in our patient group ($n = 12$)

Reason for surgery	Carcinoma		
Tumor stage	T2N0M0 – T3N3M1		
Lymph nodes removed	11.2	(range	2– 19)
Age (years)	63	(range	51– 82)
Duration of operation (min)	339	(range	208–500)
Blood transfusion (units)	3.4	(range	2– 6)
Intensive care stay (days)	1.5	(range	1– 3)
Postoperative hospitalization (days)	14.8	(range	11– 22)

Conversion to open surgery because of intraoperative complications was not necessary in any case. In one patient with a small very low posterior carcinoma, conventional anterior resection was possible after laparoscopic abdominal mobilisation with preservation of bowel continuity. Because we do not yet have the technical means (i. e. a bendable stapler), we do not regard this operation as entirely feasible by the laparoscopic method at present. In one 80-year-old patient with known cardiopulmonary problems, conversion to open operation was required at the time of laparoscopy because of early intraoperative anaesthetic problems.

There was an early postoperative stoma complication in two patients. In one a distal stoma necrosis 1–1.5 cm in length was treated by local resection. In another, retraction of the stoma because of inadequate mobilisation of the splenic flexure could also be corrected locally. One patient developed a stenosis of the stoma 2 years postoperatively which needed surgical enlargement. A superficial infection of a drain channel was controlled within a few days by local conservative wound treatment.

There was secondary venous haemorrhage in one case. Laparotomy was required because laparoscopic visualisation was inadequate.

A trocar incisional hernia in the upper right working trocar site occurred in one patient 2 years postoperatively. The commended operative treatment has been refused by the patient hitherto for personal reasons.

All of our patients have received further cancer treatment from us. The patient with known preoperative liver metastases died of his advanced tumor a few months postoperatively. Multiple bilateral pulmonary metastases occurred in one patient with a T3N2Mo tumor 26 months after operation. Three months after bilateral resection of metastases, the patient is currently free of tumor. All of the other patients are tumor-free after an average of 24 months follow-up (Fig. 1).

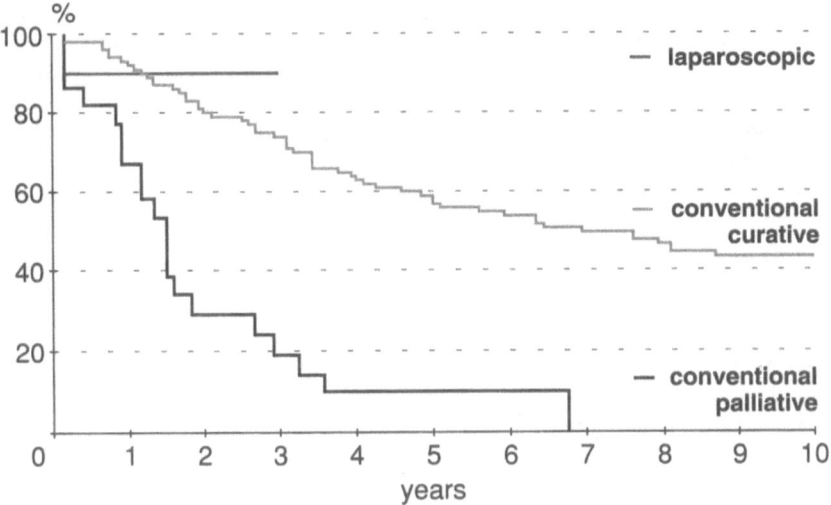

Fig. 1. Patient survival curves after the various kinds of treatment

Discussion

These experiences with a very small group of patients show that laparoscopic abdominoperineal excision of the rectum can be performed with morbidity comparable to that of the conventional operative technique. The recurrence rate does not seem higher after an average follow-up period of 2 years, which particularly underlines its feasibility with regard to the principles of cancer surgery. Our experiences are confirmed by other researchers. Regrettably, there are no experiences so far with larger groups of patients, in particular no randomised multicentre studies. Such studies are required urgently to obtain sufficient results and to prove the effectiveness of the minimally invasive operative method [2, 4, 7, 12, 18, 19, 21, 23, 26, 28].

We regard the laparoscopic procedure as particularly suitable for excision of the rectum as the tumor is not reached intra-abdominally, so that tumor cell spread should theoretically not be possible if dissection technique is adequate. Since the dissected specimen can be removed easily at the perineal stage of the operation, an additional abdominal incision can be avoided, which benefits the patient especially in the postoperative recovery phase. Because a stoma is constructed, there is no intra-abdominal anastomosis which also reduces the risk of serious complications.

Because of its different viewing angels and magnification effect, the laparoscope ensures ideal visualization of the colon, its suspension and vessels and allows better visual assessment, especially in the lower pelvis, than the conventional operation. By using 3-D systems, this advantage can probably be increased further.

Although laparoscopic abdominoperineal excision of the rectum is in our view ideally suited to laparoscopic procedure, this method has not become as popular, in Germany and in the rest of the world, as, for example, laparoscopic cholecystectomy. At present, only 1% – 3% of all excisions of the rectum are performed by this method. This is partly because the laparoscopic technique is not widely used in colorectal procedures and partly because this operation accounts for 30% – 40% of all rectal operations in smaller hospitals, and these hospitals do not perform either very low coloanal and intersphincteric resections or laparoscopic excisions.

References

1. Berman JR (1992) Sutureless laparoscopic rectopexy for procidentia – technique and implications. Dis Colon Rectum 35 : 689 – 693
2. Bleday R, Babineua T, Forse RA (1993) Laparoscopic surgery for colon and rectal cancer. Semin Surg Oncol 9 : 59 – 64
3. Buess G, Manncke K, Merhan J, Lirici M (1993) State of the art of laparoscopic colorectal surgery. Endosc Surg 1 : 3 – 12
4. Chinadasub S, Charntaracharmnong C, Nimitvanit C, Akkaranurukul P, Santitarmmanion B (1994) Laparoscopic abdominoperineal resection. J Laparoendosc Surg 4 : 17 – 21
5. Darzi A, Hill ADK, Henry MM, Guillou PJ, Monson JRT (1993) Laparoscopic assisted surgery of the colon. Operative technique. Endosc Surg 1 : 13 – 15
6. Darzi A, Lewis C, Goldin R, Menzies-Gow N, Guillou P, Monson J (1993) Laparoscopic abdomino-perineal resection of the rectum – an assessment of the adequacy of excision. 5th International Meeting of the Society for Minimally Invasive Therapy Orlando, 1993, Abstract book, p 29 S – 11
7. Decanini C, Milsom JW, Böhm B, Fazi VW (1994) Laparoscopic oncological abdominoperineal resection. Dis Colon Rectum 37 : 552 – 558
8. Falk PM, Beart RW, Wexner SD, Thorson AG, Jagelman DG, Lavery IC, Johansen OB, Fitzgibbons RJ (1993) Laparoscopic colectomy: a critical appraisal. Dis Colon Rectum 36 : 28 – 34
9. Franklin ME, Ramos R, Rosenthal D, Schuessler W (1993) Laparoscopic colonic procedures. World J Surg 17 : 51 – 56
10. Gall FP (1991) Die tiefe Rektumresektion – transabdominaler Zugang. Chirurg 62 : 1 – 7
11. Jacobs M, Verdeja JC, Goldstein HS (1991) Minimally invasive colon resection (laparoscopic colectomy). Surg Laparosc Endosc 1 : 144 – 150
12. Kmiot W, Reiver D, Binderow S, Cohen S, Nogueras J, Jagelman D, Wexner S (1994) prospective comparison of laparoscopically assisted and open colorectal surgery. Br J Surg 81 : 747 – 771
13. Köckerling F, Gastinger I, Remmel E, Gall FP (1992) Die laparoskopische tubuläre Reaktum- und Kolonresektion. Eine tierexperimentelle Untersuchung. Zentralbl Chir 117 : 103 – 110
14. Köckerling F, Gastinger I, Schneider B, Krause W, Gall FP (1992) Laparoskopische abdomino-perineale Rektumexstirpation. Anwendung mit erweiterer Lymphknotendissektion durch stammnahes Absetzen der A. mesenterica inferior. Laparoendosk Chir 1 : 99 – 113
15. Köckerling F, Gastinger I, Schneider B, Krause W, Gall FP (1992) Laparoskopische abdominoperineale Rektumexstirpation mit hoher Durchtrennung der Arteria mesenterica inferior. Chirurg 63 : 345 – 348
16. Köckerling F, Gastinger I, Reck T, Schneider B (1993) Laparoskopische Eingriffe am Rektum. Langenbecks Arch Chir [Suppl] 378 : 111 – 116

17. Köckerling F, Gastinger I, Schneider B, Krause W, Gall FP (1993) Laparoscopic abdomino-perineal excision of the rectum with high legation of the inferior mesenteric artery in the management of rectal carcinoma. Endosc Surg 1 : 16 – 19
18. Larach SW, Salomon MC, Williamson PR, Goldstein E (1993) Laparoscopic assisted abdominoperineal resection. Surg Laparosc Endosc 3 : 115 – 118
19. Meyer HJ, Ebert KH (1994) Die laparoskopische abdomino-perineale Rectumexstirpation mit hoher Durchtrennung der A. mesenteric inferior. Chirurg 65 : 1136 – 1139
20. Monson JRT, Darzi A, Carey PD (1992) Prospective evaluation of laparoscopicassisted colectomy in an unselected group of patients. Lancet 340 : 831 – 833
21. Morris EF, Ramos R, Rosenthal D, Schuessler W (1993) Laparoscopic colonic procedures. World J Surg 17 : 51 – 56
22. Mortensen NJM, Ramirez JM, Takenchi N, Smilgin Humphreys MM (1995) Colonic Y-pouch-anal anastomosis after rectal excision for carcinoma: functional outcome. Br J Surg 82 : 611 – 613
23. Phillips EH, Franklin M, Carroll BJ, Fallas MJ, Ramos R, Rosenthal D (1992) Laparoscopic colectomy. Ann Surg 216 : 703 – 707
24. Reissman P, Cohen SM, Weiss EG, Wexner SD (1994) Simple technique for pelvic drain placement in laparoscopic abdominoperineal resection. Dis Colon Rectum 37 : 381 – 382
25. Sackier JM, Berci G, Hiatt JR, Hartunian S (1992) Laparoscopic abdominoperineal resection of the rectum. Br J Surg 79 : 1207 – 1208
26. Sackier JM, Slutzki MB, Wood C, Negri M, Moor EV, Halevy A (1993) Laparoscopic endocorporal mobilization followed by extracorporeal sutureless anastomosis for the treatment of carcinoma of the left colon. Dis Colon Rectum 36 : 610 – 613
27. Scholefield JH, Northover JMA (1995) Surgical management of rectal cancer. Br J Surg 82 : 745 – 748
28. Wexner SD, Cohen SM, Johansen OB, Nogueras JJ, Jagelman DG (1993) Laparoscopic colorectal surgery: a prospective assessment and current prospective. Br J Surg 80 : 1602 – 1605

Laparoscopic Rectopexy

H.-P. Bruch, A. Herold, A. Woltmann, and T. Schiedeck

Intussusception and prolapse of the rectum are due to a change in the statics of the small pelvis. This change may be caused by insufficiency of the suspension of the rectum in the sacral cavity by very loose connective tissue or it may be caused by chronic obstipation over many years, leading to straining during defaecation which in its turn results in descending perineum and rectal prolapse. It may be initiated by a hysterectomy, with subsequent impairment of the anchoring structures in the small pelvis, or by a psycho-motor-social disorder, usually a pelvic outlet obstruction which is induced by a reversed rectoanal inhibitory reflex. Last, but not least, it may be related to traumatic alterations of the pelvic floor, especially in women who have borne many children. These women can suffer from descending perineum and disorders of the perineal innervation with rectal prolapse and often severe incontinence. From these data polyetiologic causes of intussusception and rectal prolapse may be derived, ranging from intestinal mobility disorders through idiopathic and psychological problems to squelae of birth and injury. No wonder that over the years a variety of surgical operation techniques have been developed and employed for complete or incomplete rectal prolapse. However, as yet no universally accepted preeminent treatment has appeared [12, 15, 16, 18, 19, 21, 25, 31].

Preoperative Investigations

Our method of management is based on extensive preoperative examinations. Depending on the functional disorder of the distal rectum and anus, the following are carried out preoperatively:

1. Personal history and continence score
2. Colonoscopy
3. Evaluation of transit time
4. Defaecography
5. Sphincter manometry
6. Neurological studies of the innervation and function of the pelvic floor muscles

Before diagnosis and treatment of rectal prolapse, a careful personal history and continence score must be obtained. In all patients total colonoscopy must be performed to identify any concomitant diseases such as diverticulosis, polyps or neoplasms. Defaecography reveals functional disorders in the hind gut and detects intussusception, cul-de-sac phenomena, rectocoele and descending perineum. Rectal manometry, which can be combined with a vector-volume diagram, provides further details of resting pressures, squeeze pressure, reflex mechanisms, rectal compliance and perception.

Where there is a history of straining or constipation, intestinal transit time must be tested. If colonic motility disorders with extremely prolonged passage times are detected, gastric emptying time and the passage time through the small intestines should be studied to reveal any intestinal neurological dysplasia. All of these data need to be made available as a basis for the decision whether to perform rectopexy alone or in combination with – for example – levator plasty, pre-post-anal repair and resection of the sigmoid colon or extended colonic resection [12, 16, 34].

Operative Procedure

We recommend carrying out rectopexy combined with sigmoid resection or more extended resections in patients with a delayed transit time in the descending and sigmoid colon and in those who have extreme elongation of the left and sigmoid colon, especially if causing outlet obstruction.

Laparoscopic rectopexy demands only an abdominal access, but for reasons of safety it seems advisable nevertheless to be prepared for an anal maneuver as well. The patient is placed in a lithotomy position on the operation table. The buttocks should be positioned at the lower edge and the legs in Lloyd-Davis stirrups. The patient should be fixed to the table by tapes and the shoulders held by supports, so that the table can be tilted to each side. The laparoscopic operation is facilitated by using the Trendelenburg position. Four 12-mm laparoscopic trocars are inserted. The camera trocar is positioned in the midline about 5 cm above the umbilicus. This provides a better view to the sigmoid and facilitates intra-abdominal suturing. Two trocars are positioned on the right and one in the lower left quadrant of the abdomen, outside the rectus muscle. This avoids bleeding complications from the epigastric vessels. A standard insufflation pressure of 12 mmHg with CO_2 used.

Avoiding traumatic grasping instruments and using bipolar current helps to minimize inadvertent bowel injuries. First the abdomen is inspected and obstructing adhesions are meticulously removed. Laparoscopic exposure of the sigmoid colon and the rectum can be facilitated by gravity displacement of the small bowel loops – a lateral tilt to the right is usually helpful – and the small bowel loops can be positioned in the upper right quadrant of the abdomen using two or three atraumatic swabs.

Dissection is performed with a pair of bipolar coagulation tweezers and laparoscopic scissors. The sigmoid colon is held with light tension to the right by atraumatic swabs. First it needs to be removed from its lateral fixations. To do this, the secondary fusion line of the descending and the sigmoid colon is transected, care being taken to preserve Gerota's fascia which covers the ureter. The ureter must be identified, but it is not necessary and not advisable to remove the ureter from the adjacent tissues.

The sigmoid colon is now retracted to the left abdominal wall, and in a second step the peritoneum of the right aspect of the mesosigmoid is incised. The retromesenteric and retrorectal space can easily be exposed by cephalad traction of the sigmoid colon with two laparoscopic swabs. This facilitates tunneling of the sigmoid colon. A window is created in the plane of the retrorectal space in between Gerota's fascia and the mesentery. A special atraumatic retractor, which articulates, is inserted via the left trocar through the sigmoid window, and the colon is lifted to the anterior abdominal wall.

The retrorectal space is now opened down to the pelvic floor by sharp dissection. The middle hemorrhoidal vessels are identified and saved. As the rectal intussusception and prolapse through the pelvic floor are in most cases due to a poorly supported rectum, the whole rectum has to be mobilized, and if a perineal sliding hernia can be identified, plication of the puborectalis and the levator muscles, either anteriorly or posteriorly or both, can be undertaken, at once or secondarily by a perineal approach. In females the prerectal peritoneum is incised and the rectum dissected down to the pelvic floor and stretched. In males one should be very careful anteriorly, for there is a great risk of affecting sexual function by prerectal dissection.

Having completed the preparation of the sigmoid colon and the rectum, there are two possible ways to continue the operation.

Rectopexy Combined with Sigmoid Resection

For laparoscopic-assisted resection with double stapler anastomosis; the sigmoid colon is freed of the mesenteric fat by laparoscopic dissection, the rectum is transected by an endostapler, and the sigmoid and descending colon are pulled through a 4-cm-wide incision in the lower left quadrant of the abdomen at the trocar site. The sigma is resected and the anvil of a stapler is inserted into the descending colon. A pursestring suture is tied. The colon is replaced in the abdominal cavity and the small laparotomy wound closed. A cytocidal wash-out of the rectum must be performed. After this, the circular stapling instrument is introduced into the lumen of the rectum without the anvil. The tip of the centre rod is placed under laparoscopic control into the centre of the endostapler suture line, and after the anvil has been placed on the center rod and the instrument closed, the staples are fired.

Alternatively, the whole sigmoid colon is pulled through the small incision in the lower left abdomen in the shape of a sigma loop, the mesentery is removed, the sigmoid colon resected, and the anastomosis is performed with running sutures.

To fix the rectum we favour the Sudeck procedure over others, as it avoids the implantation of foreign material such as Teflon mesh or Ivalon sponge. This gives it a distinctive advantage over other methods. The pouch of Douglas is now elevated by 5–15 cm and the prerectal peritoneum is sutured to the uterus or the round ligaments. The rectum itself is stretched and a Sudeck rectopexy is carried out. This means pleating the cut edges of the parietal peritoneum to the rectum and sigmoid colon.

Rectopexy Without Sigmoid Resection

If there is no indication of sigmoid resection, the sigmoid colon is folded and the mesosigmoid fixed with running sutures, so that a sigmoid loop results.

Patients and Methods

Laparoscopic rectopexy has so far been carried out in 55 patients. The Sudeck method was used in 54, the Wells procedure in 1. In 25 patients it was combined with sigmoid resection, and in one patient with resection of the proximal rectum. The indications for laparoscopic rectopexy were prolapse, outlet obstruction or a combination of both. A summary of patient data is given in Table. 1.

Our own experience in laparoscopic rectopexy is still very small. Between September 1992 and March 1996, 55 patients with rectal prolapse and an age range of 23 to 88 years (mean age 61 years) have been registered in a prospective record of clinical results, complications, inadvertent effects and follow-up data. Four of these patients were men. Thirty-two patients had undergone previous surgery. Seven different operative procedures have been carried out alone or in combination.

Results

Mean duration of surgery was 231 min (range 120–360 min). An average of 0.6 unit of blood were administered during the hospital stay. The mean hospital stay was 13 days (range 6–27 days), (Table 1). Four patients developed postoperative complications relating to intra-abdominal haematoma and haemorrhage (Table 2). Three complications were managed laparoscopically, while in one patient laparotomy via a small Pfannenstiel incision was carried out (Table 3) All patients regained intestinal function as documented by passed flatus after an average of 48 h.

Table 1. Summary of data on 55 patients undergoing laparoscopic rectopexy

	Mean	Range
Age of patients (years)	61	23– 88
Duration of surgery (min)	231	140–360
Duration of surgery with resection (min)	281	150–380
Blood transfusion requirement (u)	0.6	0– 5
Intensive care stay (days)	0.9	0– 3
Postop. hospital stay (days)	13	6– 27

Table 2. Complications occurring in 4 out of 55 patients undergoing laparoscopic rectopexy

	n	%
Haemorrhage	4	6
Laparoscopic revision	3	6
Laparotomy	1	2
Conversion	1	2
Mortality	0	

Table 3. Management of complications of laparoscopic rectopexy

Complication	Treatment
Diffuse disturbance of coagulation	Laparoscopic lavage
Vascular haemorrhage	Laparotomy
Trocar puncture	Laparoscopic lavage
Haematoma in the small pelvis	Laparoscopic lavage

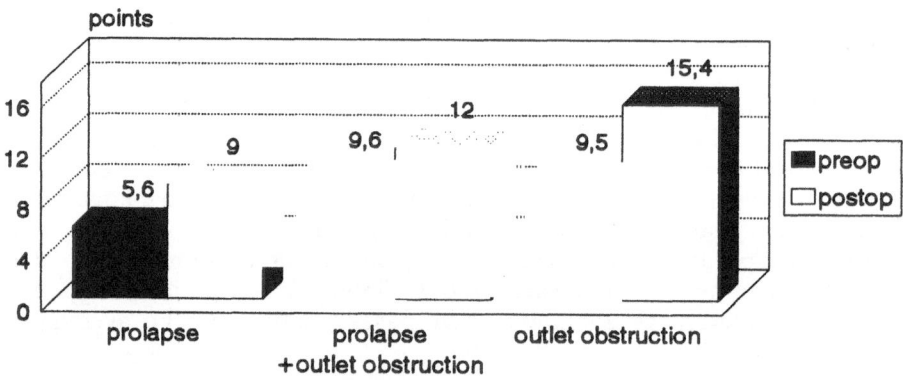

Fig. 1. Pre- and postoperative resting and squeeze pressures in 12 out of 55 patients undergoing laparoscopic rectopexy

Postoperatively there was a slight increase in continence scores, but this increase did not reach statistical significance (Fig. 1). The same is true for the resting pressure and squeeze pressure after the operation (Fig. 2). During the follow-up period of a maximum of 42 months, no recurrence of prolapse was seen. One patient suffers from moderate pain in the small pelvis; six patients complain of moderate to severe constipation [4].

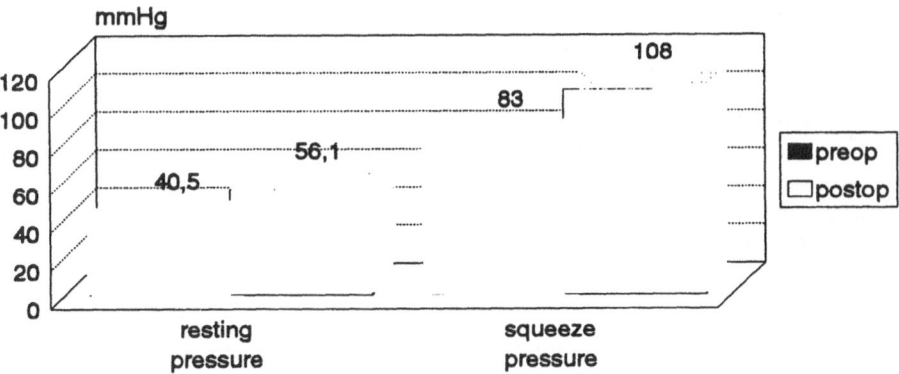

Fig. 2. Pre- and postoperative continence scores in 16 out of 55 patients undergoing laparoscopic rectopexy

Discussion

Various surgical procedures have been described for fixation of the rectum [3, 15, 27]. These procedures can be classified as posterior fixation, anterior fixation, lateral fixation, and fixation with or without resection. Most necessitate the placement of xenogenic material such a polypropylene or Malex mesh, Ivalon sponge or Teflon suspension. This foreign material makes sigmoid resection dangerous, with a considerable risk of infection [1–3, 5–7, 11, 13, 17, 22, 24, 28]. In this respect the Sudeck rectopexy provides distinct advantages [30]. It does not utilize foreign material, and simultaneous resection of the colon is possible without increasing the postoperative risk. Some authors report that there are fewer problems with constipation after the Sudeck procedure, and the continence score seems to be better in comparison to other procedures. If we look at laparoscopic rectopexy in the Sudeck modification, it must be admitted that the long rows of intra-abdominal sutures, necessary to suspend the rectum so that it is stretched, are difficult to perform. In addition, there may be a risk of insufficient scar formation, with consequent recurrence of prolapse. However, so far no prolapse recurrence has been observed in our series. This observation agrees with those of other authors.

Nevertheless the more advanced, difficult surgical procedures on the colon are still debated, and are accepted as routine only in some highly specialized centres [8–10, 20, 23, 26, 29, 32, 33]. Our own experiences with laparoscopic rectopexy and sigmoid resection show that this new surgical technique can be applied safely and effectively to manage rectal prolapse and cul-de-sac phenomena. The method is not only limited to single procedures, but seems also to be adaptable to multiple functional disorders of the sigmoid colon and rectum. All procedures which have been carried out by the abdominal or perineal route can be performed by laparoscopy. However, all these laparoscopic procedures, ranging from adhesiolysis to postanal repair and levatorplasty, are very time consuming and pose extreme technical challenges for the surgeon. Despite these technical problems and physical obstacles, however, we would like to conclude with the following hypotheses:

1. Laparoscopic rectopexy minimizes operative trauma.
2. The operative steps of conventional operations can be exactly imitated in laparoscopic maneuvers.
3. Convalescence times can be reduced.
4. The complication rate is low.
5. The long-term results are excellent.

We therefore feel that laparoscopic rectopexy should be the method of choice in patients with cul-de-sac phenomena and rectal prolapse.

References

1. Baker R, Senagore AJ, Luchtefeld MA (1995) Laparoscopic-assisted vs. open resection. Rectopexy offers excellent results. Dis Colon Rectum 38 : 199–201
2. Berman IR (1992) Sutureless laparoscopic rectopexy for procidentia. Technique and implications. Dis Colon Rectum 35 : 689–693
3. Carter AE (1983) Rectosacral suture fixation for complete rectal prolapse in the elderly, the frail and the demented. Br J Surg 70 : 522–523
4. Carter PS, Heald RJ (1995) Pain following laparoscopic rectopexy [letter]. Br J Surg 82 : 136
5. Cuesta MA, Borgstein PJ, de Jong D, Meijer S (1993) Laparoscopic rectopexy. Surg Laparosc Endosc 3 : 456–458
6. Cuschieri A, Shimi SM, Vander Velpen G, Banting S, Wood RA (1994) Laparoscopic prosthesis fixation rectopexy for complete rectal prolapse. Br J Surg 81 : 138–139
7. Darzi A, Henry MM, Guillou PJ, Shorvon P, Monson JR (1995) Stapled laparoscopic prectopexy for rectal prolapse. Surg Endosc 9 : 301–303
8. Franklin ME, Jr, Ramos R, Rosenthal D, Schuessler W (1993) Laparoscopic colonic procedures. World J Surg 17 : 51–56
9. Franklin ME, Rosenthal D, Noren RF (1995) Prospective evaluation of laparoscopic colon resection versus open colon resection for adenocarcinoma – a multicenter study. Surg Endosc 9 : 811–816
10. Geis WP, Coletta AV, Verdeja JC, Plasencia G, Ojogho O, Jacobs M (1994) Sequential psychomotor skills development in laparoscopic colon surgery. Arch Surg 129 : 206–212
11. Graf W, Stefansson T, Arvidsson D, Påhlman L (1995) Laparoscopic suture rectopexy. Dis Colon Rectum 38 : 211–212
12. Halligan S, Nicholls RJ, Bartram CI (1995) Proctographic changes after rectopexy for solitary rectal ulcer syndrome and preoperative predictive factors for a successful outcome. Br J Surg 82 : 314–317
13. Henry LG, Cattey RP (1994) Rectal prolapse. Surg Laparosc Endosc 4 : 357–360
14. Köckerling F, Gastinger I, Schneider B, Krause W, Gall FP (1993) Laparoscopic abdomino-perineal excision of the rectum with high ligation of the inferior mesenteric artery in the management of rectal carcinoma. Endosc Surg Allied Technol 1 : 16–19
15. Kodner IJ, Frey RD, Fleshman JW (1992) Rectal prolapse and other pelvic floor abnormalities. Surg Annu 24 : 157–190
16. Kuijpers JH (1989) Complete rectal prolapse is not a disorder that occurs frequently [editorial]. Neth J Surg 41 : 121–122
17. Kwok SP, Carey DP, Lau WY, Li AK (1994) Laparoscopic rectopexy. Dis Colon Rectum 37 : 947–948

18. Lowry AC, Goldberg SM (1987) Internal and overt rectal procidentia. Gastroenterol Clin North Am 16 : 47 – 70
19. Mackle EJ, Parks TG (1986) The pathogenesis and pathophysiology of rectal prolapse and solitary rectal ulcer syndrome. Clin Gastroenterol 15 : 985 – 1002
20. Mentges B, Buess G, Manncke K, Becker HD (1993) [Minimally invasive surgery of the colon and rectum]. Zentralbl Chir 118 : 746 – 753
21. Metcalf AM, Loening Baucke V (1988) Anorectal function and defecation dynamics in patients with rectal prolapse. Am J Surg 155 : 206 – 210
22. Munro W, Avramovic J, Roney W (1993) Laparoscopic rectopexy. J Laparoendosc Surg 3 : 55 – 58
23. Phillips EH, Franklin M, Carroll BJ, Fallas MJ, Ramos R, Rosenthal D (1992) Laparoscopic colectomy. Ann Surg 216 : 703 – 707
24. Ratelle R, Vollant S, Peloquin AB, Gravel D (1994) [Abdominal rectopexy (Orr-Loygue) in rectal prolapse: celioscopic approach or conventional surgery]. Ann Chir 48 : 679 – 684
25. Ryan P (1980) Observations upon the aetiology and treatment of complete rectal prolapse. Aust N Z J Surg 50 : 109 – 115
26. Sackier JM, Berci G, Hiatt JR, Hartunian S (1992) Laparoscopic abdominoperineal resection of the rectum [see comments]. Br J Surg 79 : 1207 – 1208
27. Sarin YK, Sharma AK (1993) Posterior sagittal rectopexy for rectal prolapse. Indian Pediatr 30 : 541 – 542
28. Senagore AJ, Luchtefeld MA, MacKeigan JM (1993) Rectopexy. J Laparoendosc Surg 3 : 339 – 343
29. Simons AJ, Anthone GJ, Ortega AE et al. (1995) Laparoscopic-assisted colectomy learning curve. Dis Colon Rectum 38 : 600 – 603
30. Sudeck P (1922) Rektumprolapsoperation durch Auslösung des Rektum aus der Excavatio sacralis. Zentralbl Chir 20 : 698 – 699
31. Wassef R, Rothenberger DA, Goldberg SM (1986) Rectal prolapse. Curr Probl Surg 23 : 397 – 451
32. Wexner SD, Cohen SM, Johansen OB, Nogueras JJ, Jagelman DG (1993) Laparoscopic colorectal surgery: a prospective assessment and current perspective. Br J Surg 80 : 1602 – 1605
33. Wexner SD, Johansen OB, Nogueras JJ, Jagelman DG (1992) Laparoscopic total abdominal colectomy. A prospective trial. Dis Colon Rectum 35 : 651 – 655
34. Yang A, Mostwin JL, Rosenshein NB, Zerhouni EA (1991) Pelvic floor descent in women: dynamic evaluation with fast MR imaging and cinematic display. Radiology 179 : 25 – 33

Laparoscopic Intracorporeal End-to-End Colonic Anastomosis by Means of Singly-Placed Staples

G. Meyer, H. M. Schardey, A. Holker, A. Nerlich, W. Steiner, V. Lange, and F. W. Schildberg

Intracorporeal Anastomoses – Why?

Four years after the first colon resection [12], restoration of continuity following laparoscopic resection of the gastrointestinal tract is still a problem and therefore a subject of discussion. The main debate about employing an intracorporeal, extracorporeal, or half-open technique turns on the safety and practicability of the each technique. The particular circumstances of laparoscopic operations – working with special instruments via trocars in a limited three-dimensional space with a comparatively narrow field of vision – make both conventional suturing and stapling of an anastomosis more difficult. Owing to these problems, anastomoses following colon resections are performed almost exclusively completely extracorporeally or using a half-open technique via a minilaparotomy after evisceration of the bowel end [5, 10, 18, 29, 31]. In most cases the minilaparotomy is only required for the anastomosis; extraction of the specimen can be done via a 15- to 18-mm trocar incision, especially if the resection has been carried out for a benign lesion or for palliation in patients with metastatic disease. These minilaparotomies at the end of operations forfeit some of the advantages of the minimally invasive surgical technique over conventional surgery, and this is why, in our opinion, "laparoscopically assisted" operations are not a very satisfying compromise with respect to the basic idea of minimally invasive operations. They can only be an interim solution on the way to a completely and exclusively laparoscopic surgical technique [13].

Apart the primary goal of avoiding a minilaparotomy, there are several other reasons supporting the idea of a completely intracorporeal anastomosis. These relate to the safety and practicability of the operation. Completely intracorporeal anastomosis may be safer, because the bowel ends intended for anastomosis do not need to be eviscerated. Unnecessary mobilization, wound contamination, and lesions to the mesentery or bowel wall can be avoided. It is therefore not surprising that higher stenosis and insufficiency rates have been reported in relation to anastomoses fashioned extracorporeally [27]. These complications may be the consequence of ischemia resulting from compression trauma during handling or dissection of mesenteric vessels. In obese patients with a short mesentery it may not be possible to mobilize the bowel sufficiently to allow exteriorization, so that the "mini" laparotomy becomes larger and larger, or else if the incision is inadequate an unnecessary increase in risk may arise.

Types of Intracorporeal Anastomosis

Among the presently available intracorporeal anastomosing techniques, only one has been to any degree widely adopted, especially by English and American surgeons. This is the functional end-to-end anastomosis created using a side-to-side technique with a linear stapler [1, 23, 27], which clinically has been repeatedly carried out after right colonic resections. On the basis of myographic and functional propulsive characteristics this anastomosis is the most unfavorable one available [2]. Because of the small blind sacs arising through this technique, there always is a danger of blind loop colitis [24]. In conventional surgery we have always avoided using this anastomosis whenever possible and preferred that biologically more favorable end-to-end anastomosis. In our opinion, laparoscopic anastomosis should therefore also be performed using the end-to-end technique.

For resections in the region of the left colon, with anastomoses at the level of the rectum, sigmoid and lower descending colon, there is the modified triple stapling technique for end-to-end anastomoses. Here the purse-string suture is fashioned with the help of a special laparoscopic purse-string suture clamp. The anvil is introduced into the proximal bowel end still connected to the circular stapler via a 33-mm trocar [14]. Since circular inverted anastomoses are created with the stapler introduced by the transanal route this technique can be employed only in the lower left colon and rectum. It is not used in the right colon because an additional enterotomy would be required to introduce the circular stapler, and because of the difficulties arising from the handling of the large instrument, which was developed for conventional surgery, not for laparoscopy. Most laparoscopic surgeons opt for a laparoscopically assisted operation with a half open anastomosing technique, because the creation of an intracorporeal purse-string suture on the human colon even with a specially designed clamp is not easy, and the 33-mm retrieval trocar comes rather close to a minilaparotomy. In the half-open technique the colon is exteriorized for a sufficient length to expose the proximal transection, where a purse-string is applied and the anvil of the circular mechanical stapler is placed. The proximal colon with the anvil in place is then returned to the abdominal cavity and the minilaparotomy is closed. By the transanal route, the base of the circular stapler is inserted and, using special graspers, brought into contact with the anvil components under laparoscopic view. The anastomosis is performed by firing the stapler. The overwhelming majority of anastomosises carried out in connection with laparoscopic operations have been done in this way for the above-mentioned reasons, and they are therefore not truly intracorporeal anastomoses [8, 23]. In our department also, anastomoses in suitable locations are created using this technique.

Whatever the location, anastomoses can in principle be carried out laparoscopically using conventional hand suturing technique. An all-layer single-row interrupted or running suture technique can be used. Clinically this has only been done in a few cases [23, 30]. Even for the trained laparoscopic surgeon, an anastomosis performed by intracorporeal handsuturing and knotting is a special challenge and is associated with higher risk than standard techniques. From the viewpoint of a laparoscopic surgeon, a running suture seems preferable to the interrupted technique, because it requires fewer intracorporeal knots. Few animal experimental data are available about handsuturing techniques [26]. The dramatically elevated risks of complications, with leakage rates of up to 50%, have been pointed out repeatedly [7]. In laparoscopic surgery, standardized mechanical suture techniques with instruments adapted to laparoscopy may come to be preferred because they are probably safer and faster to carry out [20]. This is in contrast to conventional surgery in Europe, where the manual suture techniques are preferred.

The biofragmental anastomotic ring (bar) represents an alternative to the different stapler techniques. In contrast to the latter, this system has not become widespread in conventional surgery. Overall experience with it is limited, and it must be regarded as a recent development [9]. For the laparoscopic surgeon there seem to be several problems: the requirement for two purse-string sutures, the problem of introducing the two rings via a 33-mm trocar or enlarged trocar incision, and the litherto unsolved problem of safely reconnecting the two rings. These problems have been examined in animal experimental studies [25], but have not yet been solved convincingly. It is therefore doubtful whether a circular inverted anastomosis with a biofragmental ring is the solution to the problem of intracorporeal anastomosis. That is at least the present view of the situation. Reports of clinical experiences of laparoscopic use of the biofragmental anastomotic ring are not yet available.

Intracorporeal End-to-End Anastomosis with Singly Placed Staples

In our opinion, the procedures discussed so far have in common the disadvantage that they are not adequately adapted to the special requirements of laparoscopic surgery or the other disadvantages have to be accepted. The anastomosing technique should be adapted to the limited access and take account of the special circumstances of laparoscopic surgery (Table 1). One obvious prerequisite is that the basic requirements of an anastomosis are fulfilled (Table 2). From a theoretical view, two techniques seem suitable. Both

Table 1. Special requirements of laparoscopic performance of anastomoses	Intracorporeal performance of the anastomosis End-to-end technique Instruments adapted to laparoscopy Technique adapted to laparoscopy Technique as simple as possible Technique as standardized as possible Technique applicable to the entire gastrointestinal tract Technique usable in different clinical situations

Table 2. Basic requirements of an anastomosis	Air- and watertightness Immediate good physical resistance Safety (low rate of leakage and stenosis)

can be employed to create intracorporeal end-to-end anastomoses with instruments developed especially for laparoscopic surgery. One is a modification of a technique taken from conventional open surgery, which has been tested in several different animal experiments using singly placed staples [4, 11, 22, 28]. We have investigated laparoscopic application of two variants. One is the two-thirds inverted, one-third everted as well as the completely circularly everted technique employing singly placed staples from the hernia stapler (Endo Hernia). The second method is the completely everted triangulation anastomosis with a linear stapler (Endo-TA 60), which has been clinically tested in conventional surgery on a large number of patients [3, 6, 17, 19].

Animal Studies

The three laparoscopic anastomoses were compared. In addition there was a comparison with two standard techniques from conventional surgery. These were anastomoses carried out with the circular stapler (CEEA) and manual suturing using Albert's modified technique. The circular stapler produces an all-layer, double-row, inverted suture line, while the Albert technique gives an interrupted, all-layer, single-row suture line with end-to-end approximation of the different tissue layers. Anastomoses employing singly placed staples functionally imitate a single-row, all-layer, interrupted suture line. Depending on the approach, which is either from the serosa side or the mucosa side, an everted or inverted suture line emerges. As for triangulation anastomosis with the linear stapler, this produces a circular, everted, triple-row, all-layer suture line. In the singly-placed staple anastomosis the staples are in line with the longitudinal axis of the intestine, as with annual sutures; the individual staples from circular and linear staplers are at a right angle to it.

Methods

Postoperative observation periods of 14 days and 3 months were chosen in order to answer the main clinical questions concerning the physical properties, adequacy of healing, and rate of stenosis of the anastomoses. On the 14th postoperative day and after 3 months the newly developed and the established types of anastomoses could also be compared. Altogether 78 anastomoses were fashioned on the small bowel and colon in domestic pigs.

Along with the questions already mentioned, the main objective of the first series carried out was to evaluate the laparoscopic feasibility of these new anastomoses. These initial trails were carried out on the *small bowel* of the pig, because it is markedly smaller than the colon and the laparoscopic operation is therefore technically more demanding. Six anastomoses using each laparoscopic technique were created and explanted after 14 days. The small bowel anastomoses using the conventional techniques were created following conventional laparotomy.

In a second trial, the healing and physical properties of the different anastomoses were tested in the unprepared *colon*. In a randomized trial six anastomoses were created with each of the laparoscopically tested techniques and explanted after 14 days. In a long-term observation trail six anastomoses were fashioned with all techniques and explanted after 3 months. All anastomoses on the colon were created following conventional laparotomy.

As clinical parameters that correlate with possible complications, body weight and temperature were monitored. In addition, serum chemistry, microbiological, and radiological variables were investigated. During explanation, adhesions between the anastomoses and adjacent organs were observed and documented, the surgical site was evaluated macroscopically, the watertightness of the anastomosis were examined, and its patency and width were determined using an anastomotic index. The mechanical resistance of the anastomosis was investigated by measuring bursting pressure and tensile strength [21]. Neovascularization was examined by angiography (Table 3). Biopsy samples of the anastomosis were analyzed for hydroxyproline content. All anastomoses were evaluated macroscopically and microscopically (Table 4).

Results

The techniques using singly placed staples and the Endo-TA instrument were both successfully employed to create completely intracorporeal end-to-end anastomoses. All the small bowel anastomoses were successfully carried out laparoscopically at the first attempt; no conversions were required. This means that all tree techniques are basically suitable for performing intracorporeal laparoscopic anastomoses [15, 16, 21]. All animals whether with laparoscopic or conventional anastomoses of the small intestine or colon, survived the operation and the observation period until they were sacrificed for further

Table 3. Scoring system for evaluation of the microangiograms

	Score		
	0	1	2
Quality of the Angiogram	Not useable	Medium	Good
Avascular regions	Present	Absent	–
Neovascularization at 14 days	Not detected	Moderate	Marked
Neovascularization at 3 months	Marked	Moderate	Not detected
Parenchymal contrast	Marked	Moderate	Not detected
Transanastomotic vascular regeneration	Not present	Moderate	Marked
Similarity to normal vascular system	Not detected	Moderate	Marked

Table 4. Criteria and scoring of the histological examination

Epithelium	Submucosa, muscularis, subserosa	Serosa
Reepithelialization	Inflammation: superficial	Inflammation
Hyperplasia	deep	
Inflammation	Connective tissue	
	Proliferation	
	Vascularization: superficial	
	deep	
	Fistulas	
	Islets of mucosa	
	Giant cell reaction	
	Foreign bodies	

Scoring: In top half of table: 0, not present; 1, merely detectable; 2, moderate; 3, severe.
In bottom half of table (fistulas etc.) 0, no; 1, yes.

evaluation of the anastomoses. Leakage was not observed in any case. Neither the postoperative "clinical" course nor the serum tests gave any indications of complications of anastomotic healing due to leakage. The only relevant complications were two significant stenoses that developed by the 14th post-operative day in two animals with small bowel anastomoses created using the two-thirds inverted, one-third everted, singly placed staple technique. After reviewing the video recordings of these two operations, we formed the opinion that both stenoses were the result of iatrogenic ischemia due to uncontrolled electrocoagulation for hemorrhage control after transection of the bowel. All other anastomoses healed during both the short and the long observation periods without any sign of stenosis.

The minor differences in anastomotic diameter observed between the different techniques within the first 14 days (Fig. 1) disappeared during the first 3 months postoperatively, resulting in an almost normal anastomotic lumen for all techniques. Adhesions between the anastomoses and adjacent organs or structures were found after 14 days and after 3 months for all techniques on small bowel and colon with almost equal frequency and degree of severity. Only for the two-thirds inverted, on-third everted, singly placed staple technique were no adhesions found after 3 months.

After both 14 days and 3 months, the bursting pressure and tensile strength of small and large bowel anastomoses were practically identical. The same held true for the comparison between the anastomosis-carrying bowel segments and the control segments in the same animals. In no case did the rupture of the intestine occur at the anastomosis, neither during bursting pressure nor during tensile strength measurements.

After 14 days – and even more after 3 months – the hydroxypyroline/proline quotient, a measure of collagen synthesis, was clearly elevated above the level at the time the anastomosis was carried out. There were no relevant differences between the techniques.

The microangiographic findings for the different anastomoses were also fairly similar (Fig. 2).

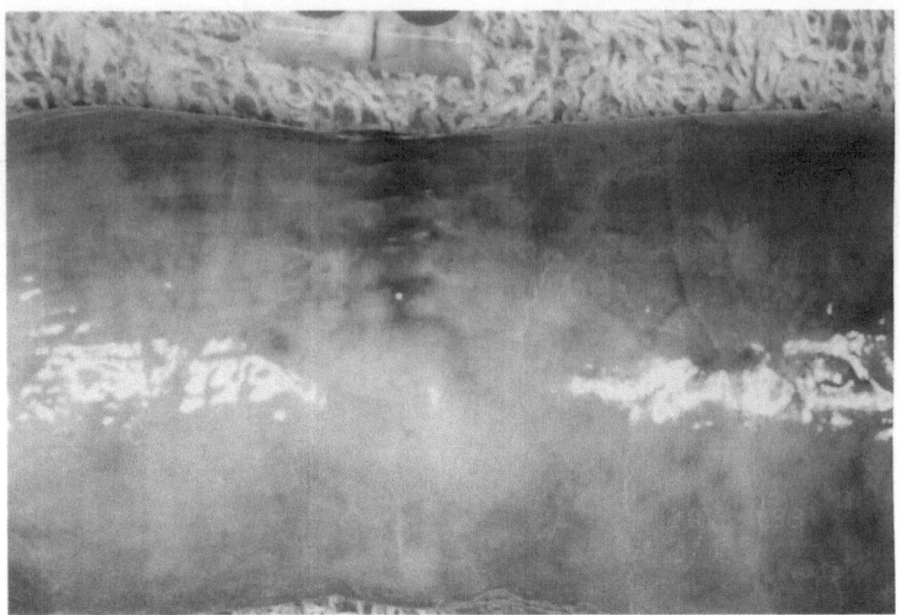

Fig. 1. Animal studies. Two-thirds inverted, one-third everted, singly placed staple technique, colon, 14th postoperative day. Anastomotic index 0.83

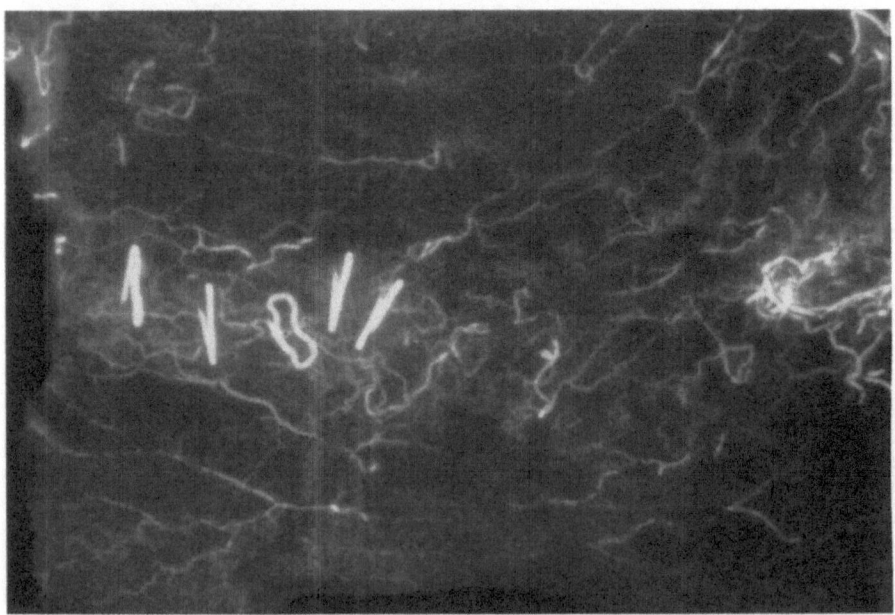

Fig. 2. Animal studies. Two-thirds inverted, one-third everted, singly placed staple technique, colon, 3 months after operation. Microangiogram without avascular regions and without parenchymal contrast uptake showing moderate neovascularization, well-developed transanastomotic vascular regeneration, and increasing similarity to the genuine vascular system

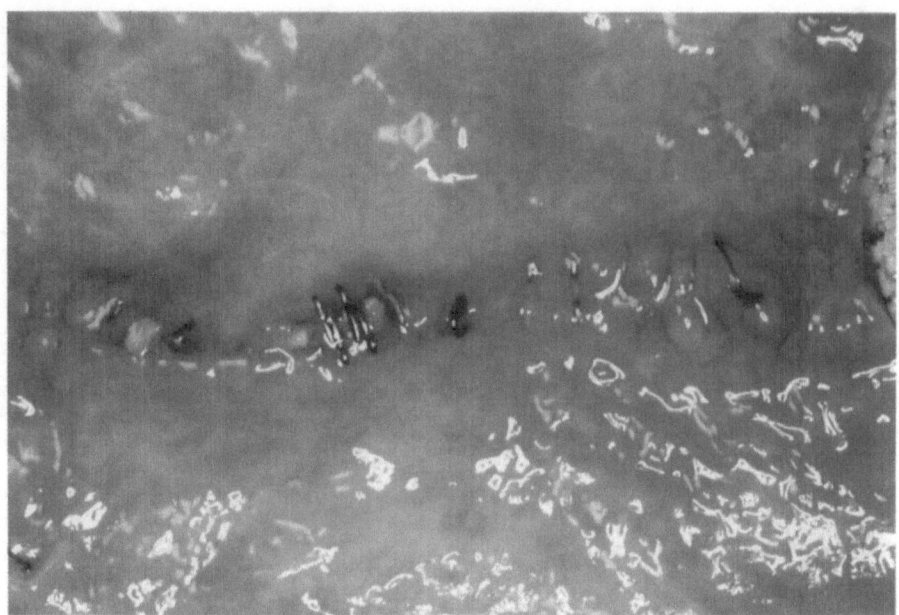

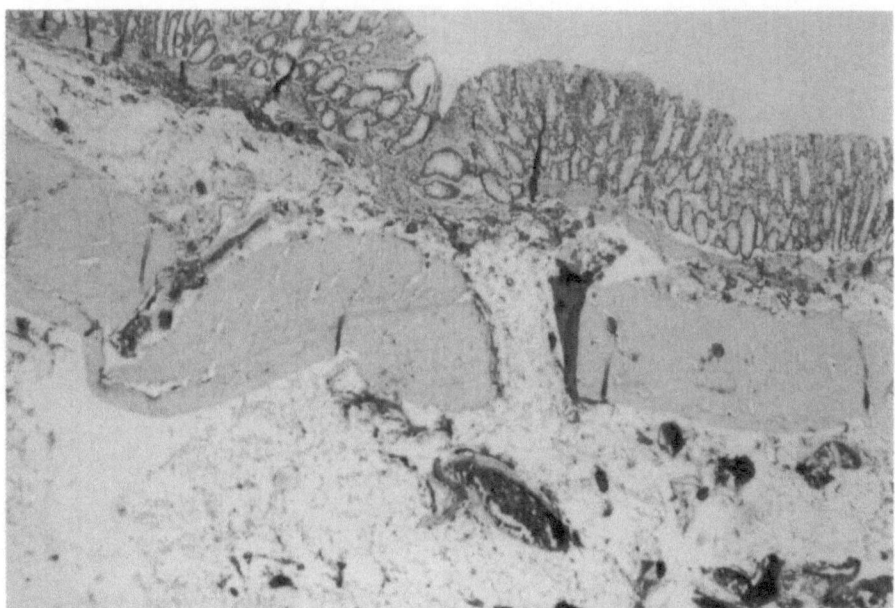

Fig. 3a, b. Animal studies. Two-thirds inverted, one-third everted, singly placed staple technique, colon, 14th postoperative day. **a** Macroscopic view. **b** Histologic section from the inverted part of the suture line. The anastomosis is situated at the level of the bowel wall

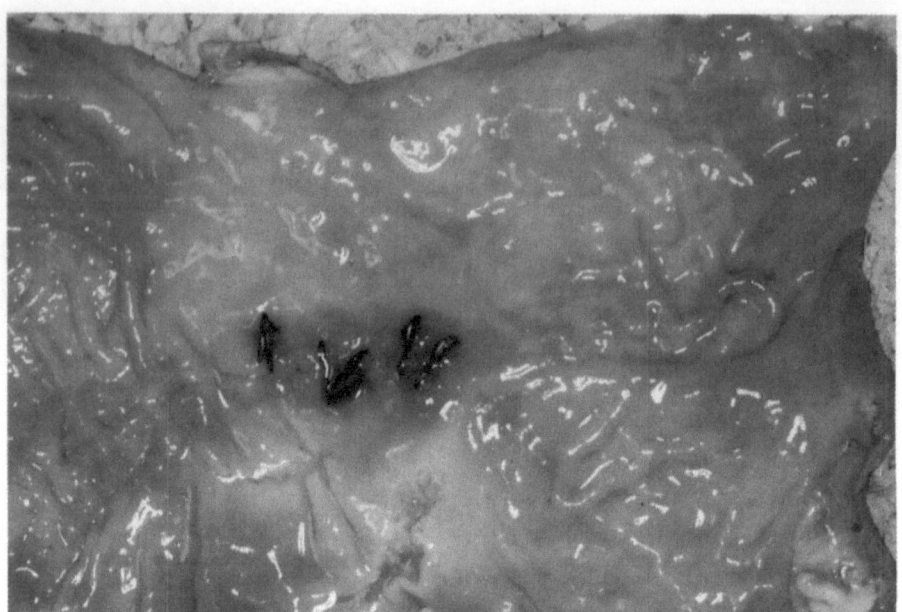

a

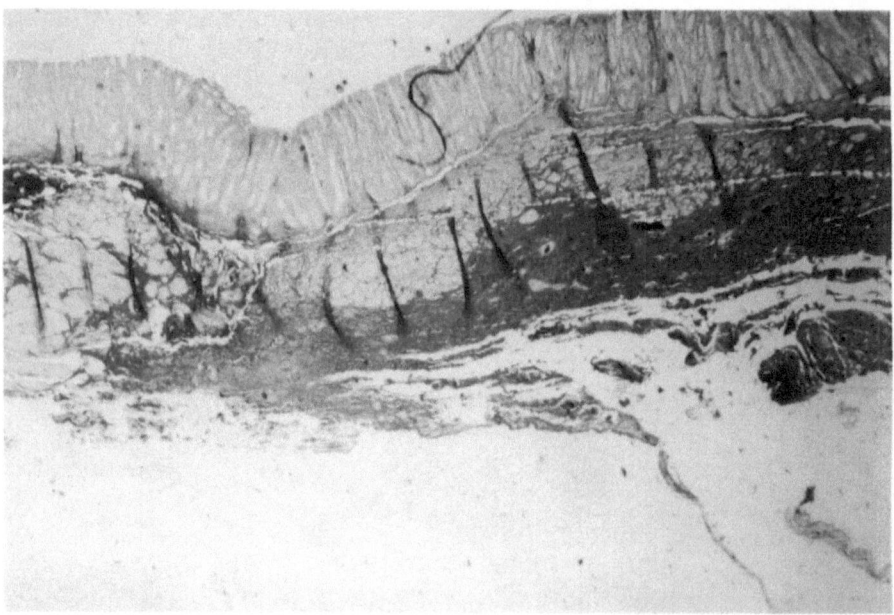

b

Fig. 4a, b. Animal studies. Two-thirds inverted, one-third everted, singly placed staple technique, colon, 3 months after operation. **a** Macroscopic view. Healed anastomosis with a few residual staples. **b** Histologic section showing completion of scar tissue formation and complete epithelialization

From anastomoses created using the singly placed staple technique in small and large bowel, spontaneous loss of staples was noted after 14 days. More were lost from the inverted segments of the anastomosis than from the everted ones. Many more staples were lost from small bowel than from colon, although as a result of the continuous loss of staples, after 3 months only about one-third of the staples originally placed could be retrieved even from colon anastomoses (Figs. 3a, 4a), and at this stage there was no longer any difference between inverted and everted suture lines.

Macroscopically the 14-day-old small bowel anastomoses showed more imperfections than the colon anastomoses of the same age. Mucosa defects could be detected in only a few anastomoses created laparoscopically, with the exception of the two stenotic anastomoses. The everted singly placed staple rows and the everted Endo-TA anastomoses showed broader reaction zones than the inverted singly placed staple row, the inverted CEEA anastomoses, and the Albert sutures. Although the everted singly placed staple rows showed broader reaction zones than the other suture techniques after 3 months, there were actually no macroscopically detectable differences between any of the anastomoses at that time. All were completely healed and reeptihelialized (Fig. 4a). We had the impression that inverted and Albert sutures heal less reactively than everted suture lines.

After both 14 days and 3 months, histological examination of the small and large bowel anastomoses showed a relatively homogeneous picture with only small differences between the techniques (Figs. 3b, 4b). The differences were more pronounced after 14 days than after 3 months. After 3 months the anastomoses had healed which explains why inflammatory reactions could no longer be detected, except for low-grade connective tissue proliferation (Fig. 5). Islets of discontinuous epithelium in distant wall layers were only found in everted anastomoses or everted segments of anastomoses.

Summarizing our animal studies, we were able to show that laparoscopic intracorporeal end-to-end-anastomoses can be successfully created with singly placed staples and with a linear stapler using the triangulation technique. Using these semistandardized techniques, anastomoses can be produced fast and safely. Apart from the two small bowel stenoses which were caused by electrocoagulation and were not attributable to the suture technique, the postoperative course of all the experimental anastomoses – i.e., 76 of them – was without complications. There were no significant differences in quality between the different anastomosing techniques. However, the laparoscopic performance of the singly placed staple anastomosis seemed technically easier than the anastomosis made with the Endo-TA instrument [21]. This was because of the problem caused by the large size of the instrument in the restricted space available within the abdomen of the pig, especially during alignment of the bowel margins for suturing. The hernia stapler is a much smaller and more elegant instrument, which can also be angled, so that during laparoscopic use impaired accessibility and restricted mobility of bowel ends is much less of a problem, than it is when using the larger, rigid linear or circular staples [16]. Although anastomosis using the circular everted singly placed staple technique is technically easier and therefore faster to create,

Scale

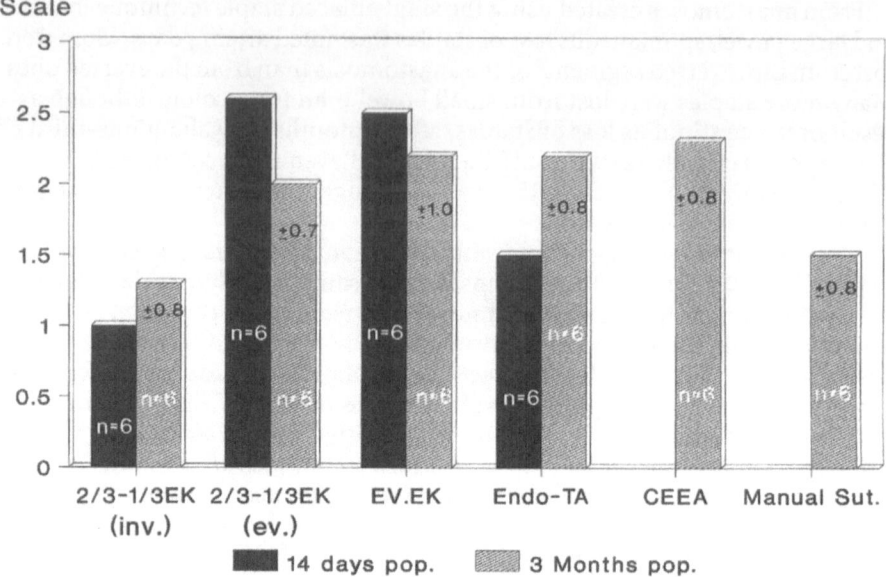

Fig. 5. Animal studies. Connective tissue proliferation of different anastomoses of the colon after 14 days and 3 months. Pronounced proliferation in the everted singly placed staple lines after 14 days and moderate proliferation in the inverted singly placed staple lines as well as the manual suture lines after 3 months. The differences must be interpreted as quite small. *EK*, Singly placed; *EV.EK*, everted singly placed

there have been some qualitative disadvantages in comparison to the two-thirds inverted, one-third everted technique. For these reasons, we consider the combination of inverted and everted singly placed staples to be best suited to clinical use. When creating these anastomoses, the inverted segment of the suture line should be clearly the greater.

Clinical Experience

Technique

The bowel ends, sealed with a staple line , were opened with the scissors. Any differences in lumen size were equalized by an antimesenteric longitudinal incision of the smaller bowel end. Transmural inverting stay sutures were placed to ensure inversion of the mucosa at 4 and 8 o'clock (mesentery at 6 o'clock). While keeping the stay sutures taut, the bowel ends were inverted and transmurally stapled (Endo-Hernia stapler; Fig. 6a). The distance between staples (Fig. 6b) corresponded to the thickness of the stapler tip, which was approximately 2–3 mm. The distance between staples was considered to be correct when the tip of a dissecting instrument was unable to pass

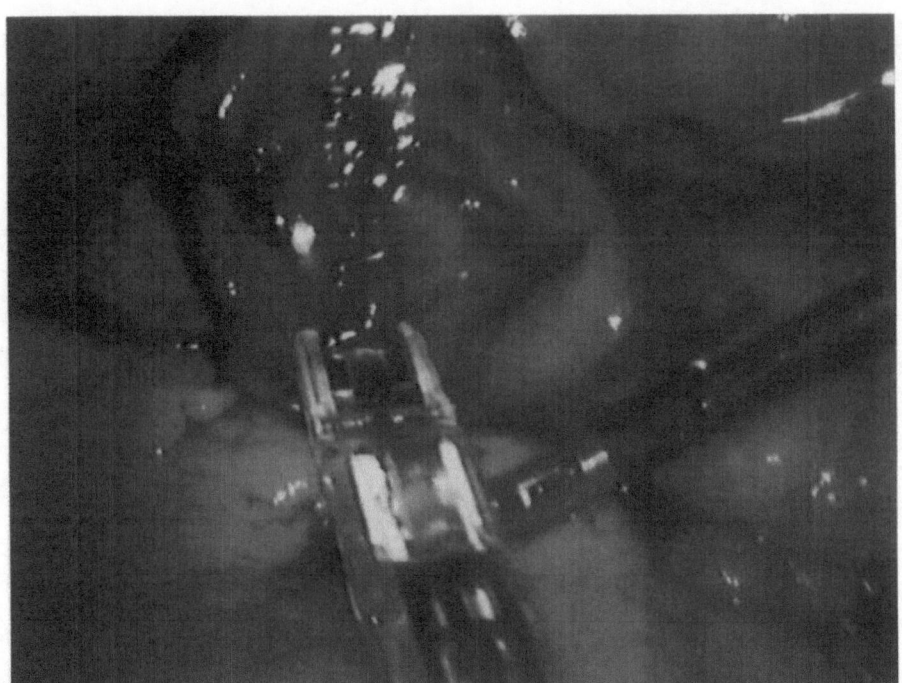

a

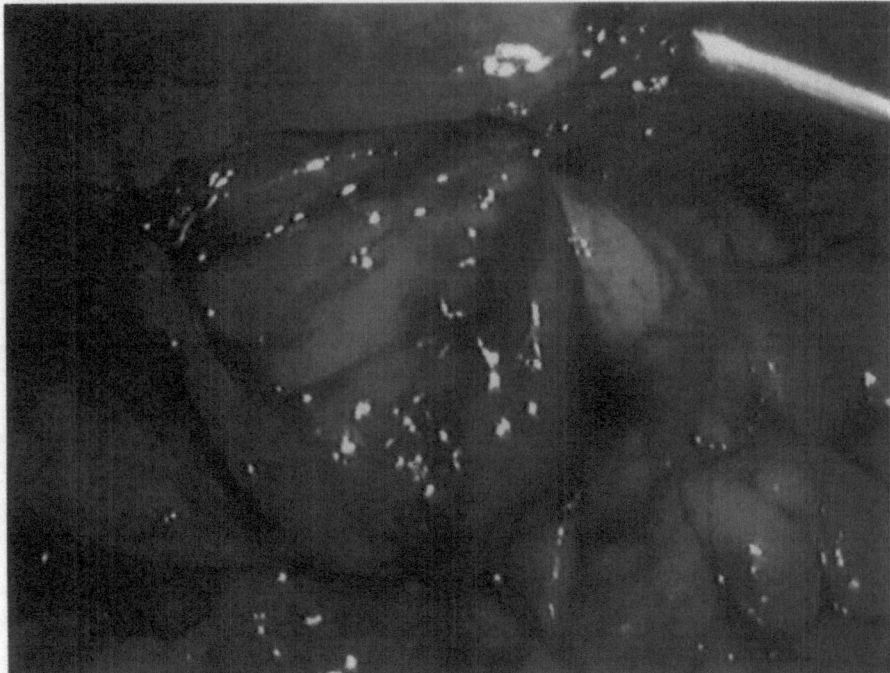

b

Fig. 6a–d. Clincal case. End-to-end anastomosis in combined everted-inverted singly placed staple technique after laparoscopic segmental resection of the descending colon because of a broad-based adenoma. **a** Inverted staple line of the first quarter of the circumference. **b** Finished suture line of the first two quarters

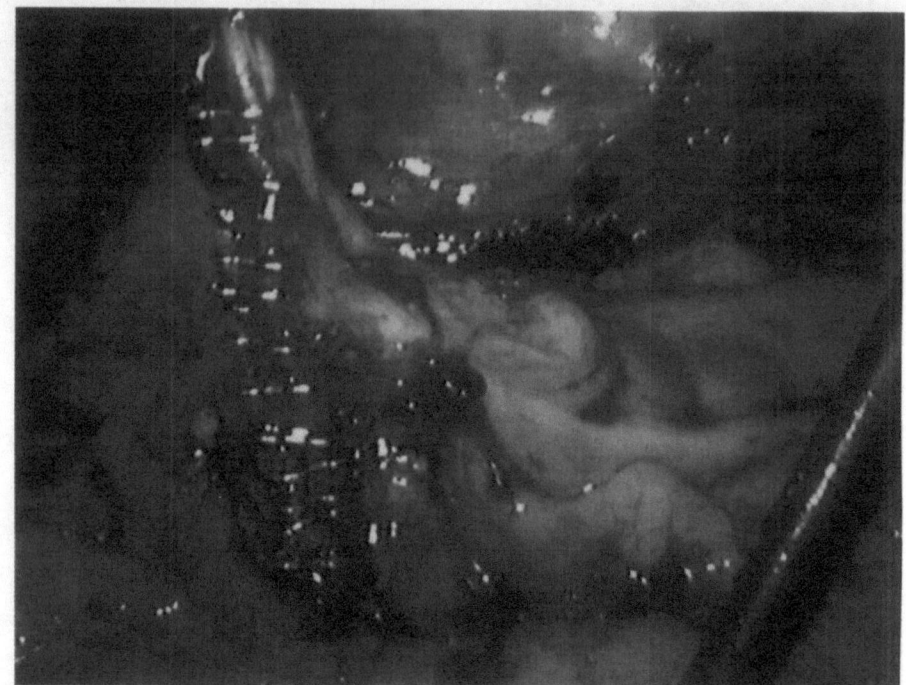

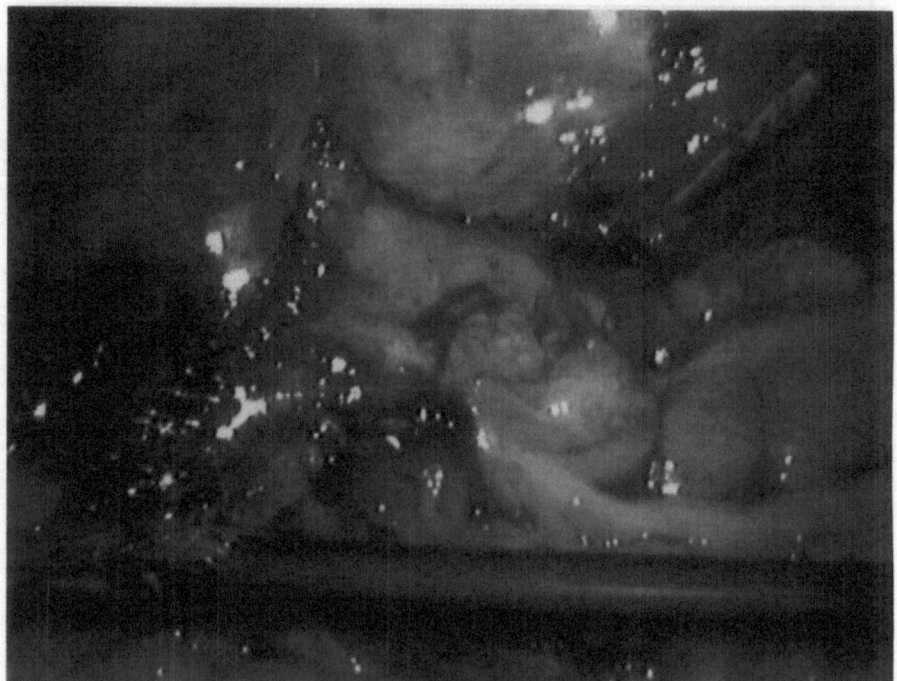

Fig. 6c–d **c** Finished third and fourth quarters of the suture line, everted. **d** Finished anastomosis suspended between stay sutures. *Left,* the everted suture line

between the staples. After completing one-third of the circumference a third stay suture was placed with the bowel ends inverted and was tied at 12 o'clock. By keeping the last and one of the previously placed stay sutures taut, the second leg of the triangle could be stapled with the bowel ends inverted. The stay suture remaining in the middle of the completed two-thirds of the circumference was now cut off. The remaining leg of the triangle was then closed with eversion (Fig. 6c, d). The mesenteric defect was also closed with hernia staples. In some cases where bowel circumference was very large, e.g., in the ascending colon, we took to a quadrangulating technique using four stay sutures to facilitate the handling. It must be emphasized that the larger part of the circumference is stapled inverted. The mesenteric part of the anastomosis is always stapled inverted.

Patients and Methods

Using the above-described technique, eight anastomoses were created in different segments of the gastrointestinal tract, six of them in the colon (Table 5). These were two ileoascendostomies, two transversotransversostomies, one descendodescendostomy, and 1 sigmoidosigmoidostomy. All laparoscopically produced anastomoses were endoscopically checked intraoperatively for hemorrhage, patency, and airtightness. A final irrigation of the abdomen was carried out. After suctioning the irrigant a Robinson drain was placed near the surgical site in the civinity of the anastomosis and passed out through one of the trocar incisions. All patients received preoperative single-shot antibiotic prophylaxis with 2 g cefotaxime i.v. Postoperatively patients were put on parenteral nutrition for 5–7 days. We began oral fluid intake between the 1st and 3rd postoperative day and enteral nutrition between the 5th and 7th day.

In addition to general clinical monitoring, a radiological check of the anastomosis by Gastrografin enema was carried out between the 7th and 9th postoperative day. Alternatively, endoscopy was carried out (Fig. 7). Six to 8 weeks postoperatively, a clinical examination and a colonoscopic check-up of the colon anastomosis were carried out. These examinations were repeated after 1 year, at which time a barium study of the anastomosis was done. In addition to the diameter of the anastomosis, the remaining staples were reviewed. The anastomotic index was determined by reference to the experimental animal studies. Follow-up presently ranges from 5 to 24 months.

Results

All operations were carried out without a minilaparotomy (Fig. 8). Creation of the anastomosis took between 39 and 65 min. On the colon, the triangulation technique was used in two cases and quadrangulation in four.

There were no intraoperative complications. After opening of the bowel, no spillage of bowel content into the abdomen cavity was observed in any case. We considered this to be a result of the preoperative bowel lavage and

Table 5. Clinical details of eight patients who underwent laparoscopic intracorporeal anastomosis with individually placed staples

Patient no.	Age (years)	Diagnosis	Operation	Anastomosis	Technique Inverted	Everted
1	51	Stomach outlet obstruction	B-II resection	Gastrojejunostomy	$^1/_2$	$^1/_2$
2	16	Peutz-Jeghers polyp	Sigmoid resection	Sigmoidosigmoidostomy	$^2/_3$	$^1/_3$
3	62	Adenoma	Tansverse colon resection	Transversotransversostomy	$^1/_2$	$^1/_2$
4	74	Cancer, metastases	Segmental ileum resection	Ileoileostomy	$^1/_3$	$^2/_3$
5	74	Cancer, metastases	Transverse colon resection	Transversotransversostomy	$^1/_2$	$^1/_2$
6	63	Adenoma	Ileocecal resection	Ileoascendostomy	$^2/_3$	$^1/_3$
7	70	Adenoma	Descending colon resection	Descendodescendostomy	$^1/_2$	$^1/_2$
8	38	Crohn's disease, stenosis	Ileocecal resection	Ileoascendostomy	$^3/_4$	$^1/_4$

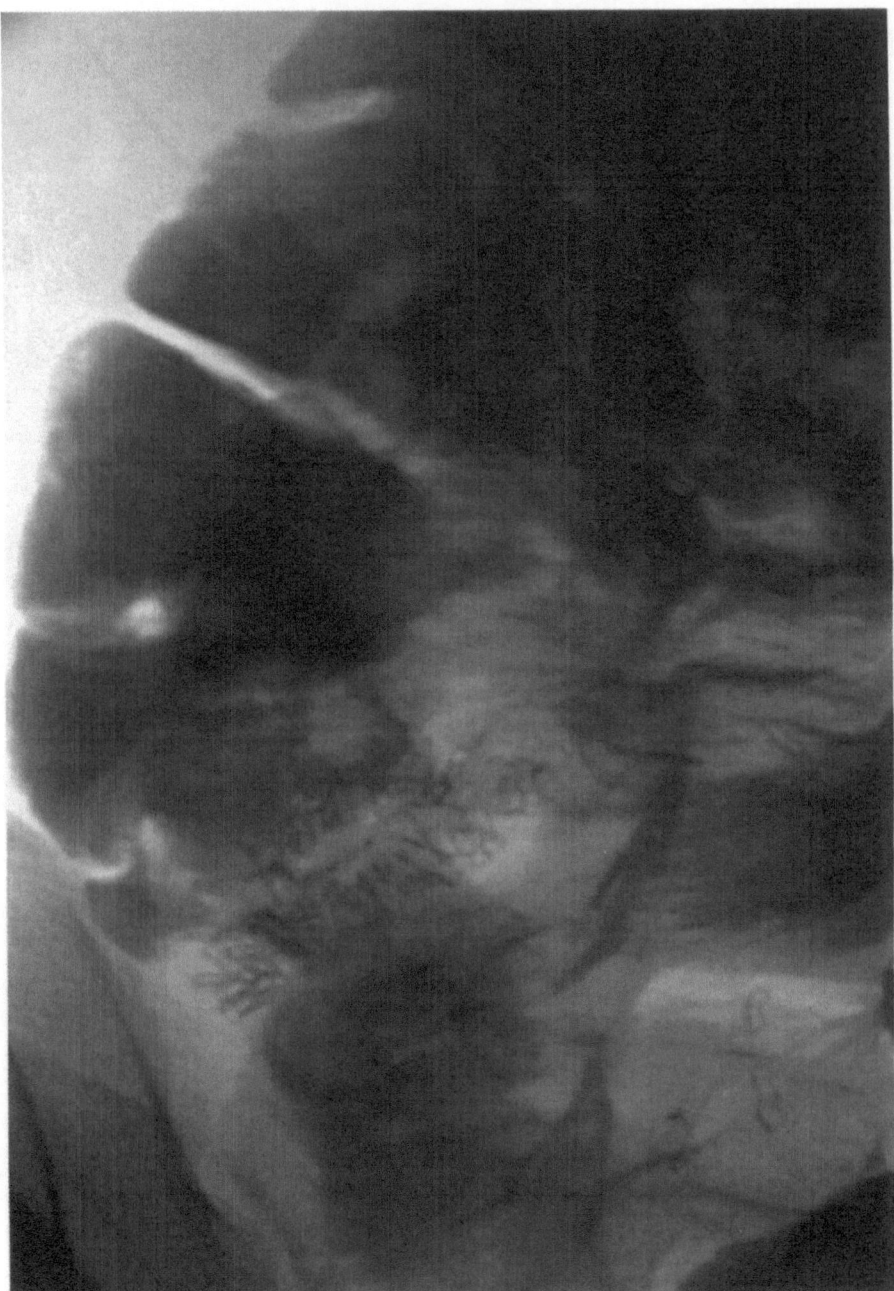

Fig. 7. Patient 8. Gastrografin X-ray 8 days after laparoscopic ileocecal resection. Wide, watertight anastomosis

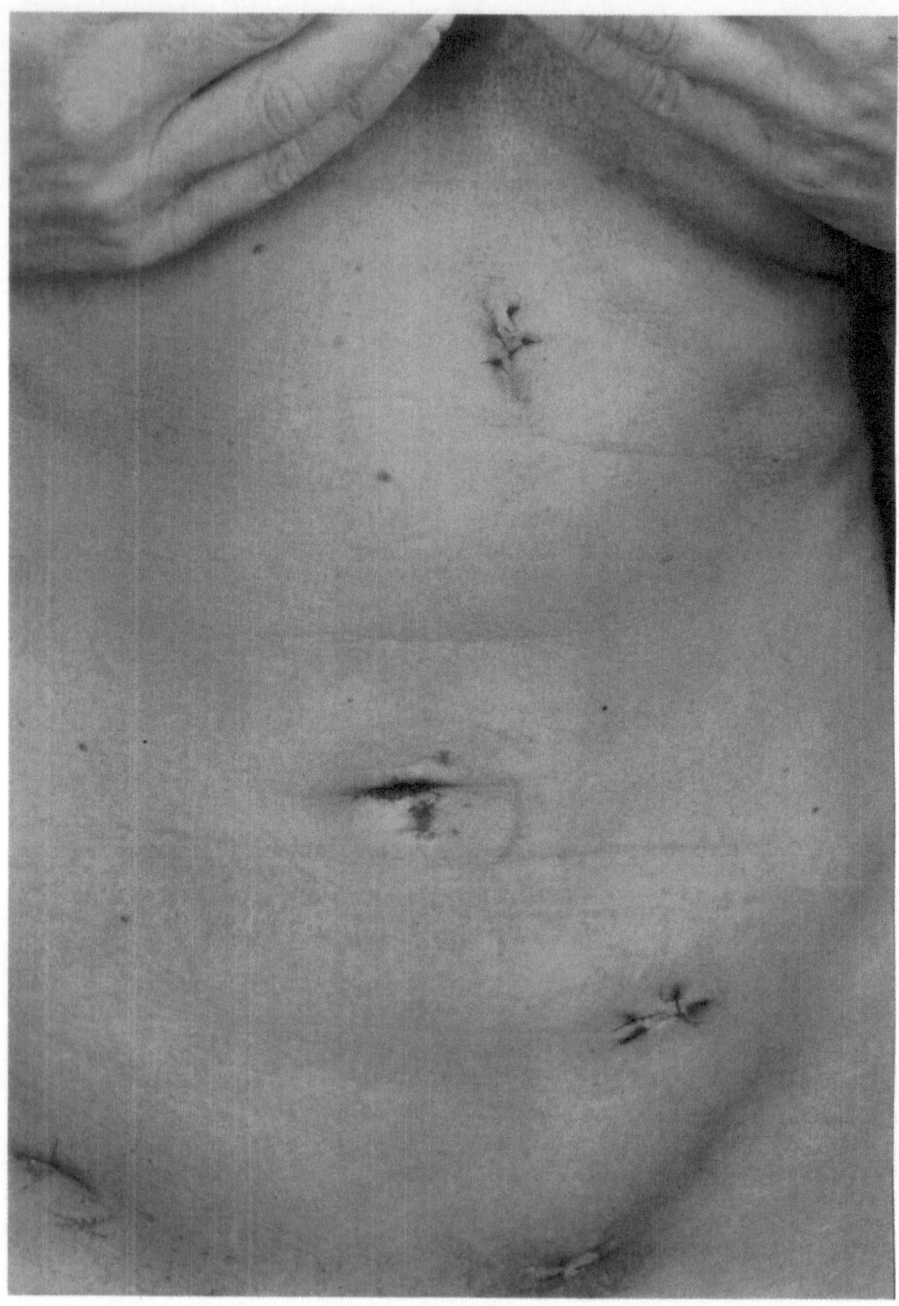

Fig. 8. Patient 8, 9 days after laparoscopic ileocecal resection with singly placed staple anastomosis

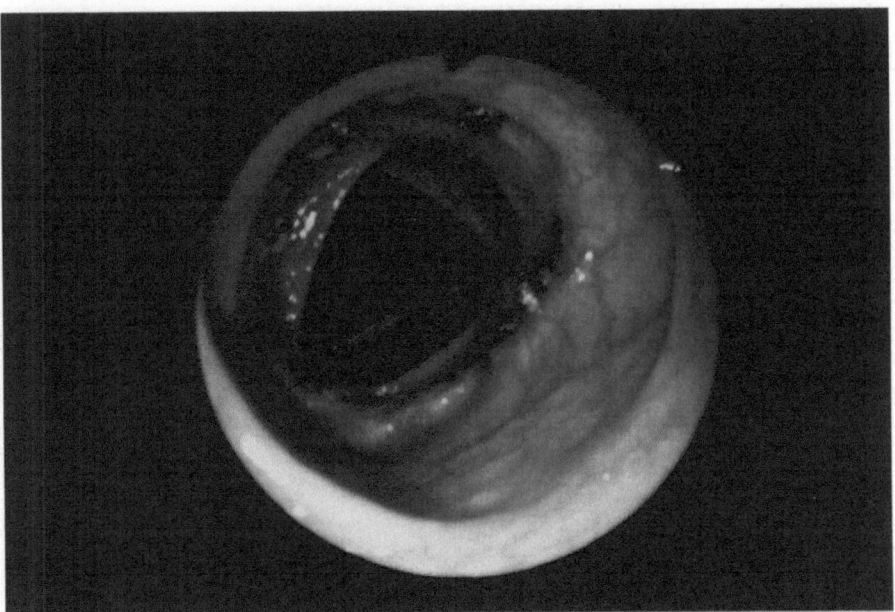

Fig. 9. Patient 3, 12 months after segmental resection of the transverse colon. Transverso-transversostomy with residual staples

the elevated intra-abdominal pressure. None of the patients required blood transfusion. The postoperative course of all patients was uneventful. The Robinson drains from the colon anastomoses were extracted 5.0 ± 2.0 days after surgery. The first stool was passed 4.4 ± 2.4 days after surgery. In all patients, peristalsis could be detected on the 1st postoperative day.

In neither the short- nor the long-term follow-up were any anastomosis-related complications such as leakage, hemorrhage, or stenosis. At the follow-up examinations, all patients were free of complaints concerning the anastomosis. At least same of the staples had been released into the bowel lumen over time. This process seemed chiefly to involve the staples in the inverted segments first; after 1 year, there were larger graps in inverted staple lines (Fig. 9). However, gaps and loosely fixed staples could be observed in the everted anastomotic segments as well (Fig. 10). The anastomotic index for all anastomoses after 1 year was 0.93 ± 0.01, compared to the ideal value of 1.0, showing that practically no stenoses were detectable.

Summarizing, the first positive clinical experiences [20] support the result of the animal studies. In different segments of the human gastrointestinal tract, anastomoses can be created laparoscopically with singly placed staples from the hernia stapler and without any complications. This semistandardized suture technique proved to be especially suitable for laparoscopic use in different surgical situations. It allows intracorporeal fashioning of an end-to-end anastomosis employing an instrument specially developed for laparoscopic

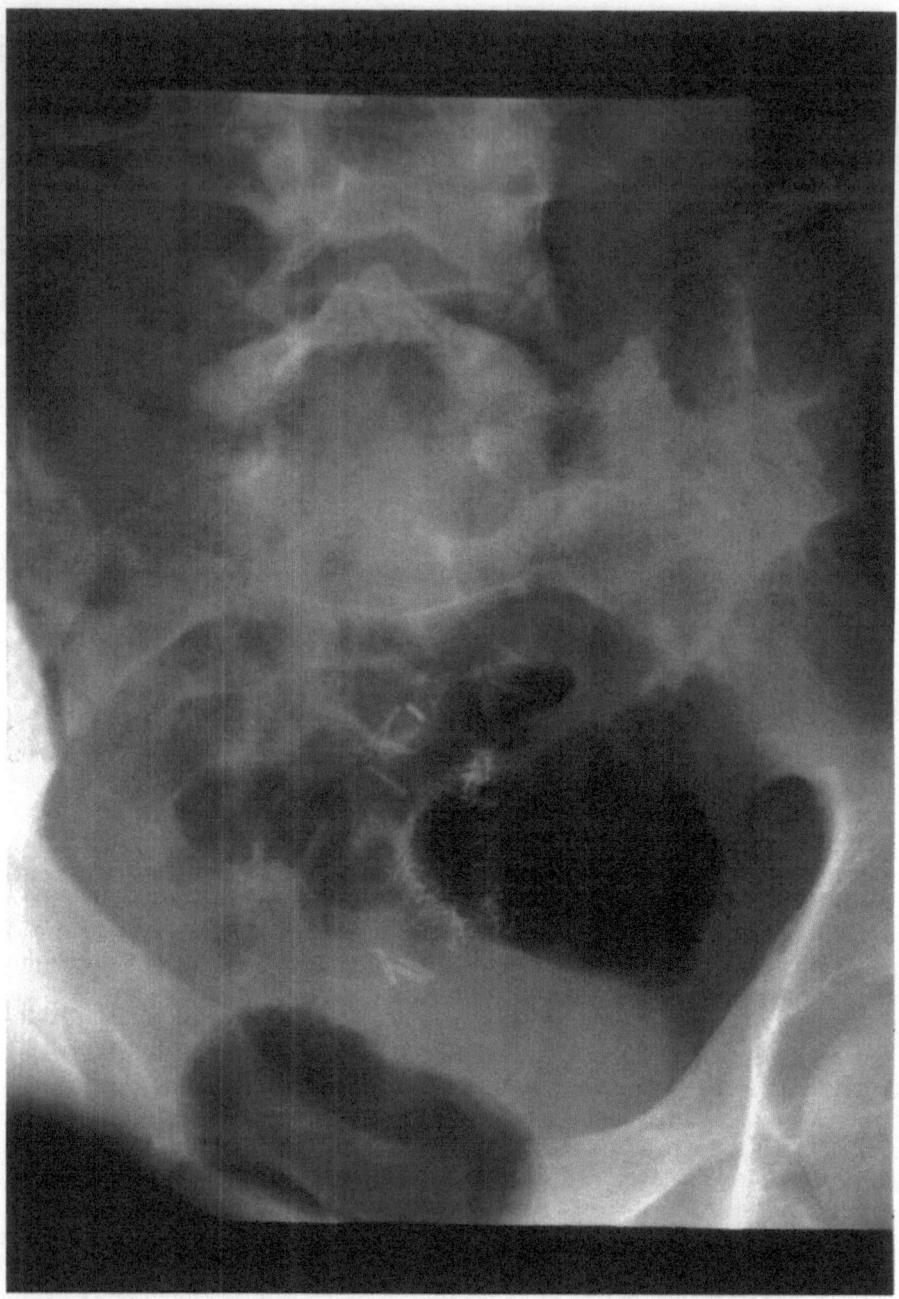

a

Fig. 10a, b. Patient 2. Sigmoidosigmoidostomy. **a** Circular staple ring 4 weeks after creation of the anastomosis. **b** Twelve months postoperatively staples remain only in the everted suture line. Endoscopically these could be seen to be only loosely fixed to the mucosa

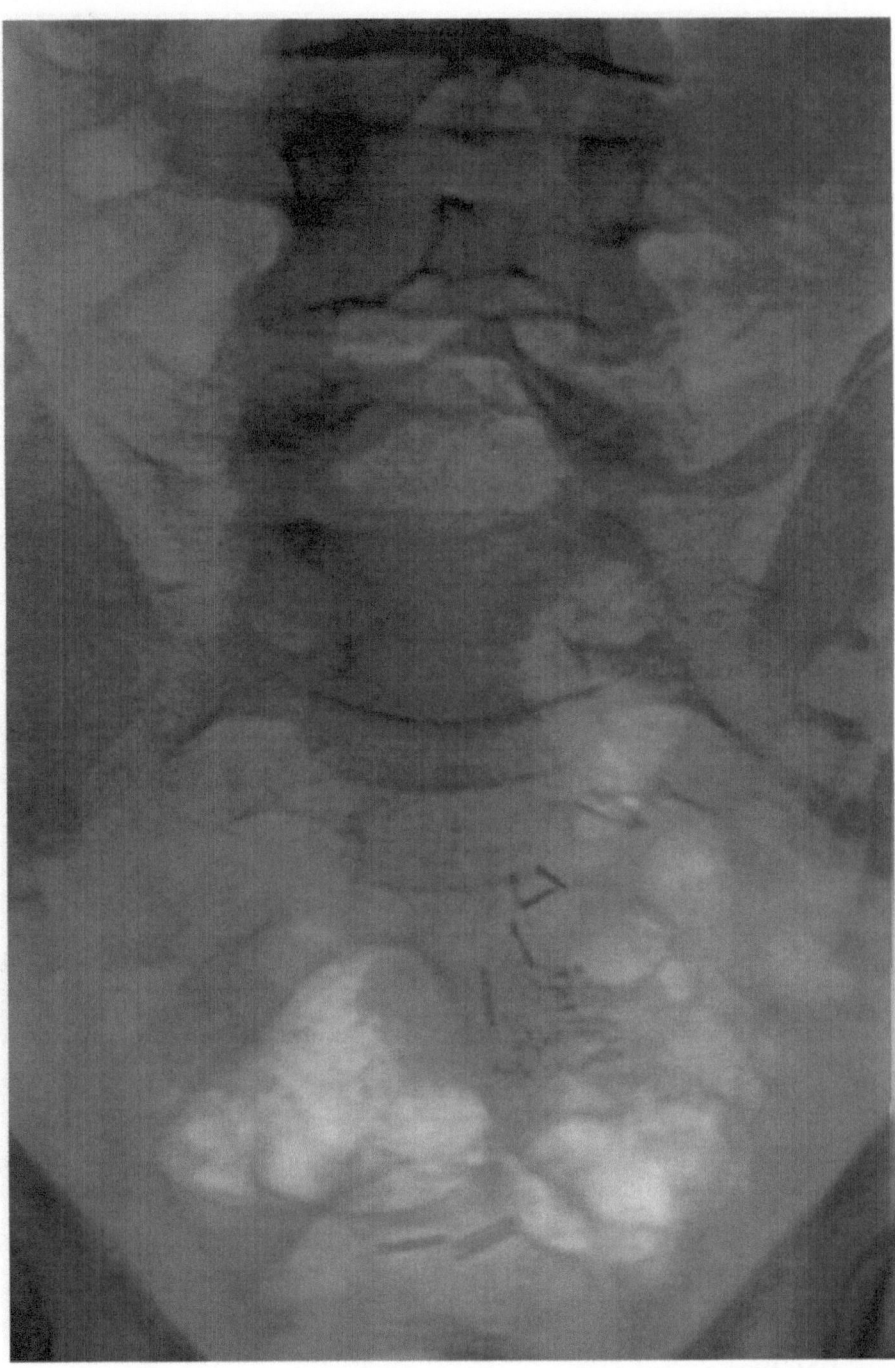

b

surgery. We are therefore convinced of the value of this anastomosis for laparoscopic routine, created by us for the first time with the staples from the hernia stapler. For a final evaluation, however, further clinical experience is required.

References

1. Böhm, B, Milson JW, Fazio VW (1994) Laparoskopische Ileocoecalresektionen beim M. Crohn. Zentralbl Chir 119: 420 – 427
2. Bruch HP (1994) Kommentar auf Anforderung der Schriftleitung zum Beitrag „Laparoskopische Ileocoecalresektionen beim M. Crohn". Zentralbl Chir 119: 426 – 427
3. Castrup HJ (1986) Triangulationsanastomosen. In: Ulrich B, Winter J (eds) Klammernahttechnik in Thorax and Abdomen. Enke, Stuttgart, pp 112 – 116 (Praktische Chirurgie, Vol 99)
4. Chung RS (1980) Gastrointestinal anastomoses constructed with singly placed staples. Am J Surg 139: 876 – 879
5. Darzi A, Hill ADK, Henry MM, Guillou PJ, Monson JRT (1992) Laparoscopic assisted surgery of the colon. Operative technique. End Surg 1: 13 – 15
6. Ferguson EF Jr, Houston H (1975) Simplified anterior resection: use of the TA-stapler. Dis Colon Rectum 18: 311 – 318
7. Fourquier P (1995) Bowel anastomoses through laparoscopy: an experimental study. Paper presented at the Third International Congress of New Technology and Advanced Techniques in Surgery, Luxembourg, June 11 – 17
8. Franklin ME Jr, Ramos R, Rosenthal D, Schuessler W (1993) Laparoscopic colonic procedures. World J Surg 17: 51 – 56
9. Hardy TG, Pace WG, Maney JW, Katz AR, Kaganov AL (1985) A biofragmentable ring for sutureless bowel anastomosis. Dis Colon Rectum 28: 484 – 490
10. Hildebrandt U, Pistorius G, Lindemann W, Kreissler-Haag D, Ecker KW (1995) Laparoskopische Resektionen bei Morbus Crohn, Chirurg 66: 807 – 812
11. Howell GP, Ryan JM, Morgans BT, Cooper J (1991) Assessment of the use of disposable skin staples in bowel anastomoses to reduce laparotomy time in penetrating ballistic injury to the abdomen. Ann R Coll Surg Edinb 73: 87 – 90
12. Jacobs M, Verdeya JC, Goldstein HS (1991) Minimally invasive colon resection (laparoscopic colectomy). Surg Laparosc Endosc 1: 144 – 150
13. Klaiber Ch, Tschudi J, Metzger A, Wagner M (1993) Minimal-invasive Chirurgie in Kombination mit offener Chirurgie. Langenbecks Arch Chir Suppl Kongressbd 117 – 123
14. Köckerling F, Schneider I, Gastinger I, Schneider B, Gall FP (1993) Laparoskopische Tabaksbeutelnahtklemme für die minimal invasive kolorektale Chirurgie. Minim Invasive Chir 2: 68 – 75
15. Lange V, Meyer G, Schardey HM, Gutschow Ch, Schildberg FW (1993) Verschiedene Techniken für die laparoskopische Dünndarmanastomosierung. Eine vorläufige Mitteilung. Chirurg 64: 408 – 411
16. Lange V, Meyer G, Schardey HM, Holker A, Lang R, Nerlich A, Schildberg FW (1995) Different techniques of laparoscopic end-to-end small-bowel anastomoses. Surg Endosc 9: 82 – 87
17. Latimer RG, Doane WA, McKittrick JE, Shepherd A (1975) Automatic staple suturing for gastrointestinal surgery. Am J Surg 130: 766 – 771
18. Marema RT (1993) Die laparoskopische Kolonresektion. Eine Übersicht über 50 Fälle, Chir Gastroenterol 9: 20 – 23
19. McGinty CP, Kasten MC, Kinder JL, Hunt RS (1979) Update on stapled bowel anastomosis. M Med 76: 145 – 150, 159
20. Meyer G, Lange V, Rau HG, Schardey HM, Schildberg FW (1994) Laparoskopische Einzelklammernaht – erste klinische Erfahrungen. Chirurg 65: 361 – 366

21. Meyer G, Lange V, Schardey HM, Holker A, Gutschow Ch, Schildberg FW (1994) Laparo-skopische Dünndarmanastomosierung – drei Techniken im Vergleich. In: Thiede A, Lünstedt B (eds) Standards in der Viszerosynthese, Springer, Berlin Heidelberg New York pp 46–56

22. Okudaira Y, Kholoussy AM, Sharf H, Yang Y, Matsumoto T (1984) Experimental study of singly placed staples for an everted intestinal anastomosis. Am J Surg 147 : 234–236

23. Phillips EH, Franklin M, Carroll BJ, Fallas MJ, Ramos R, Rosenthal D (1992) Laparoscopic colectomy. Ann Surg 216 : 703–707

24. Schlegel DM, Maglinte DDT (1982) The blind pouch syndrome. Surg Gynecol Obstet 155 : 541–544

25. Schneider IHF, Schneider C, Thaler K, Reck T, Köckerling F (1994) Intrakorporale Kolon-anastomosen mit laparoskopischer Tabaksbeutelnahtklemme und Valtrac-Ring. Langen-becks Arch Chir 379 : 188–192

26. Schüder G, Pistorius G, Plusczyk T, Hildebrandt U (1995) Technik und Qualität laparo-skopisch handgenähter Darmanastomosen im Experiment. Zentralbl Chir 120 : 409–414

27. Uddo JF (1995) Intestinal intracorporeal anastomosis. Paper presented at the Third Inter-national Congress of New Technology and Advanced Techniques in Surgery, Luxembourg, June 11–17

28. Wetherall AP, Cooper GJ, Ryan JM, Taylor DEM, Howell GP, Rice P (1992) Use of disposable skin staples for bowel anastomosis to reduce laparotomy time in war. Ann R Coll Surg Edinb 74 : 200–204

29. Wexner SD, Johansen OB (1992) Laparoscopic bowel resection: advantages and limi-tations. Ann Med 24 : 105–110

30. Wolharn R, Reuter F, von Kenne R, Clotten M, Szabo Z, Coburg AJ (1995) Laparoscopic hand-sewn Colon Anastomosis. Surg Endosc 9 : 242

31. Zucker KA, Pitcher DE, Martin DT, Ford RS (1994) Laparoscopic-assisted colon resection. Surg Endosc 8 : 12–18

Ultrasonography of Adhesions Prior to Laparoscopic Procedures After Previous Abdominal Operations

H. O. Steitz, G. Meyer, and F. W. Schildberg

Introduction

The risk of trocar-induced injuries of the abdominal organs during laparoscopic operations is 0.2%. In patients who have previously had a laparotomy, this risk rises by a factor of 10 to 2%, because of the development of adhesions between the abdominal organs and the abdominal wall as a consequence of the surgical procedures. Positioning the first blindly inserted trocar, in particular, can cause haemorrhage or injury to hollow organs as serious complications of the laparoscopy.

When there is reason to suspect the presence of major adhesions, laparoscopy after mini (re-)laparotomy is recommended instead of a blind puncture of the abdomen with the Veress needle. The purpose of this study was to confirm the suspicion of adhesions between the abdominal organs and the abdominal wall preoperatively by means of an ultrasound examination, and, if necessary, to mark lower-risk trocar insertion sites in the light of the planned operative strategy in each case.

Method

In 124 patients with a history of one or more laparotomies, the abdomen was explored sonographically using the "nine field technique" (Fig. 1) prior to the laparoscopic operation. Without preparing the patients in any special way, the abdomen was examined sonographically on the evening before surgery. The patients were supine and nine longitudinal scans were made, three each in the two mid-clavicular lines and in the median sagittal lines and in the upper, middle and lower abdomen. If existing scars and the planned trocar positions were not sufficiently explored by these nine scans, these regions were examined further. The cranio-caudal displaceability of liver, omentum and bowel relative to the abdominal wall during maximum forced respiration was measured. This adhesion sonography was performed with an Ultramark 5 from ATL, to which a linear array of 5 MHz frequency was connected, and a 7.5 MHz array was used for thin abdominal walls.

Fig. 1. Technique of adhesion ultrasound. The cranio-caudal slide of the abdominal organs relative to the abdominal wall is examined with longitudinal scans using the nine field technique in the upper, middle and lower abdomen in both mid-clavicular lines and in the median sagittal line during maximum forced inspiration

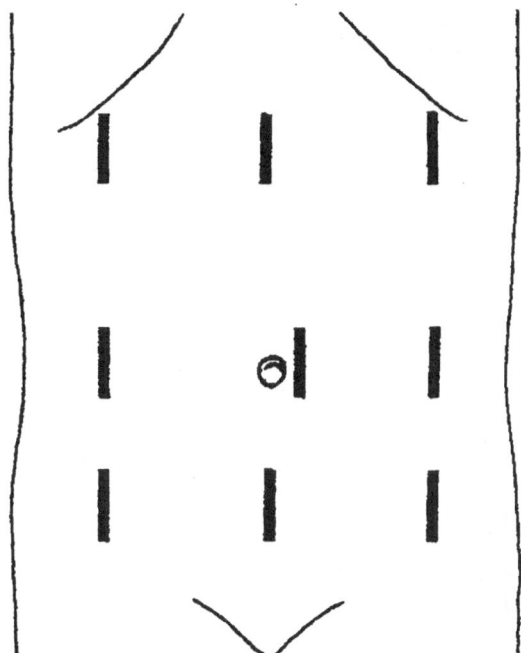

Results

It had already been shown in previous investigations that the border between the abdominal wall and the abdomen can be clearly identified during normal respiration by a fine echo-rich border lamella which does not move with respiration. This border lamella corresponds functionally to the parietal layer of the peritoneum but does not have a direct morphological correlate; it is rather an interface, which forms as an artefact due to the large jump in acoustic impedance on the border between the abdominal wall and the abdominal cavity. It is only the excursion that occurs with forced respiration, which gives information about the extent of any demonstrable restriction of cranio-caudal slide. Adhesions of the liver, bowel, omentum, and possibly of the stomach or urinary bladder also, can be clearly differentiated.

In the meantime, restrictions of the cranio-caudal displaceability of the abdominal organs relative to the abdominal wall have not only been described qualitatively but have also been classified quantitatively. The displaceability is more marked in the upper and middle abdomen than in the lower abdomen. We now define three basic degrees of restricted displaceability (Table 1). There is unrestricted displaceability in the upper and middle abdomen when there is cranio-caudal movement greater than 4 cm, while unrestricted displaceability can be assumed in the lower abdomen with cranio-caudal movement greater than 3 cm. In using this definition, it should be noted that the measurement points in the lower abdomen must be about halfway between the umbilicus

Table 1. Quantitative grading of the restricted cranio-caudal displaceability of the abdominal organs relative to the abdominal wall in the cranial two-thirds and in the lowest third of the abdomen

Degree of restriction	Cranial-caudal displaceability	
	Upper + middle abdomen (cm)	Lower abdomen (cm)
Free	≥ 4	≥ 3
Low	3–4	2–3
Medium	1.5–3	1–2
High	0–1.5	0–1

and the pubic symphysis. With low longitudinal scans cranio-caudal displaceability is slight even without adhesions to the abdominal wall, while with longitudinal scans made higher up the same displaceability can be assumed to approach that of the middle abdomen.

The restriction of cranio-caudal organ displaceability is described as slight, moderate or high. The extent of adhesions correlates directly with the severity of the limitation of movement, which we classify as first-, second- or third-degree. Low-grade restriction of displaceability is present in the upper and middle abdomen when the cranio-caudal displaceability is 3–4 cm, middle-grade restriction when displaceability is between 1.5–3 cm and high-grade restriction when a displaceabiltiy is less than 1.5 cm. In the lower abdomen, there is low-grade restriction of displaceability with cranio-caudal displaceability of 2–3 cm, middle-grade restriction with 1–2 cm and high-grade restriction with less than 1 cm.

Precise evaluation of cranio-caudal displaceability is only possible when the patient is able to cooperate and can inspire maximally when requested, with slow inspiration using the diaphragm and avoiding the accessory respiratory muscles. The correct breathing technique must be practiced with the patient before beginning the examination. For each measurement point, if there is doubt about the correctness of the rating and examination method, the measurement must be repeated until the patient has actually performed the desired maximum diaphragmatic ventilation. Slow inspiration is necessary in order to determine both the displaceability of the loops of bowel and, in particular, the exact quantitative displaceability of the omentum.

The grading of the severity of the adhesions has the following morphological correlates (Table 2): a first-degree adhesion is usually due only to the omentum, which is attached to the abdominal wall as a single strand or in moderately cribriform fashion. Second-degree adhesions can also involve adhesions of the omentum only which are either strongly cribriform or moderately extensive. In these cases, the bowel is only passively restricted in its movement. However, it can also be directly adherent with a single loop. Third-degree adhesions correlate with broad adhesions between the omentum and the abdominal wall. In general, the bowel is also involved and is fixed to the abdominal wall either at several points or over a broad area.

Table 2. Correlation between the degree of restriction of cranio-caudal displaceability and the morphological appearance of the adhesion

Degree of adhesion	Morphological correlate
First:	Omentum: single strand, slightly cribriform
Second:	Omentum: very cribriform, somewhat dense
	Bowel: single strand, passive with omental adhesion
Third:	Omentum: broad band, bowel usually involved
	Bowel: extensive, multiple single strands

There are often mixed findings in patients with variably marked restriction of displaceability at the different measurement points. Classification of the patient in these cases depends on the highest degree of adhesions measured. Operative logistics, however, are defined exclusively by the degree of adhesions at the planned trocar sites or possible alternatives to these.

Of the 124 patients studied, 89 had surgically relevant adhesions (Table 3). This corresponded to a prevalence of 71.8 % (Table 4). These adhesions were correctly identified ultrasonographically in 85 patients. The 35 patients without adhesions could be identified. However, in 4 other patients with adhesions, no ultrasound evidence of an adhesion was found. These data yield a sensitivity of 95.5 % with a specificity of 100 %. The positive predictive value (pV +) was 100%, the negative (pV –) 89.7 %.

Table 3. Results of qualitative diagnosis of adhesions in 124 patients in the four-quadrant table

Sonographic findings	Operative findings		Total
	Adhesions present	Adhesions absent	
Adhesions present	85	0	85
Adhesions absent	4	35	39
Total	89	35	124

Table 4. Accuracy of sonographic assessment of abdominal adhesions

	n	N	%
Prevalence of adhesions	89	124	71.8
Sensitivity	85	89	95.5
Specificity	35	35	100
Positive predictive value	85	85	100
Negative predictive value	35	39	89.7

Table 5. Summary of sonographic misdiagnoses

Location	Ultrasound findings	Operative findings
Middle abdomen[a]	Second-degree adh.[c]	First-degree adh.
Middle abdomen[a]	0[d]	Second-degree adh.
Lower abdomen[b]	0[e]	Second-degree adh.
Lower abdomen[b]	0[d]	Third-degree adh.
Lower abdomen[b]	0[e]	Second-degree adh.

[a] Periumbilical.
[b] Middle of lower abdomen after Pfannenstiel's incision.
[c] Overestimation of an omental adhesion with inadequate demonstration of the echoes reflected by the omentum.
[d] Failure to demonstrate adhesions due to inadequate patient cooperation.
[e] Adhesion only in the lowest part of the abdomen due to scars following Pfannenstiel's incision.

The false sonographic interpretations (Table 5) were due in two cases to the fact that in patients who had had a gynecological operation performed by a Pfannenstiel's incision, adhesions in the area of the scar over the pubic symphysis could not be differentiated from high-grade restricted craniocaudal displaceabiltiy in the lower segments of the abdomen. In two other cases, the adhesions were not recognised, because of insufficient cooperation by the patients. As a result, a third-degree adhesion in the lower abdomen and a second-degree adhesion in the middle abdomen were not identified sonographically. In one case, a first-degree adhesion in the middle abdomen was overestimated as second-degree, because the reflections from the omentum could not be distinctly differentiated and their movability was therefore underestimated.

Quantitatively (Table 6), a first-degree adhesion was diagnosed correctly by ultrasound in 20 of 21 patients and a third-degree adhesion in 35 of 36 patients. This corresponds (Table 7) to a sensitivity of 95.2% (grade I) and 97.2% (grade III). A second-degree was described in 30 patients sonographically, but

Table 6. Quantitative assessment of the degree of severity of the adhesions in 89 patients

Sonographic findings	Operative findings				
	None	First-degree	Second degree	Third-degree	Total
None	35	–	3	1	39
First-degree	–	20	–	–	20
Second-degree	–	1	29	–	30
Third-degree	–	–	–	35	35
Total	35	21	32	36	124

Table 7. Sensitivity of the quantitative assessment of the degree of severity of the adhesions

Degree of adhesion	Ultrasound findings	Operative findings	Sensitivity
First	20	21	95.2%
Second	30(29)[a]	32	93.8%
Third	35	36	97.2%
Total	85	89	95.5%

[a] A second degree adhesion was described in 30 of 32 patients, but one of these was a false-positive one.

Table 8. Operative consequences of the ultrasound findings in 124 patients

	n	%
Trocar position modified	14	16.5
Trocar sequence altered	10	11.8
Primary laparotomy	8	9.4
Trocar-induced injury	0	0

a first-degree adhesion was overestimated in one case. A second-degree adhesion was found in 32 patients at operation, correctly identified sonographically in only 29 patients. This corresponds to a sensitivity of 90.6%; when the one false-positive is taken into account, this would give a sensitivity of 93.8%.

The operative logistics were influenced by the preoperative sonography as follows (Table 8): the originally planned trocar position was modified in 14 cases (16.5%) and the sequence of trocar positioning was altered in 10 cases (11.8%). On the basis of the sonographic findings, it was decided in 8 patients (9.4%) not to perform laparoscopy and they underwent laparotomy. None of the patients in this group sustained a trocar-induced injury of the abdominal organs.

Discussion

In the series of examinations presented here, the preoperative sonography and the subsequent laparoscopy were performed by two different surgeons. It was possible to show that cranio-caudal restriction of slide of the abdominal organs can be ascribed qualitatively to adhesions on the abdominal wall, and that the degree of severity of these adhesions can be defined quantitatively by the extent of the reduction in displaceability. Quantitative analysis of the adhesions allows more differentiated operative planning, since the primary puncture can nearly always be performed with the Veress needle when there are first-degree adhesions, and even with second-degree adhesions, which arise only from attachment of the omentum, an attempt can be made with only slightly increased risk to produce the pneumoperitoneum and to position the primary trocar without resorting to a minilaparotomy.

Quantitative diagnosis of adhesions requires a patient who is able to co-operate. The examiner must be prepared to repeat the investigation when there is even a small doubt about optimum abdominal respiratory excursion until an unequivocal assessment of displaceabiltiy can be made.

The degree of severity of adhesions of the omentum only can be under-estimated, if bowel displaceability is well preserved, which can sometimes lead to haemorrhage from the fixed omentum, if a minilaparotomy is not performed in these cases. At the end of the laparoscopic operation, at the latest, the insertion site of the primary trocar must therefore be inspected for haemorrhage.

From the predicted values obtained, the following conclusions can be drawn for operative planning: if adhesions between the abdominal wall and abdomi-nal organs are described qualitatively in a patient, the presence of such adhesions can be confidently anticipated (pV+ = 100 %). Exclusion of an adhesion by ultrasound currently correlates with a probability (pV–) of 89.7 %. The part of the abdomen adjacent to the pubic symphysis in particular (e. g. following Pfannenstiel's incision) remains diagnostically "blind", but this is usually not of any significance for initial trocar positioning.

V Results: Morbidity, Mortality, Long-Term Results

Our Experience with Laparoscopic Colorectal Surgery

P. Petropoulos

Introduction

Since October 1993, we have been carrying out large bowel and rectal surgery laparoscopically in Fribourg Cantonal Hospital. Together with ten other Swiss hospitals (Table 1), we have treated over 160 patients using this technique since then. We perform laparoscopic surgery predominantly in patients with benign disease, and also patients with small malignant tumors, tumours requiring excision of the rectum or those that have already metastasized.

It is a basic postulate that a new technique must not alter the established method of a surgical operation without reason. In other words, we should not make any concessions to the new technique. The basic requirements of classical colon surgery must be met: operate cleanly, ensure vascularization, avoid traction on the anastomosis and ensure sufficiently radical resection. The cost must also be borne in mind.

Table 1. Swiss hospitals carrying out laparoscopic colorectal surgery

	No. of cases
Fribourg	76
Aarau (Klinik im Schachen)	2
Baden	12
Bern (Clinique Beau Site)	18
Geneva (HCUG)	1
Lugano (Ospedale Regionale)	1
Montreux	21
Morges	6
Payerne	4
Vevey	10
Yverdon	9
	160

Patients

In the period from October 1993 to September 1995, our group operated laparoscopically on 160 patients with colorectal disease. Forty patients had malignant and 120 patients had benign disease. Fifty-seven percent were men, with a mean age of 62 years; 42 % were women, with a mean age of 65 years. Tables 2 and 3 show the diagnoses and the operations carried out.

Table 2. Diagnoses in the
160 patients undergoing
laparoscopic colorectal
surgery

Diagnosis	No. of cases
Nonmalignant disease (*n* = 120)	
Crohn's disease of terminal ileum	1
Large polyps in right colon	3
Large polyps in left colon	6
Dolichocolon	2
Rectal prolapse	3
Sigmoid diverticulitis	98
Diverticulitis with sigmoidovesicular fistula	5
Sigmoid injury	2
Malignant disease (*n* = 40)	
Carcinoma of ascending colon	3
Malignant polyps	10
Sigmoid carcinoma (< 2 cm)	9
Rectal carcinoma	18
	160

Table 3. Laparoscopic
colorectal procedures carried
out

Procedure	No. of cases
Ileocaecal resection	1
Right hemicolectomy	6
Left hemicolectomy	6
Sigmoid resection	117
Low anterior resection	12
Anastomosis	2
	160

Laparaoscopic Technique

Our laparoscopic technique is as follows (this example is a sigmoid resection):

Position of Patient

The patient lies supine with the legs apart, and with the right leg a little lower than the left. The buttocks extend about 10 cm over the distal edge of the operating table, which makes operation of the circular stapler easier. The left buttock is raised by a pad and shoulder supports are attached to permit a Trendelenburg position. An armrest is secured over the patient's chest for the surgeon and the assistant.

Operating Team and Video Equipment

The surgeon, the first assistant and the instrument nurse stand on the patient's right. The second assistant stands between the patient's legs. The video equipment is to the left of the patient's feet and a second television monitor is to the left of his head.

Position of Trocars

The trocars are inserted in a circle, the centre of which is the left suprapubic region. Five trocars are inserted in total, two of 10 mm diameter, two of 10 – 12 mm diameter and one of 5 mm diameter.

Surgical Technique

After producing a pneumoperitoneum with CO_2 (10 – 12 mmHg), the trocars are inserted under visual control. The operation begins with inspection of the abdominal cavity. The patient is then put in the Trendelenburg position and the table is rotated towards the right. The small intestine thus lies cranially on the right. The coloparietal adhesions from the splenic flexure to the pelvis are divided. The left ureter is demonstrated and preserved. The median peritoneum is then incised and the vessels going to the bowel segment that is to be resected are clipped and divided. The proximal and distal resection levels of the colon are prepared, ensuring that a secure tension-free anastomosis is possible. The bowel is divided distally with an Endo GIA instrument. The prepared bowel is delivered through a 4- to 6-cm incision in the left suprapubic region. The bowel is now divided proximally outside the abdominal cavity and the head of a stapler with a diameter corresponding to the bowel lumen is introduced. The 2 – 0 Prolene suture inserted in the bowel wall is tied and the bowel is replaced inside the abdomen. The wound is closed in layers with continuous sutures. The pneumoperitoneum is restored. The circular stapler is inserted through the anus. The head of the stapler is joined to the trocar incorporated in the body of the stapler so that the anastomosis is made under laparoscopic vision and can be inspected for intactness. If there is a leak, it can be sutured laparoscopically. A drain is placed only if the surgeon regards it as necessary. The pneumoperitoneum is released, the instruments are withdrawn and the wounds are closed in layers.

Results

Conversion Rate

Changeover to the classical open technique was necessary in only 15 of the 160 patients (9.4%). The reasons are listed in Table 4.

Table 4. Conversions to open surgery among 160 laparoscopic colorectal procedures

	No. of cases
Problems with instruments	4
Inability to push the stapler up	4
Abscess formation in diverticulitis	3
Extensive tumor with uterine invasion	1
Left ureter injured	1
Trocar injury of transverse colon	1
Injury of wall of rectum	1
	15 (9.4%)

Operating Time

Laparoscopic procedures generally last about a third longer than the open procedure (65–300 min).

Postoperative Course

It is striking how quickly patients recover after this operation. Good bowel activity can be observed only a few hours later and complete oral nutrition is resumed by the 2nd postoperative day at the latest.

Analgesic Requirement

We analysed the requirement for analgesics and compared it with cases from conventional surgery. The requirement was exactly halved after the laparoscopic operations.

Duration of Hospitalization and Unfitness for Work

Compared with patients undergoing open surgery, the duration of hospitalization and unfitness for work was also reduced by at least one third.

Morbidity and Mortality

All recorded complications and the mortality are shown in Table 5. It should be mentioned that both are higher in cancer patients than in those with benign disease. For instance, we observed a massive haemorrhage on the 5th postoperative day which was treated in conventional operative fashion. An anastomotic leak with ileus occurred in two patients and was treated by laparotomy on both occasions. One patient who had rectal excision and who had had radiotherapy a year previously for prostatic carcinoma developed a urethro-

Table 5. Morbidity and mortality in 160 patients undergoing laparoscopic colorectal surgery

Complications ($n = 16$, 10%)	
Haematoma, seroma	5
Mural abscess	1
Anastomatic leak	2
Anastomotic stenosis[a]	1
Haemorrhage[b]	1
Postop. ileus with anastomotic leak	3
Urethroperitoneal fistula	1
Trocarsite metastases	1
Urinary incontinence	1
Deaths ($n = 2$, 1.2%)	
Septic shock (cancer)	1
Heart failure (cancer)	1

[a] Three months after surgery.
[b] Five days after surgery.

peritoneal fistula which was treated operatively 3 months later. A woman who had had amputation of the rectum developed urinary incontinence; this was treated with Cystofix products for suprapubic bladder drainage Regrettably, we noted metastases in the trocar puncture sites 8 months after surgery in a patient who had liver metastases prior to operation.

Conclusions

The laparoscopic technique as the method for resecting the colon and rectum cannot yet be indicated generally. We regard it increasingly as the surgical method of choice for all benign diseases but would be cautious in considering it for cancer patients. The metastases noted at the trocar puncture sites and in the peritoneum, in particular, as described in the literature even in patients with stage A disease, are on obstacle.

The significant advantages of the laparoscopic technique for colorectal procedures are that less pain is caused, the incisions are smaller, hospitalization is shorter, and the patient can return to work earlier.

The training of the surgeon in laparoscopic procedures is a task to be taken seriously and requires continuous training, whether in the laboratory or in collaboration with experienced surgeons.

Laparoscopic Rectosigmoid Resection for Carcinoma

E. Bärlehner, B. Heukrodt, and R. Schwetling

Introduction

There are very few stages in the development of surgery which have changed the field as profoundly as the laparoscopic operating technique. The break with a great deal of tradition, the technical demands and the difficulty in learning this operation skill have led to polemical discussions and arguments. In spite of considerable resistance, cholecystectomy and, in laparoscopic centres, appendicectomy and hernia repair procedures have become standard laparoscopic operations.

The advantages of minimally invasive surgery can be reproduced in procedures on all organs and can be demonstrated with large numbers of cholecystectomised patients [15, 16]. The main advantages relate to improved patient comfort owing to the

- Very small wounds,
- Reduced pain,
- Rapid mobilisation,
- Short hospital stay, and
- Short period of unfitness for work

associated with this kind of surgery. The reduction in morbidity is explained by a reduction in the various factors influencing morbidity:

- Less postoperative stress reaction syndrome
- Very little blood loss
- Low tissue trauma (peritoneum)
- Low fluid losses
- Low bacterial contamination
- Rare wound infections
- Rare herniation
- No wound dehiscence

Laparoscopic colorectal surgery was introduced by Cooperman et al. [1] and Zucker et al. [27] in 1991 and was given significant momentum in Germany by Köckerling [11–13)]. The great difficulty of these procedures and the particular problems with malignant disease make particular demands of the surgeon. Competence in abdominal surgery, cancer surgery and laparoscopic technique are all required, so that operative involvement is limited to a few centres [3, 13, 17].

There are three groups of problems to be dealt with in laparoscopic colorectal surgery:

1. Technical operative problems:
   - Identification of the lesion
   - Mobilisation
   - Resection
   - Anastomosis technique
   - Removal of specimen
2. Cancer Surgery problems:
   - Extended lymph node dissection with division of named vessels near their origin
   - En bloc operation (specimen consisting of primary tumor and lymph drainage area)
   - No incision of tumor
   - No perforation of tumor
3. Problems of recurrence:
   - Local recurrence
   - Atypical recurrence (trocar site recurrence)
   - Systemic recurrence

In order to answer to outstanding questions, we have analysed our own patients operated on laparoscopically with 82 colorectal procedures and 45 laparoscopically assisted rectosigmoid resections for carcinoma, performed in a standardised way.

Patients

From November 1992 to June 1995, 82 laparoscopic colorectal procedures were performed in the Klinikum Buch. There were 44 men and 38 women with an average age of 65 years (range 53–84 years). Thirty-four patients had benign disease; in these, the laparoscopically assisted sigmoid resection was the predominant operation ($n = 22$). Forty-eight patients underwent an operation for carcinoma with curative intent. The carcinomas were situated in the rectum ($n = 25$), sigmoid ($n = 18$), caecum ($n = 3$), ascending colon ($n = 1$) and descending colon ($n = 1$).

A standardised rectosigmoid resection was performed in 45 patients, in 3 of the cases as a laparoscopically assisted abdominoperineal resection of the rectum.

The extended histopathological examination of the resected tumor specimens was in accordance with the guidelines of the German Tumor Centres Working Group [2]. All tumor patients were recruited prospectively. The laparoscopically operated carcinoma patients were analysed without being selected according to oncological features and the extent of operative radicality was assessed. The operating time, transfusion requirement, clinical course and the results of follow-up were recorded. All patients who had a resection with restoration of continuity underwent radiological examination of the anastomosis between the 7th and 10th postoperative days. In a median follow-up of 11 months, rectoscopy and investigation of continence were performed.

Methods

The patients receive a liquid diet for 2 days preoperatively, and have bowel preparation with Prepacol (Guerbet) on the day before operation. All patients are operated on the lithotomy and extreme Trendelenburg position. Two monitors are required, one placed at the foot of the patient and one over the left shoulder. The surgeon stands on the right side, two assistants on the left. The optical trocar is positioned three finger-breadths above the umbilicus. Two operating trocars are inserted each side two finger-breadths below the umbilicus pararectally and medial to the iliac spine. The trocar in the right lower abdomen is 12 or 18 mm in size, and all the other trocars are 10 mm. The sigmoid is mobilised from the left after division of fetal adhesions with exposure of the ovarian or spermatic vessels and clear identification of the left ureter. The peritoneum is incised on the right of the root of the sigmoid mesocolon. Division of the sigmoid mesocolon is continued down to Gerota's fascia. The inferior mesenteric artery and vein are exposed and isolated. In cancer, the artery is divided high up with the 30-mm stapler. The inferior mesenteric vein is divided below the pancreas between clips. The mesocolon is skeletonised as far as the intended resection line in the distal descending colon. The peritoneum is incised pararectally as far as the rectovesical or rectouterine pouch. Mobilisation of the rectum on Waldeyer's fascia and ventrally in the rectovaginal space or on Denonvilliers' fascia is followed by division of pararectal tissue close to the pelvic wall with clipping or coagulation of the median rectal artery.

Distal dissection depends on the level of the lesion, with complete removal of the mesorectum in tumors of the middle and distal rectum. Careful preservation of the neurovascular bundle anterior to the rectum is particularly required [12, 13]. Distally, the rectum is divided with the linear stapler; we have found the 30-mm instrument best because it is the easiest to manoeuvre. The deepest division from above was 2 cm above the dentate line. The specimen is covered with the removal bag. The left colon is mobilised after division of the peritoneal reflection. The phrenocolic ligament is divided and the splenic flexure mobilised with division of the greater omentum. The trocar channel in the left lower abdomen is extended to a minilaparotomy. The laparotomy is protected with an adhesive ring film. The resected specimen is guided out and divided proximally. A pursestring suture is placed in the proximal bowel limb and the ILS press-on disc is tied in place (29–33 mm, Ethicon). The bowel is returned to the abdomen und the minilaparotomy is closed. The capnopneumoperitoneum is restored. The stapler shaft is introduced transanally. The row of staples is perforated by the central spike, it is joined to the press-on disc and the anastomosis is made. Integrity of the anastomosis is tested with methylene blue solution, and it is checked to ensure that it is not under tension. A Robinson drain is always placed in the presacral space. When the rectum is amputated, the proximal limb of bowel is sutured in the extended trocar channel in the left lower abdomen as a colostomy and the resected specimen is removed distally after perineal excision.

Results

All 45 cancer patients undergoing a standardised rectosigmoid resection survived the laparoscopic procedure. We recorded complications in six patients (13.3%), as follows: two intraoperative complications (one injury to a ureter, one injury to the rectal stump with the stapler) and four postoperative complications (one sacral ileus/distal obstruction, one small bowel fistula and two anastomotic leaks). The ureteric injury was repaired through the mini-laparotomy and the rectal stump performation was repaired transanally. The anastomotic leak required proximal diversion in the first case; in the second it was sutured transanally. Two complications (4.4%) required open revision (small bowel fistula in a necrotic carcinoma, sacral ileus/distal obstruction after rectal amputation).

Operating time was 217 min on average. All laparoscopic procedures concluded laparoscopically. In three cases, the operation had to be continued openly after laparoscopic diagnosis (two patients with anaesthetic-induced air insufflation of the bowel, one patient with a large carcinoma of the descending colon and extension into the retroperitoneum). The conversion rate was 6.7%.

Advanced tumor stages predominated according to the histopathological report (stage N1–3 in 56% of patients). UICC stages are indicated in Table 1.

Ro resections were achieved in 98% of patients; there was one R2 resection. The R2 specimen was from a laparoscopically assisted amputation of the rectum which was incurable distally. Table 2 shows the length of the resected

Table 1. ICC tumor stages of 45 rectosigmoid carcinomas

Stage	No. of patients	%
I	10	22.2
II	10	22.2
III a	9	20.0
III b	16	35.6
	45	100.0

Table 2. Number of lymph nodes, length of resected specimens and number of patients who received transfusions in 45 rectosigmoid resections

Tumor site	No. of patients	Length of resected specimen (fixed, median) (cm)	No. of lymph nodes (median)	Transfusion (no. of patients)
Sigmoid	22	23.7	26.3	1
Rectum	23	23.6	25.2	4

specimens, number of lymph nodes and the number of patients requiring blood transfusion.

Follow-up for a median of 11 months included 85 % of the patients. Seventy-four percent of the anastomoses were in the middle third, 23 % in the lower third and 3 % in the upper third of the rectum. Ninety percent of patients stated that they were fully continent. Mild incontinence and stool leaking each occurred in 5 %. Tumor progression was found in four patients: one case of atypical recurrence at a trocar site in a patient with peritoneal carcinomatosis, and three cases of metachronous liver metastases (one in a patient with a second carcinoma). There was no local recurrence.

Discussion

Since the first laparoscopically assisted sigmoid resection for carcinoma was performed by Fowler and White [5], minimally invasive surgery has been developing increasingly as a procedure in competition with the open technique. The predominant location of benign and malignant lesions in the rectum and sigmoid colon, the fairly constant vascular anatomy and the transanal approach for the anastomosis have favoured the laparoscopic technique for this region of the bowel.

The benefits of laparoscopic technique are stated as shorter hospitalisation, less pain, early return of gastrointestinal function and fewer wound infections [9, 18]. The technical feasibility of the laparoscopic operation in colon cancer has been confirmed by several large series of cases [3, 7, 8, 24, 25, 27]. Identification of the malignant lesion in the rectosigmoid region was possible using the palpating laparoscopic instrument in the majority of our 45 patients. In 5 cases, orientation was achieved endoscopically. Primary mobilisation of the sigmoid colon from the left has proved worthwhile because of the early exposure of the left ureter. Irritation of the tumor is not inevitable if the area is marked by a clip or suture. Early on in the learning phase we recorded one division of the ureter when the inferior mesenteric vein was divided. It was noticed immediately and repaired through the minilaparotomy.

In accordance with the general principles of cancer surgery [2, 8], high division of the mesenteric vessels was performed in all patients, for which adequate mobilisation of the splenic flexure is always required. Dissection in the pelvis follows anatomical tissue planes [11 – 13] and is seen more easily and in more detail when done laparoscopically than in the open technique. During division of the pararectal tissues close to the pelvic wall, the median rectal artery can be demonstrated as a rule and is divided between clips. Preservation of the prerectal neurovascular bundle also seems more secure to us. With proximal rectal carcinomas and the sigmoid carcinomas, resection was regularly done in the middle third of the rectum. This guarantees problem-free placing of the stapled anastomosis in addition to sufficiently radical excision while maintaining perfusion intact.

We have used a 30-mm stapler repeatedly for the distal division and have encountered the problems reported by other authors to only a limited extent

[3]. With adequate distal mobilisation and steering of the instrument from the right lower abdomen, nearly perpendicular division of the rectum is possible. The deepest row of staples was 2 cm proximal to the dentate line. In three cases, the rectum was divided transanally at the level of the dentate line after deep laparoscopic dissection, and a coloanal anastomosis was fashioned. A technical improvement of the linear stapler with a greater branch opening for the distal rectum, which is often voluminous, would simplify handling considerably; with currently available instruments, an injury occurred deep in the rectum in one case, which could be repaired adequately by transanal suturing.

Secure anastomosis technique is the most important prerequisite for low morbidity rates. Since unproblematic removal of the specimen is at present only possible through a minilaparotomy, the double row stapling technique appears currently to be the best method of anastomosis in the left colon [5, 9, 10, 24, 25]. Out of 42 anastomoses in the region of the rectum after resection of carcinoma, we saw 2 cases of anastomotic leak (4.7%). The clinical leak rate with the open stapled method is given as between 4.1% [25] and 12.1% [6]. Jansen observed a clinically apparent anastomotic leak in only 1 of 51 laparoscopically assisted colon resections. The perioperative complication rate of 13.3% with a mortality rate of 0% in an unselected group of patients shows no disadvantages compared to the open technique [21, 22, 23]. Data in this regard relating to laparoscopic colorectal operations varied between 6.1% and 24% for morbidity [10, 19, 27] and 0% and 1.9% mortality.

Our conversion rate at 6.7%, was comparatively low; conversion rates between 13.7% and 22% [10,19] have been given in reports of laparoscopic experience. In our three cases, conversion took place after diagnostic laparoscopy, and all operations which began laparoscopically were concluded in the same way.

The particular features of laparoscopic cancer operations are due to the high vessel ligation and the resected safety margins. On no account should a compromise be made in favour of the laparoscopic technique at the expense of radical resection. The length of resected specimens, injuries to the tumor and the number of lymph nodes are measurable criteria of quality [7, 8] and should be analysed by critical histopathology. Our numbers of lymph nodes, with a median of 25.2 for rectal cancer and 26.3 for sigmoid cancer, meet the standard requirements; the average specimen length of 23 cm average is similar to comparable reports from other authors [7]. Tumor injury was not found in any case.

The histopathological report confirms Ro resection in 44 of 45 patients. Current standards in the surgery of rectal and sigmoid carcinoma should be met laparoscopically without qualification. Subsequent examination with a median follow-up time of 11 months yielded tumor recurrence in 4 of the 45 patients (8.9%), localised in the liver in 3, and 1 patient with peritoneal carcinomatosis developed a recurrence in the trocar channel (working trocar). No local recurrence has been observed so far. All recurrences resulted from tumors in stages pT3N1 – 3; the peritoneal carcinomatosis with port recurrence occurred with a pT4N2 tumor. At 55.6% the advanced cancers (pT3, pT4) are overrepresented in our patient group. In UICC stages I and II, there have been no recurrences so far. In the series reported by Safi [23], recurrences were diagnosed 13 months postoperatively on average, and the recurrence rate was 35% in rectal carcinoma. The incidence of local recurrence is given as 10.5% in all stages and 18.9% in stage II in the CRCSG (Colorectal Carcinoma Study Group) study.

While the metachronous liver metastases result from occult tumor dissemination at the time of the operation [14], local recurrence rates depend in part on the operative procedure [2]. An assessment of our results is not possible because of the short oberservation period, but at any rate there is no disadvantage apparent compared to experiences in conventional tumor surgery.

Trocar channel or abdominal wall recurrences are particularly emphasized in the discussion on laparoscopic tumor surgery, but are also observed in laparotomy scars after open surgery. In the majority of cases, they can be attributed to advanced tumor stage and diffuse peritoneal carcinomatosis. Ramos et al. [20] have recorded port recurrences in 3 cases out of 208 patients (1.4%) and came to the conclusion that the rate is very low and are to be attributed less to the technique than to the extent of the cancer.

Subsequent examination of 85% of all patients showed an anastomotic stenosis in two cases (4.4%) which could be treated by dilatation. Fingerhut et al. [4] observed a stenosis rate of 16% in their study, no clear causes for which were apparent. Finally, the inverted part of the anastomosis with implanted metal staples is subject to secondary healing with fibrosis and a tendency to shrink. The continence of our patients in view of the low rectal anastomoses in 25% was very satisfactory: 90% were fully continent, while 10% had an occasional disturbance of continence.

In conclusion, our experiences with 45 laparoscopic carcinoma operations in the rectosigmoid area do not show any disadvantages compared to the conventional technique. However, we do not have long-term observations. This very demanding operating method should be restricted to special centres for the present and should be monitored in studies.

References

1. Cooperman, AM, Katz V, Zimmon D, Botero G (1991) Laparoscopic colon resection: a case report. J Laparoendosc Surg 1:122–224
2. Hermanek P (ed) Diagnostische Standards in der Onkologie. Zuckschwerdt, Munich
3. Faust H, Reichel K (1995) Laparoskopische Kolonresektion – ist eine onkologische Resektion auf laparoskopischem Wege möglich? Zentralbl Chir 120:392–395
4. Fingerhut A, Elhadad A, Hay JM, Lacaine F, Flamant Y (1994) Infrapreritoneal colorectal anastomosis, hand-sewn versus circular staples. A controlled clinical trial. Surgery 116:484–489
5. Fowler DL, White SA (1991) Laparoscopy-assisted sigmoid resection. Surg Laparosc Endosc 1:183–188
6. Mc Ginn FP, Gartell PC, Cliffort PC, Brunton FJ (1985) Staples or sutures for low colorectal anatomoses. A prospective randomized trial. Br J Surg 72:603–608
7. Gray D, Lee H, Schlinkert R, Beart RW (1994) Adequacy of lymphadenectomy in laparoscopic-assisted colectomy for colorectal cander: a preliminary report. J Surg Oncol 57:8–10

8. Hermanek P, Wittekind Ch (1994) Inwieweit sind laparoskopische Verfahren in der onkologischen Chirurgie vertretbar? Chirurg 65 : 23 – 28
9. Jacobs M, Verdeja JC, Goldstein HS (1991) Minimally invasive colon resection (laparoscopic colectomy). Surg Laparosc Endosc 1 : 144 – 150
10. Jansen A (1994) Laparoscopic-assisted colon resection. Evolution from an experimental technique to a standardized surgical procedure. Ann Chir Gynaecol 83 : 86 – 91
11. Köckerling F, Gastinger I, Schneider B, Krause W, Gall FP (1992) Laparoskopische kolorektale Chirurgie: Kolon- und Rektumanastomosen in Triple-Stapling-Technique. Minim Invasive Chir 1 : 44 – 50
12. Köckerling F, Gastinger J, Schneider B, Krause W, Gall FP (1992) Laparoskopische abdomino-perineale Rektrumexstirpation mit hoher Durchtrennung der A. mesenterica inferior. Chirurg 63 : 345 – 348
13. Köckerling F, Gall FP (1994) Chirurgische Standards beim Rectumcarcinom. Chirurg 65 : 593 – 603
14. Lindemann F, Schlimok G, Dirschedl P, Witte J, Rithmüller G (1992) Prognostic significance of micrometastatic tumor cells in bone marrow of colorectal cancer patients. Lancet 340 : 685 – 689
15. Löhde E, Raude H, Kleine U, Schairer W, Kraas E (1994) Erfahrungen nach 2200 laparoskopischen Cholecystektomien als Behandlungskonzept des Gallensteinleidens. Zentralbl Chir 119 : 371 – 377
16. Morlang T, Umscheid T, Stelter WJ (1995) Laparoskopische Cholecystektomie: eine prospektive Studie an 1775 unselektierten Patienten. Zentralbl Chir 120 : 353 – 359
17. Müller G, Herold A, Schiedeck T, Bruch HP (1995) Laparoskopische Rektumchirurgie. Minim Invasive Chir 4 : 33 – 40
18. Plasencia G, Jacobs M, Verdeja JC, Viamonto M (1994) Laparoscopic-assisted sigmoid colectomy and low anterior resection. Dis Colon Rectum 37 : 829 – 833
19. Puente J, Sosa JL, Sleeman D, Desai U, Tranakas N, Hartmann R (1994) Laparoscopic assisted colorectal surgery. J Laparoendosc Surg 4 : 1 – 7
20. Ramos JM, Gupta S, Anthone G, Ortega AE, Simons AJ, Bearth RW (1994) Laparoscopy and colon cancer. Is the port site a risk? A preliminary report. Arch Surg 129 : 897 – 899
21. Riedl S, Wiebelt H, Bergmann U, Hermanek P (1995) Postoperative Komplikationen und Letalität in der chirurgischen Therapie des Coloncarcinoms. Chirurg 66 : 597 – 606
22. Safi F, Beger HG (1994) Morbidität und Letalität der operativen Therapie des colorektalen Carcinoms. Chirurg 65 : 127 – 131
23. Safi F (1995) Recurrence and survival rates after surgical therapy of rectal cancer. Symposium of Rectal Cancer, Berlin, September 1995
24. Senagore AJ, Luchtefeld MA, Mackeigan JM, Mazier WP (1993) Open colectomy versus laparoscopic colectomy: are there differences? Am Surg 59 (8) : 549 – 553
25. Szinicz G, Beller S, Zerz A, Erhardt K (1992) Laparoskopisch unterstützte Sigmaresektion. Chirurgische Technik und erste Erfahrungen. Chir Gastroenterol 9 : 24 – 27
26. West of Scotland and Highland Anastomosis Study Group (1991) Suturing or stapling in gastrointestinal surgery: a prospective randomized study. Br J Surg 78 : 337 – 341
27. Zucker KA, Pitcher DE, Martin DT, Ford RS (1994) Laparoscopic assisted colon resection. Surg Endosc 8 : 12 – 18
28. Hermanek P Jr, Wiebelt H, Riedl S, Staimmer D, Hermanek P et al. (1994) Langzeitergebnisse der chirurgischen Therapie des Coloncarcinoms. Chirurg 65 : 287 – 297

Laparoscopically Assisted Colorectal Surgery: A Review of 87 Cases

I. Baca and V. Götzen

The obvious advantages of laparoscopic surgery, such as less postoperative pain, short hospital stay and earlier return to normal activities [1], have led to an increase in the performance of laparoscopic procedures besides the now established laparoscopic cholecystectomy [2–6]. A new generation of instruments has been developed which enable us to perform even complicated operations [7]. This, together with important technological advances in the management of colon and rectal diseases in recent years – such as the development of video colonoscopy and stapling devices – has led us to use laparoscopic techniques in various types of colon resection as well.

First reports about the application of laparoscopic colorectal surgery were published in 1991 [8, 9]. Since then a number of medical centers have reported their experience [10, 14], but no detailed analysis are yet available to document significant savings over open laparotomy procedures. The present study analyzed our experience and results in 87 patients who underwent attempted laparoscopic-assisted colorectal surgery in the course of nearly 3 years in our hospital.

Patients

The diagnoses for which laparoscopic surgery was performed, and the types and number of colonic procedures carried out between the beginning of 1993 and the end of September 1995, are shown in Table 1. All patients with malignant disease and the majority of patients with benign disease were carefully selected for laparoscopically assisted colorectal surgery, and all operations except one were elective. Patients were informed of the nature of their disease and the proposed surgery and recorded in a protocol prospectively. Data recorded in the study related to the type of operation attempted, conversion to open laparotomy, operative parameters, duration of operation, pathologic findings, complications, postoperative analgesic requirements, length of postoperative stay, and, in malignant disease, follow-up examination findings.

Fifty-three patients were women and 44 were men, with a mean age of 64 ± 6 years. Of the successfully completed laparoscopically assisted colorectal operations, 49 were for benign disease and 32 for malignancy.

Table 1. Laparoscopically completed colorectal procedures ($n = 81$)[a]

Diagnosis	Procedure	n
Diverticulitis	Sigmoid resection	29
	Hartmann's procedure	1
	Reversal of Hartmann's	8
Crohn's disease	Ileocecal resection	4
	Repeat operation	1
Ulcerative colitis	Proctocolectomy	1
Rectal prolapse	Rectopexy	2
Colon adenoma	Sigmoid resection	2
	Right hemicolectomy	1
Sigmoid carcinoma	Sigmoid resection	10
Rectal carcinoma	Low anterior resect.	2
	Abdomino perineal resection	5
Cecal carcinoma	Right hemicolectomy	6
Ascending colon carcinoma	Right hemicolectomy	9
		81

[a] Six procedures were converted to open surgery.

Operative Techniques

All operations were performed with laparoscopical assistance with intracorporeal anastomosis for left colon procedures and extracorporeal anastomosis for right colon procedures. Apart from two operations, all were done by one surgeon.

Sigmoid Resection

For sigmoid and rectal resection we perform a laparoscopically assisted operation with intracorporeal anastomosis. As preoperative preparation for elective procedures, patients receive 4 l electrolyte solution for orthograde bowel lavage. The patient is placed in the lithotomy and Trendelenburg position. In addition to the operating surgeon there are two assistants. Usually the surgeon stands on the right of the patient. Four trocars are used, one for the lens and three to work. The 30° lens is inserted through a 10-mm trocar above the umbilicus. One 12-mm trocar is placed in the left side, a 15-mm trocar on the right side of the lower abdomen, and a 5-mm trocar close by over the symphysis. First the resection margins are determined. Then the sigmoid is mobilized free of embryonal attachments and any inflammatory adhesions, the left ureter being exposed in all cases. In benign colon disease the bowel is now dissected in the area of the proximal resection level using a linear stapler. Next the mesosigmoid is dissected near the bowel wall using the 30-mm linear stapler. Now it is possible to luxote the bowel gradually from the pelvis. At the end of the dissection the bowel is transected using a 60-mm linear stapler at the distal resection level below the affected segment. In malignant sigmoid and rectal disease, after mobilization the mesocolon together with vascular and lymphatic tributaries is first divided proximally, usually using a linear vascular stapler. To avoid contamination, the resected portion of colon is placed in a bag. The pneumoperitoneum is released and the left trocar incision is enlarged (recently we have started to use the suprapubic trocar incision). Through this incision the resected bowel segment is withdrawn. In cancer cases, the specimen is removed en bloc with the entire corresponding mesentery, including vessels and lymph nodes. Anastomosis is effected by means of a double stapling technique. When the left colon is withdrawn from the abdomen the anvil of a circular stapler is placed extracorporeally into the proximal bowel. The prepared stump is returned to the abdomen, a drain is placed, and the incision is closed in layers. After reestablishment of pneumoperitoneum, the circular stapler is introduced transanally. Under direct vision the anvil and shaft are connected and then the anastomosis is created in the standard fashion inspection of the donuts and checking for integrity.

Right Hemicolectomy

For right side lesions an extracorporeal anastomosis is performed in all patients. The procedure requires placement of three or four laparoscopic cannulas. The surgeon stands on the left and the assistants on the right side of the patient. After placement of a left paraumbilical cannula, two other trocars are placed suprapubically in the upper and lower right quadrants. After the cecum, ascending colon, and hepatic flexure have been mobilized from their attachments, the peritoneum overlying the mesocolon is incised and the mesenteric vessels are clipped and divided. After the bowel is mobilized laparoscopically, a small incision (4–7 cm) is made at the site of the port in the right upper quadrant. The bowel is grasped and drawn trough the wound. If necessary the mesenteric dissection is completed extracorporeally. After the bowel is transected, the anastomosis is done by the hand-sewing technique. The bowel is then returned to the abdomen and the wound is closed, usually without a drain.

Colostomy Closure and Anastomosis After Hartmann's Procedure

We start our procedure for reversal of Hartmann's procedure with three trocars placed as in sigmoid resection except the left one, where usually the colostomy is sited. After laparoscopic adhesiolysis, the Hartmann stump is located using a rectoscope or dilatator. The colostomy is excised and after fixation of the anvil of the stapler the colon is returned to the abdomen. The wound is closed and pneumoperitoneum is reestablished. The rest of the procedure is similar to that of sigmoidresection.

Rectopexy

One 10-mm and three 12-mm trocars were placed near the umbilicus, bilaterally in the abdomen and suprapubically. Mobilization of the distal sigmoid is started, as in open operation, with incision of parietal attachments and identification of the left ureter. Posterior and lateral mobilization of the rectum is completed using blunt and sharp dissection and electrocoagulation as needed. After that the pelvis is well visualized down to the levator musculature. A 4 × 10-cm polypropylene mesh is introduced and placed in the presacral space. The mesh is fixed with a hernia stapler in the midline below the sacral promontory, after which the rectum is secured in a suspended position by suture with Endo stitching to the mesh edges.

Results

Of the 87 patients in whom laparoscopically assisted colorectal surgery was attempted, 6 required conversion from laparoscopic to open technique. Conversion was necessary in four cases for inflammatory sigmoid colon disease and in two cases because of the presence of adhesions.

Operative time and length of postoperative stay are shown in Table 2. The mean age of patients with benign disease was 59 years and that of patients with malignant disease was 70 years. Average operative time in the 81 patients in whom laparoscopically assisted colorectal surgery was completed was 150 ± 60 min. Average time cases of benign disease was 160 ± 62 min in cases of malignancy 145 ± 52 min. The longest operation lasted 360 min; this was a protocolectomy with ileum pouch. The overall average length of postoperative stay was 12 days, the averages varying with the different types of procedure

Table 2. Operative times and postoperative hospital stay according to reason for surgery

	n	Average ages (years)	Average operative time (min)	Average postop. stay (days)
Diverticulitis	38	62	160	12
Crohn's disease	5	35	145	8
Ulcerative colitis	1	50	360	10
Rectal prolapse	2	72	97	10
Colon adenoma	3	63	110	9
Sigmoid carcinoma	10	73	160	15
Rectal carcinoma	7	64	180	16
Cecal carcinoma	6	68	105	11
Ascending colon carcinoma	9	72	125	12
	81	64	150	12

(Table 2). Patients with benign disease were often earlier discharged than those with malignancy, but this was not statistically significant.

The nasogastric tube was removed on the 1st day in 60 patients and on the 2nd in 21. Gastrointestinal function, defined as intake of solid food with flatus or bowel movements, returned in an average of 3 days after surgery. On average, parenteral narcotics were used for 2 days.

Complications of surgery were noted in 12 patients (Table 3). Two patients developed a wound infection of the incisions used for a facilitated anastomosis. Two patients developed manifest anastomostic leakage, one after sigmoid resection for diverticulitis and one after reversal of Hartmann's procedure. One patient suffered from postoperative bleeding, which was successful treated laparoscopically. Another developed pneumothorax 2 days after surgery. Ileus with absence of bowel activity, and nasogastric decompression for 3 or more days, occurred in four patients. There were two deaths, one in the laparoscopically assisted colorectal group and one in the converted open colectomy group, caused by anastomotic leakage.

The histological diagnoses of patients with colorectal tumor were adenoma in 3 cases and carcinoma in 32 (Table 4). The average number of lymphnodes harvested was 10 ± 3. Patients undergoing sigmoid and rectum resection had an average of 8 lymph nodes removed and those undergoing right hemicolectomy an average of 11. In nine patients the procedure was palliative because of distant metastasis. In six cases lymph nodes showed signs of metastatic spread.

Table 3. Perioperative and postoperative complications in 87 patients

	n
Wound infection	2
Ileus	4
Anastomosis insufficiency	2
Hemorrhage	1
Pneumothorax	1
Death	2

Table 4. Histological diagnoses of patients with colorectal tumors

	n	Lymph-nodes (average no.)	Adenoma	Cancer stages		
				T1-T3N0M0	T1-T3N1M0	TNM1
Sigmoid and rectal resection	14	8	2	8	2	2
Rectal amputation	5	9	–	1	1	3
Right hemicolectomy	16	11	1	8	3	4
Total	35	10	3	17	6	9

Table 5. Postoperative follow-up for colorectal cancer ($n = 32$)

	Stage T1-T3N0M	Months of follow-up (average)	Stage T1-T3N1M0	Months of follow-up (average)	Stage TNM1	Months of follow-up (average)
Patients alive	17	12	6	24	5	7
Recurrence (port-site metastasis)			1			
Distant metastasis			1			
Deaths						4

Follow-up time (Table 5) was on average 13 months. Seventeen patients with stage 1 and 2 tumors are well without complaints. Four patients with stage 3 tumors are also well, while one showed distant metastasis after 24 months and received chemotherapy. One 84-year-old women developed a port-site metastasis 2 years after laparoscopic sigmoid resection. After local removal of the metastasis, she is now alive 32 months after the primary operation. Of the nine patients who underwent palliative operation, four died within 7 months.

Discussion

Reports from other groups [11–13, 15, 16] and our own experience with 87 laparoscopic procedures in colorectal surgery have shown that this procedure can be performed with an operative risk equal to that of conventional surgery.

Laparoscopic surgery can be used in benign and malignant disease if the patients are selected carefully [13, 16, 17]. We performed nearly the whole spectrum of colorectal procedures with a conversion rate of 7%.

We described the technical procedure precisely. Newly developed instruments enable us to perform the operations better, more safely and more quickly. Under certain circumstances a large inflammatory tumor forces conversion to an open procedure.

The use of laparoscopic techniques in malignant disease is hotly debated [18, 19]. The benign disease, it seems that the risk are not greater than those of conventional procedures [12–14]. Generally, laparoscopic surgery is more difficult and more complex, which is expressed in a longer operation time.

We achieved an acceptable complication rate in our group of patients. One of the two patients who died suffered from diverticulitis, the other from carcinoma. The 80-year-old woman with diverticulitis sustained a perforation of the anastomosis intraoperatively after a successfully completed laparoscopic procedure when a rectal tube was placed. She died 5 weeks later of prolonged sepsis caused by a retroperitoneal phlegmon which developed from perforation with contamination. The second patient, who had a small tumor of the sigmoid colon, died 48 h postoperatively of a septic shock due to anastomotic leak. The patient underwent conventional open reoperation and the anastomosis was renewed. We found an early anastomotic leak which was difficult to explain, because the integrity of the anastomosis was confirmed intraoperatively and the donuts of the circular stapler found to be intact.

It must be remembered in a critical evaluation that our patients were carefully selected and that nearly all operations were performed by the same surgeon. On the other hand, this was a new operative technique being introduced with a corresponding learning phase [20]. In our opinion, the operation time and the complication rate will be reduced with experience. This is what has happened with other groups [13, 20].

At present, the equipment available for laparoscopic colon resection makes it three times as expensive as conventional surgery. Shorter hospitalization should compensate for the intraoperative costs [12], but we failed to obtain a meaningful reduction of the hospital stay with our patients. One reason for this was that we chose to have patients stay longer while this new technique was being introduced, in order to exclude all possible postoperative complications.

There are working groups who have shown that laparoscopic colectomy is a cost-efficient procedure. The decrease in costs, as with laparoscopic cholecystectomy, is related to the decrease in the need for inpatient care [12, 13, 16]. Undoubtedly it is a fact that the hospital stay can be reduced as experience increases, and that market forces will decrease the cost of instrumentation in the future. Greater experience and better handling will minimize the use of single-use instruments, so that the costs will match those of the conventional procedure.

It seems that our observations confirm the benefits of this method during the postoperative period, which have meanwhile been proven for other laparoscopic procedures [1, 2, 6]. Patients recover more quickly and with few complications, and feel less pain, which is reflected in reduced analgesic requirements. Experience shows that bowel function returns 4–5 days after in conventional surgery. Despite initial caution, were able to start oral nutrition, 2 days after laparoscopic surgery, as opposed to 4 days after conventional surgery. Leaving the nasogastric tube in place for longer than 24 h was exceptional. Only in four patients did we see mild ileus for a short period.

We closely followed the colorectal carcinoma group postoperatively. The major controversy associated with laparoscopically assisted resection is whether this allow sufficiently radical resection with removal of lymph nodes for staging and for treatment [21]. In view of the debate on this subject, we mainly performed laparoscopic procedure for tumors in early stages or with palliative intention. In regard to the number of lymph nodes and the size of the specimen, pathohistological results showed no difference from the conventional method, as other groups have also shown [11, 13, 16, 18].

In this group of patients we saw one special feature during the average follow-up of 13 months: in the group of six patients we operated on with tumor stage C, one port-site metastasis occurred in a 84-year-old patient after 24 months. This was one of our first operations and we did not use an endobag, so this complication can be explained by our technique at the time. Nevertheless, the literature contains reports of the frequent occurrence of metastases at port sited after laporoscopic treatment of the colon [20], and also at other incisions, even if the specimen is retrieved using a bag [19].

Specific questions relating to technique focus on the pneumoperitoneum that is required and the attendant increased intra-abdominal pressure (15 or 16 mmHg), which exceeds the pressure in capillaries, lymphatics, and possibly event terminal venules. The question is, if gas can enter the bloodstream, under pressure can tumor cells be spread by this increased pressure?

A number of medical centers have reported their experience [4, 11, 13, 16] but no detailed analyses are yet available to document significant savings over open laparotomy. These questions must be answered in a prospective randomized study. Until such studies are available, in our opinion colorectal carcinoma should only be operated on laparoscopically at an early stage or with palliative intent. From our experience, a laparoscopic procedure can at present recommended in patients with uncomplicated benign diseases of the colon. Our patients confirm us in our policy, specially mentioning the early painlessness and the early commencement of normal nutrition, besides cosmetic aspects, as reasons to continue this procedure.

References

1. The Southern Surgeons Club (1991) A prospective analysis of 1518 laparoscopic cholecystectomies. N Engl J Med 324:1073–1078
2. Dallemagne B, Weerts JM, Jehaes C, Markiewicz S, Lombard R (1991) Laparoscopic Nissen funduplication. Surg Laparosc Endosc 1:138–143
3. Kathouda N, Mouiel J (1991) A new technique of surgical treatment of chronic duodenal ulcer without laparotomy by videocoelioscopy. Am J Surg 161:361–364
4. Berman IR (1992) Sutureless laparoscopic rectopexy for procidentia. Technique and implications. Dis Colon Rectum 35:689–693361–364
5. Klotz HP, Schlumpf R, Weder W, Largarder F (1993) Minimal invasive surgery for treatment of symptomatic liver cyst. Surg Laparosc Endosc 3:351–353
6. Fitzgibbons RJ, Camps J, Cornet DA, Nguyen NX, Litke BS, Annibali R (1995) Laparoscopic inguinal herniorrhaphy. Result of a multicenter trial. Ann Surg 221:3–13
7. Brune IB, Schönleben K (1993) Laparo-Endoskopische Chirurgie. Hans Marseille, Munich
8. Jacobs M, Verdeja JC, Goldstein HS (1991) Minimally invasive colon resection. Surg Laparosc Endosc 1:144–150
9. Fowler DL, White SA (1991) Laparoscopy assisted sigmoid resection. Surg Laparosc Endosc 1:183–188
10. Phillips EH, Franklin M, Carroll BJ, Fallas MJ, Ramas R, Rosenthal D (1992) Laparoscopic colectomy. Ann Surg 216:703–707
11. Franklin ME, Ramos R, Rosenthal ID, Schuessler W (1993) Laparoscopic colonic procedures. World J Surg 17:51–56
12. Musser DJ, Boorse RC, Madera F, Reed JF (1994) Laparoscopic colectomy: at what cost? Surg Laparosc Endosc 4:1–5
13. Hoffmann GC, Baker JW, Fitchett CW, Vansant JH (1994) Laparoscopic-assisted colectomy. Initial experience. Ann Surg 219:732–774
14. Baca I, Götzen V, Schultz Ch (1995) Laparoskopische Eingriffe bei akuter und chronischer Divertikulitis. Zentralbl Chir 120:396–399
15. Senagore AJ, Luchtefeld MA, Mackeigan JM, Mazier WP (1993) Open colectomy versus laparoscopic colectomy: are there differences? Am Surg 59:549–554
16. Van Ye TM, Cattey RP, Henry LG (1994) Laparoscopically assisted colon resection compares favorably with open technique. Surg Laparosc Endosc 4:25–31
17. Guillou PJ, Darzi A, Monson JRT (1993) Experience with laparoscopic colorectal surgery for malignant disease. Surg Oncol 2 [Suppl 1]:43–49

18. Ramos JM, Gupta S, Antone GJ, Ortega AE, Simons AJ, Beart RW Jr (1994) Laparoscopy and colon cancer. Is the port site at risk? A preliminary report. Arch Surg 129 : 897 – 909
19. Wexner SD, Cohen SM (1995) Port site metastasis after laparoscopic colorectal surgery for cure of malignancy. Br J Surg 82 : 295 – 298
20. Larach SW, Salomon MC, Williamson PR, Goldstein E (1993) Laparoscopic assisted colectomy:experience during the learning curve. Colo Proctology 1 : 38 – 41
21. Hermanek P, Wittekind Ch (1994) Inwieweit sind laparoskopische Verfahren in der onkologischen Chirurgie vertretbar. Chirurg 65 : 23 – 28

Accelerated Recovery After Laparoscopic Colorectal Surgery for Cancer in Old Patients

L. Bardram

Introduction

Laparoscopic surgery for colorectal cancer still is a controversial matter and a subject of lively discussion [1–4]. Are the benefits we obtain for the patients great enough to make up for the fact that as yet the long-term outcome is unknown and there may be an increased risk of port-site metastases? [4–6].

Our contribution to the evaluation of laparoscopic surgery for colorectal cancer has been to try to obtain the most possible benefits from the use of the minimally invasive technique. We have tried to do this by combining laparoscopic surgery with an intensified postoperative care regime. This includes continuous epidural infusion of local anesthetics for 48 h, opioid-free pain treatment, early enteral nutrition and enforced mobilisation [7].

Patients and Methods

Patients

Patients, aged over 75 years (or over 70 years and with complicating cardiopulmonary disease) scheduled for colon resection for cancer were included in the trial. They had to be able to take care of themselves at home with perhaps some help from the homecare service before they were admitted for surgery. Patients with rectal cancer (less than 15 cm from the anus) were not included.

Preoperative Information to Patients

Patients were informed both verbally and in writing about the perioperative program. They were told that they would receive sufficient continuous pain relief to allow early mobilisation. Oral food intake should be normal on the day after operation. Finally, they would be expected to stay in hospital for about 2 days.

Anesthesia

All patients were premedicated with diazepam 0.2 mg/kg 1 h to surgery. A thoracic epidural catheter was inserted between T_7 and T_9. The position was verified by the injection of 6-9 ml bupivacaine 0.5%. During operation bupivacaine 0.5% 4 ml was injected every hour and a continuos epidural infusion of bupivacaine 0.25% was given. General anaesthesia was induced with i.v. midazolam 0.15 mg/kg and maintained with N_2O/O_2 2:1, enflurane and i.v. fentanyl (0.1-0.25 mg). Tracheal intubation was facilitated with atracurium 0.5 mg/kg i.v.

As the peritoneal cavity was not exposed, intravenous administration of fluids was restricted to about 1500 ml during the operation and the first few immediately postoperative hours.

Surgical Procedures

After CO_2 insufflation to an abdominal pressure of 12 mmHg, four trocars (10-12 mm) were inserted in a semicircular fashion opposite the tumor. In right-sided hemicolectomy the ileum and the right colon were mobilised from the lateral wall, retroperitoneum and duodenum/antrum. The ileocalic vessels were isolated close to the third part of the duodenum and divided with an endo-GIA stapler. The mesentery was dissected by electrocautery and clips to the terminal ileum, which was transected with an endo-GIA. The terminal ileum and right colon was then delivered through a small incision in the right hypochondrium. The transverse colon was divided and a one-layer hand-sewn anastomosis performed extracorporally.

In sigmoid resection the colon was dissected from the lateral and retroperitoneum. The vessels were divided centrally by endo-GIA. The distal resection was performed using an endo-GIA as well. After delivery of the bowel through a small incision in the left fossa, the proximal bowel transection was performed extracorporally. The head of the circular stapler was inserted and the anastomosis was performed intracorporally with the circular stapler inserted through the anus. No drains were used.

A single dose of antibiotics (metronidazole 1.5 g and cefuroxime 3 g) was given.

Postoperative Analgesia

At the end of surgery 20 ml bupivacaine 0.25% was injected in the largest of the abdominal incisions. Postoperative pain treatment consisted of continuous epidural infusion of bupivacaine 0.25%, 4 ml/h for 48 h, and oral paracetamol 1 g four times daily. Opioids were avoided but NSAIDs could be given if needed.

Postoperative Regime

Gastric tubes were not used postoperatively. Normal oral food intake was allowed immediately following surgery. It was enriched by supplements of enteral protein solution (Fortimel) providing about 1000 kcal and 80 g protein daily.

If the anastomoses in left-sided resections ended up being below 12 cm from the anus, the patients followed a more conservative postoperative regime in which solid food was not given until bowel function was re-established (defecation).These patients ($n = 3$) are not included in the present report.

Cisapride 20 mg twice daily was given from the day of operation.

The bladder catheter was removed after 24 h. Early mobilisation was enforced according to a fixed schedule. The peridural catheter was removed after 48 h and discharge was planned to take place some hours later. An appointment was arranged in the out-patient clinic on postoperative day 10 for removal of the stitches, registration and final information about the operation.

Recording of Postoperative Symptoms

Pain at rest and during mobilisation, nausea and fatigue were all assessed for the first 10 postoperative days on a four-point scale on which 0, 1, 2, 3 signified none, slight, moderate and severe respectively. Any additional analgesics used were recorded. Oral intake, defecation and hours of mobilisation were also recorded for the first 10 postoperative days. One month postoperatively the patients were asked if they had been satisfied with the information, the operation, the pain treatment and the time of discharge. They were also asked whether they would recommend this form of treatment to others.

Results

Patients

By the end of August 1995, 21 patients with a median age of 81 years (range 71–92 years) had entered the trail: 15 women and 6 men. One patient with severe cardiac disease was 71 years old; the rest were over 75.

In four patients the operation had to be converted to open surgery. This was due to growth of the cancer into neighboring organs in three patients. In the fourth patient the resection was all done laparoscopically, and the anastomosis performed intracorporally with the circular stapler. Removal of the stapler resulted, however, in a 1- to 2-cm-long tear in the anastomosis. A resection and a new anastomosis were performed after conversion.

In 17 patients the operation was completed laparoscopically. One of these developed small bowel strangulation on the 4th postoperative day and was reoperated on by open surgery. Accordingly, 16 patients followed the scheduled postoperative regime.

Complicating Diseases

Ten patients were treated with diuretics for cardiac disease, two of them also with digoxin. Two had severe cardiac disease with earlier myocardial infarction and pulmonary embolus. They were also treated with digoxin, calcium blockers and Aldactone. One patient had earlier apoplexy and stenosis of the mitral valve, but was doing well without medicine. Three others had obstructive pulmonary diseases. Only five had no signs of cardiopulmonary diseases.

Diagnoses and Surgical Procedures

Among the 17 patients whose procedures were completed laparoscopically, one had a large sessile adenoma with moderate dysplasia. Nine had adenocarcinoma Dukes' type B and seven had Dukes' type C. Thirteen had a right-sided hemicolectomy, one a left-sided hemicolectomy and in three a sigmoid resection was performed. Median duration of surgery was 180 min (range 130–260 min). This included intraoperative colonoscopy in three patients. The median abdominal incision length was 6 cm (range 5–12 cm). Median perioperative blood loss was 50 ml (range 0–200 ml). Perioperative intravenous fluids administered amounted to a median of 1300 ml (range 600–2300 ml).

Operative Complications

As mentioned, a tear in the rectosigmoid anastomosis resulted in conversion to open surgery in one patient. In a patient in whom the operation was converted due to growth of the cancer into the left ureter, a small lesion of the ileum was made by the forceps. The lesion was diagnosed immediately and closed and would not in itself have required conversion.

Postoperative Complications

One patient developed small bowel ileus and was reoperated on in an open procedure on day 4.

One patient suffered side effects of the epidural anaesthesia, with sensory disturbances and loss of motor control of both legs for several days. In this patient the rate of infusion had been 6 ml/h instead of 4 ml/h for the first night. The symptoms disappeared spontaneously, but delayed discharge till day 5.

Postoperative Pain

In two patients the epidural catheter had to be reinserted in the early postoperative period due to malfunction. In one it was impossible to insert the catheter preoperatively. This patient was treated with morphine 10 mg once during the first postoperative night and thereafter with paracetamol and nonsteroidal anti-inflammatory drugs. With this treatment the pain scores were 1–2 during the first 2 days and 1 thereafter.

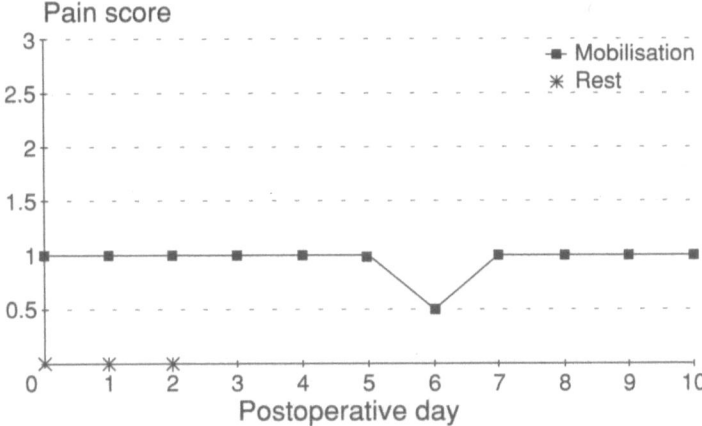

Fig. 1. Median postoperative pain scores in 16 patients with a median age of 81 years undergoing laparoscopic colonic resection. (0, none; 1, slight; 2, moderate; 3, severe)

During continuous epidural infusion of local anaesthetic, pain scores were low in all patients (0–1) both at rest and during mobilisation (Fig. 1). After discharge 11 of the patients had no or only slight pain during the whole period and needed no extra pain treatment. Median pain score was 1 during the whole period, but five patients experienced moderate pain (score 2) now and then during the first days after discharge. One patient took morphine 10 mg orally once after discharge, one needed the same three times in 10 days, and one took one 10-mg tablet of morphine every day for the first 5 days after discharge.

Postoperative Fatigue

Fatigue scores were between 1 and 2 until day 6, which the patients felt only slight fatigue (Fig. 2).

Mobilisation

The effective pain treatment allowed early mobilisation. Patients were out of bed about 5 h on the first day after surgery and 8 h on day 2. After discharge they very quickly regained their normal activity level at home and were up and about for about 12 h a day from day 3 (Fig. 3).

Gastrointestinal Function

Only few patients suffered nausea and vomiting (Table 1). Median oral intake was 2500 ml (range 1300–3200 ml) from day 1 and no intravenous fluids were given after day 1.

Fourteen patients had their first postoperative defecation on day 1 and two on day 2. Bowel function thereafter was normal except in one patient who had no function from day 3 to day 6, but was then normal again.

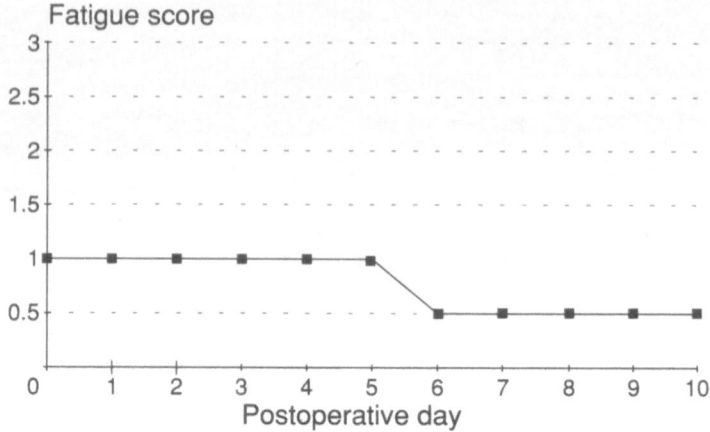

Fig. 2. Median postoperative fatigue scores in 16 patients with a median age of 81 years undergoing laparoscopic colonic resection (0, none; 1, slight; 2, moderate; 3, severe)

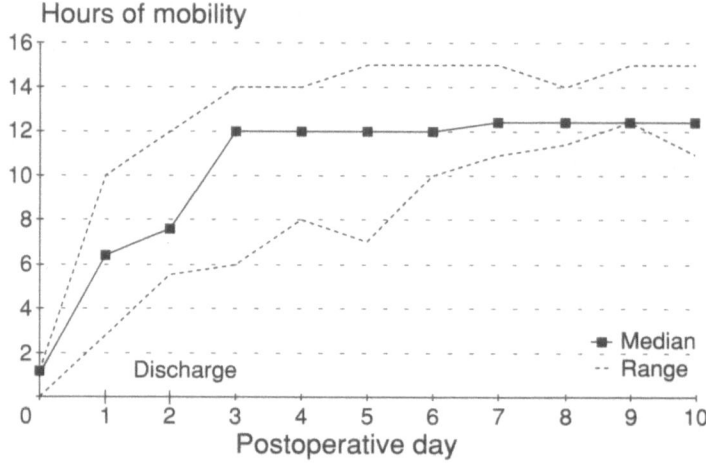

Fig. 3. Hours of daily mobility (median and range) after laparoscopic colonic resection in 16 patients with median age of 81 years

Table 1. Postoperative gastrointestinal function in 16 patients undergoing laparoscopic colonic resection	Day 1 *n*	Day 2 *n*
Nausea	2	1
Vomiting	2	6
Peroral intake more than 2000 ml	12	15
Defecation	14	16

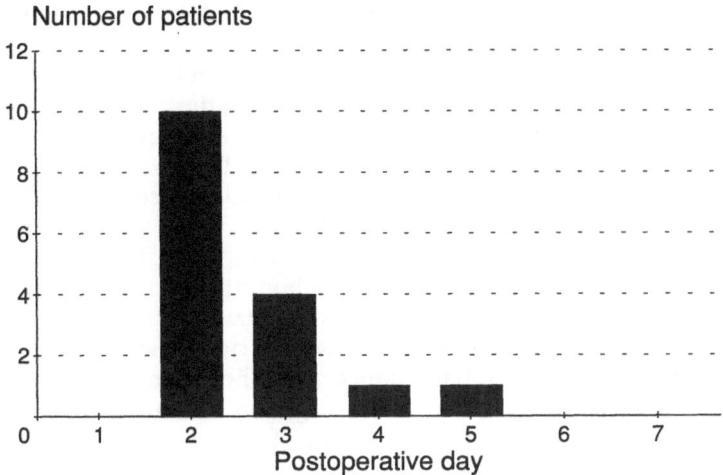

Fig. 4. Day of discharge after laparoscopic colonic resection in 16 patients with a median age of 81 years

Hospital Stay

Median hospital stay was 2 days. Ten patients were discharged according to plan on day 2. Four were discharged on day 3, mainly because their usual homecare service had not been ordered in time. One patient, who was operated on a Thursday, usually took care of his debilitated wife, who was admitted to the hospital together with him. They both stayed over the weekend and were discharged on day 4. These patients were all as well mobilised as the others and took care of themselves in the department. The patient with side effects from the epidural infusion was not discharged until day 5 (Fig. 4).

Patients' Final Opinion

One month after surgery the patients were asked for a final opinion. They were all back to normal activity at this time. They were all satisfied with the entire perioperative course, the information and the pain treatment. They would all recommend the same procedure to others. One patient thought, however, that her discharge (at day 3) was too early. She actually managed all right with her usual help from the homecare service and nurse, but she had been very worried.

Discussion

In this investigation we have shown that postoperative recovery can be accelerated considerably in old patients undergoing colon resection when laparoscopic minimally invasive surgery is combined with continuous epidural blockade, early postoperative enteral nutrition and active mobilisation.

We included only colon resections in this trial leaving out rectal resection. The reason for this was that the primary purpose of the investigation was to try to obtain the benefits possible – including very early oral nutrition – from minimally invasive surgery in high-risk patients. Due to the higher incidence of leaks in rectal anastomoses, we are still a little conservative about postoperative enteral feeding in such patients.

The most notable results were the lack of nausea, vomiting and postoperative ileus. In addition the high level of activity at home after the early discharge was remarkable in this elderly group of patients (median age 81 years).

In most laparoscopic colorectal surgery series, hospital stay has been reduced to 5–7 days [7–19]. Little information, however, is given about postoperative regimes. In the present investigation the multimodal approach makes it difficult to identify precisely the factors responsible for the accelerated recovery. An important limiting factor to early recovery after colon resection is the postoperative gastrointestinal paralysis. The use of epidural blockade probably played an important part in the lack of paralysis in our patients [20, 21]. We also used a prokinetic drug and avoided opioids. Early protein-rich enteral nutrition together with early mobilisation has an important effect on the duration of postoperative fatigue [22].

Although the number of patients in this study was low incidence of infectious, cardiopulmonary and thromboembolic complications was surprisingly low, especially since about two-thirds of the patients had cardiopulmonary disease. The small amount of bleeding, the restricted administration of intravenous fluids and the epidural blockade probably all reduced cardiopulmonary stress.

The accelerated recovery obtained in these patients shows that an active effort in the early postoperative period to reduce the surgical stress response is of great value. The stress response of our patients was reduced by the combined effects of minimised surgical trauma and epidural blockade. The patients never reached the low level of functional capacity and immobilisation often seen after major abdominal surgery in this old age group [23]. If these observations can be confirmed in larger series, this may – especially in old or higher-risk patients – be an advantage large enough to make up for the uncertainty about the long-term outcome.

References

1. Musser DJ, Boorse RC, Madera F, Reed JF (1994) Laparoscopic colectomy: at what cost? Surg Laparosc Endosc 4 : 1–5
2. Beart RW (1994) Laparoscopic surgery panel. Panel discussion. Dis Colon Rectum 37 [Suppl] 144–150
3. Guillou PJ (1994) Laparoscopic surgery for diseases of the colon and rectum – quo vadis? Surg Endosc 8 : 669–671
4. Wexner SD, Cohen SM (1995) Port site metastases after laparoscopic colorectal surgery for cure of malignancy. Br J Surg 82 : 295–298

5. Bart RW (1995) Wound and port site recurrence. Letter to the editors. Surgery 117:719
6. Cirrocco WC (1995) Letter to the editors (reply). Surgery 117:719–720
7. Bardram L, Funch Jensen PM, Jensen P, Crawford ME, Kehlet H (1995) Recovery after laparoscopic colonic surgery with epidural analgesia, and early oral nutrition and mobilisation. Lancet 345:763–764
8. Hoffman GC, Baker J, Fitchett CW, Vansant JH (1994) Laparoscopic assisted colectomy. Ann Surg 219:732–743
9. Falk PM, Beart RW Jr, Wexner SD, Thorson AG, Jagelman DG, Lavery IC, Johansen OB, Fitzgibbons RJ Jr (1993) Laparoscopic colectomy: a critical appraisal. Dis Colon Rectum 36:28–34
10. Monson JRT, Darzi A, Carey PD, Guillou PJ (1992) Prospective evaluation of laparoscopic-assisted colectomy in an unselected group of patients. Lancet 340:831–833
11. Jacobs M, Verdeja J, Goldstein H (1991) Minimally invasive colon resection (laparoscopic colectomy). Surg Laparosc Endosc 1:144–150
12. Franklin ME Jr, Rosenthal D, Norem R (1995) Prospective evaluation of laparoscopic colon resection versus open colon resection for adenocarcinoma. A multicenter study. Surg Endosc 9:811–816
13. Guillou PJ, Darzi A, Monson JRT (1993) Experience with laparoscopic colorectal surgery for malignant disease. Surg Oncol 2: [Suppl 1] 43–49
14. Wexner SD, Cohen SM, Johansen OB, Nogueras JJ, Jagelman DG (1993) Laparoscopic colorectal surgery: a prospective assessment and current perspective. Br J Surg 80:1802–1805
15. Franklin ME Jr, Ramos R, Rosenthal D, Schuessler W (1993) Laparoscopic colonic procedures. World J Surg 17:51–56
16. Vara-Thorbeck C, Garcia-Caballero M, Salvi M, Gutstein D, Toscano R, Gomez A, Vara-Thorbeck R (1994) Indications and advantages of laparoscopy-assisted colon resection for carcinoma in elderly patients. Surg Laparosc Endosc 4:110–118
17. Van Ye TM, Cattey RP, Henry LG (1994) Laparoscopically assisted colon resection compares favourably with open technique. Surg Laparosc Endosc 4:25–31
18. Tucker JG, Ambroze WL, Orangio GR, Duncan TD, Mason EM, Lucas GW (1995) Laparoscopically assisted bowel surgery. Analysis of 114 cases. Surg Endosc 9:297–300
19. Ortega AE, Beart RW, Steele GD, Winchester DP, Greene FL (1995) Laparoscopic bowel surgery registry. Preliminary results. Dis Colon Rectum 38:681–686
20. Kehlet H (1993) General vs regional anesthesia. In: Rogers M, Tinker J, Covino B, Longnecker DE (eds) Principles and practice of anesthesiology. Mosby, St Louis 1218–1234
21. Wattwil M (1988) Postoperative pain relief and gastrointestinal motility. Acta Chir Scand [Suppl] 550:140–145
22. Christensen T, Kehlet H (1993) Postoperative fatigue. World J Surg 17:220–225
23. Watters JM, Clancey SM, Moulton SB, Brier KM, Zhu J-M (1993) Impaired recovery of strength in older patients after major abdominal surgery. Ann Surg 218:380–395

Laparoscopic Colectomy: Experience and Outcomes at the Minimally Invasive Surgical Training Institute in Baltimore

W. P. Geis, H. C. Kim, and E. J. Brennan Jr

Introduction

Six years have passed since the explosive introduction of laparoscopy into the general surgical arena [1–2]. The laparoscopic approach to colon resection has given positive results as well as negative results; strong opinions to the positive and to the negative have also been generated regarding its benefits vs its drawbacks. It is clear, however, that surgeons who have persevered and who have generated development of strong laparoscopic colectomy programs have endured with excellent success [3–8]. We have personally had the opportunity to provide operative and postoperative care for 327 patients who underwent laparoscopic colectomy by ourselves during the past 60 months.

The Patients, the Experiences

Our first patient underwent laparoscopic colectomy in May 1990. She was 86 years of age at the time and was sent to the emergency department at our hospital with right lower quadrant pain, tenderness, and a loss of bowel sounds. She had fever, anorexia, and diminished mentation. We performed a diagnostic laparoscopy expecting acute gangrenous appendicitis. The laparoscopy revealed a gangrenous cecum and ascending colon due to peripheral atherosclerotic disease. We mobilized the cecum and ascending colon along with the viable distal ileum and hepatic flexure of the colon. A muscle-splitting incision was made in the right lower abdomen and the entire right colon extracted through the mini-incision. The extracted right colon was devascularized, resected and ileocolic anastomosis was performed. The anastomosis was replaced in the abdominal cavity through the muscle-splitting incision and the incision was irrigated and closed.

Since this patient had sepsis prior to surgery, was an elderly obese patient, and was a 60-year three-packs-per-day smoker, her outcome was predicted as dubious at best. However, in contrast to our expectations, the patient was extubated in the recovery room, had active bowel sounds on the 1st postoperative day and had a liquid bowel movement on the 2nd postoperative day. She walked on her own recognizance on the 1st postoperative day. Her temperature was normal throughout the postoperative period and her white blood count returned to normal after 48 h. She had a liquid diet by mouth on the 2nd postoperative day with progression to regular diet by the 4th–5th postoperative day. This elderly lady, who was at risk for abdominal sepsis, deep

Table 1. Diagnoses in 327 patients undergoing laparoscopic colectomy

Diagnosis	No. of cases	Percentage of total
Carcinoma	176	53.8
Diverticulosis	73	22.3
Polyp	33	10.1
Prolapse	10	3.1
Inertia	10	3.1
Ulcerative colitis	12	3.7
Crohn's disease	9	2.7
Angiodysplasia	1	0.3
Pseudo-obstruction	1	0.3
Incontinence	1	0.3
Lymphoma	1	0.3
Total	327	100

vein thrombosis, pulmonary embolus, and pulmonary sepsis clearly benefited in physiologic and immunologic ways not quite understood by us at the time. However, it was obvious to our surgical team that the laparoscopic environment formulated an equation which resulted in the well-being of this lady during her postoperative period.

Since that occasion, we have performed 327 laparoscopic colectomy procedures – the majority of which have been elective colon resections. There heave been 157 male and 170 female patients. The ages have ranged from 19 years to 94 years. The diagnoses have been the expected broad spectrum of disease processes (Table 1), with carcinoma and diverticulosis as the most common entities. The first 31 cases, however, were operated on for benign disease, because of our respect for the learning curve necessary to perform proper regional colon resection for cancer laparoscopically [9–10]. Further, the majority of our first 20 cases were right colon resections which confirmed our recognition from our first case that the three laparoscopic skills (mobilization, devascularization, and anastomosis) could be learned sequentially if cases were chosen judiciously early in the learning experience [11].

Once laparoscopic mobilization of the right colon for benign disease became a comfortable operative experience, the addition of intracorporal devascularization was added to the procedure. Intracorporeal devascularization for benign disease provided us with the opportunity to learn confidently to perform regional devascularization and resection for malignancy using the laparoscopic approach. Following this experience, we added intracorporal anastomosis as a third skill. These operations were most often performed as sigmoid colon resection for benign disease early in the experience. Following these learning experiences, we broadened our indications and eventually performed all of the various laparoscopic colectomy procedures (Table 2). Table 2 shows that the most frequently performed procedures continued to be laparoscopic sigmoid colectomy and laparoscopic right colon resection even when

Table 2. Laparoscopic colectomy procedures performed

Procedure	No. of cases of total	Percentage
Right colon resection	95	29.1
Sigmoid colectomy	115	35.2
Low anterior resection	25	7.6
Abdominoperineal resection	24	7.4
Abdominal colectomy	17	5.2
Anterior resection	6	1.8
Transverse colon resection	8	2.5
Segmental colon resection	6	1.8
J pouch	4	1.2
Colostomy	4	4.6
Left colon resection	15	0.6
Proctocolectomy	26	1.8
Colostomy closure Total	327	100

all patients were eventually offered laparoscopic approach. After 50 cases, we included all patients who accepted laparoscopic colectomy as a choice of surgical therapy, including those who were at risk for technical reasons, e.g. because of obesity, prior abdominal surgery, inflammatory bowel disease, and prior peritonitis or abdominal abscess.

From February 1991 through March 1995, we offered laparoscopic colectomy to all patients with colonic malignancy requiring colon resection. Table 3 identifies the anatomic location of each of the malignant lesions within the colon, and Table 4 gives a breakdown of patients based on their tumor staging. In this large series of 176 patients, we have not experienced port-site recurrences in any patient. In the patients with malignant disease, our policy is to follow these guidelines:

1. do not grasp the bowel with retractors or Babcocks, but rather grasp the mesentery;
2. ligate and divide the regional blood supply with mesentery early in the procedure;
3. transect the distal planned line of resection laparoscopically in order to place the specimen in a bag prior to removal through a mini-incision;
4. remove the specimen in a bag to protect the mini-incision and the abdominal cavity;
5. do not remove ports while carbon dioxide under pressure is within the peritoneal cavity, thus avoiding an efflux of carbon dioxide through tissue surrounding the port sites;
6. remove all carbon dioxide upon completion of the procedure through port stopcocks;
7. irrigate all incisions and ports utilizing sterile water and/or dilute Betadine.

Table 3. Tumor sites in patients undergoing laparoscopic colectomy for carcinoma

Tumor site	No. of cases	Percentage of cases
Cecum	24	13.6
Ascending colon	29	16.5
Hepatic flexure	9	5.1
Transverse colon	10	5.7
Splenic flexure	4	2.3
Descending colon	12	6.8
Sigmoid colon	46	26.1
Rectum	41	23.3
Anal canal	1	0.6
Total	176	100

Table 4. Tumor stages of patients undergoing laparoscopic colectomy for carcinoma

Stage	Percentage of cases
In situ	13
Dukes stage A	14
Dukes stage B_1	41
Dukes stage B_2	50
Dukes stage C_1	9
Dukes stage C_2	33
Dukes stage D	16
Total	176

Results

The patients have been followed for a maximum of 65 months and a minimum of 6 months following laparoscopic colectomy. As mentioned earlier, there are no patients who have encountered trocar site implantation of tumor to date. Table 5 shows a mortality of 1%. Three patients died, each in the immediately postoperative period. They were 84, 86, and 87 years of age. Each had known cardiac disease and each was well 2–6 days postoperatively when an abrupt cardiac event occurred. Each patient died immediately. We presume that cardiac arrhythmia with or without cardiac infarction was the cause.

There was a conversion rate to open procedure of 4.6% representing 15 patients. Table 6 delineates the causes of conversion in our early experience; adhesions and technical reasons were the major cause. We also have converted for metabolic reasons – a progressive rise in carbon dioxide in the blood or in the end-tidal carbon dioxide level. Tumor size was large enough to result in a mode-

Table 5. Summary of results of laparoscopic colectomy in 327 patients

Mortality (3/327)	1.0%
Complication rate	9%
Conversion rate	4.6%
Average postop. length of stay	5 days
Recurrences of malignancy at port site	0

Table 6. Reasons for conversion to an open procedure in 327 patients undergoing laparoscopic colectomy

Adhesions	3
Technical reasons	2
Tumor size	6
Rise in CO_2 levels	2
Epigastric bleeding	0
Bladder injury	2
	15 (4.6%)

rate-sized incision (10 cm or greater) which resulted in a conversion to open procedure in six patients. In the majority of the aforementioned circumstances, the conversion to open procedure maintained a distinct laparoscopy-related benefit for the patients. In each of these cases, the choice of the incision was strategic, the location and size of the incision was carefully planned, and the length of time the abdomen was open to the atmosphere was markedly reduced when compared to an open procedure. Therefore, the majority of these patients continued to proceed postoperatively as if they had undergone a laparoscopic procedure rather than an open procedure. In two patients, diverticulitis had directly involved the wall of the urinary bladder. In both of these cases, we intentionally resected a segment of free wall of the bladder. A small incision was made in the suprapubic space to accommodate removal of the specimen, but also to allow closure of the bladder defect under direct vision.

Complications following our laparoscopic procedures are listed in Table 7. There were 29 complications or a 9% complication rate. The majority of the complications were wound infections. These wound infections were all super-

Table 7. Complications encountered in 327 patients undergoing laparoscopic colectomy

Wound infection	16
Small bowel obstruction[a]	6
Anastomotic leak	2
Fistula	1
Bowel strangulation	1
Bladder perforation (operative)	2
Small bowel perforation	1
	29 (9%)

[a] Port site obstruction (SB): 2.

ficial and did not require maintenance of the patient in the hospital. It was impossible for these wound infections to cause major wound dehiscences since they occurred in port sites and mini-incisions only. Six patients experienced small bowel obstruction. Five were reoperated upon. Two had adhesive small bowel obstruction and one had an incarceration of the small bowel through a mesenteric defect (partially closed small mesenteric defect). Two patients experienced anastomotic leaks. In both of these patients, the operative procedure was a low anterior resection and the anastomosis was a circular stapled end-to-end anastomosis. In both of these cases, the leak was a contained leak and treatment consisted of a temporary colostomy and diversion until healing occurred. One patient experienced formation of a small bowel fistula to the right lower abdominal port site. In this patient, radiation to the pelvis had previously performed for malignant disease of the uterus. The fistula was treated with hyperalimentation and closed spontaneously. One patient exhibited strangulation of the small bowel due to an adhesive portion. The patient experienced the adhesive complication approximately 3 months postoperatively and had a small bowel resection performed successfully. A final patient experienced small bowel perforation 5 days after a successful subtotal colectomy. This small bowel perforation is thought to have been due to a bovie electrical injury causing a nontransmural injury to the small bowel, which necrosed over an interval of days. The two patients who had bladder perforations in the operating room were discussed above. Each of these bladder perforations was in order to remove diseased tissue. It should be noted that two of small bowel obstructions were secondary to small bowel incarceration into port-site hernias at the site of 10-/12-mm ports in the lateral abdomen (lower abdomen). Each of these were successfully treated with reduction and repair of the abdominal wall defect.

Discussion

We conclude over this 5 year experience that laparoscopic colon resection is safe and effective. It is also reasonable to assume that the cost of these surgical health care experiences and the length of the operative procedures are similar or superior to those for open procedures and they are described elsewhere in this volume [12]. The average discharge is currently at 4.9 days. However, it is clear that 15% of the patients have been discharged on the 2nd, or 3rd postoperative day and the majority of the patients are currently discharged on the 3rd or 4th postoperative day. The gradual improvements in modification of postoperative care of the patient as well as the introduction of early discharge planning by the hospital personnel continue to move in the direction of diminished cost and diminished use of resources as well as providing clear evidence that patients have experienced less trauma and less physiologic insult during the operative procedure.

The large number of patients in our series who have been treated with laparoscopic colectomy for malignant disease provides evidence that this approach is safe and effective for this subset of patients in our hands. Further, the lack of port-site tumor implants in our patients (both those with early stage disease and those with advanced stage disease) suggests that mechanical aspects of the operative procedure and technical aspects of the procedure must play some role in the avoidance of these postoperative events. We have earlier delineated the safeguards which empirically would favor absence of port-site seeding with tumor. It is also reasonable to assume that the biology of the individual tumor and the stage of the disease must play a role in the implantation of tumor in port sites as well as other local metastatic sites [13, 14].

Small bowel obstruction occurring in small mesenteric defects in our experience raises the issue as to whether the mesentery should be closed. Most of these cases of small bowel obstruction occurred in the first 150 cases of laparoscopic colectomy, and they all occurred in patients in whom we "closed" the mesentery. In each case, the reoperation showed that the mesentery was not closed entirely or had opened during the postoperative interval. Therefore, we have in the last 150–200 cases not closed port sites in any of the laparoscopic colon resections. There have been no bowel obstructions or adverse sequelae secondary to a persistent large defect in the mesentery.

The occurrence of two bowel obstructions in incarcerated hernias in 12-mm port sites in the lower lateral abdomen underlines the need to address the 12-mm port-site defect at the end of the operative procedure [15]. For approximately 30 months, we have closed these port sites using a large mass ligature to approximate all layers of fascia. However, in the most recent 9 months, we have used an Optiview port (Ethicon Endo-Surgery, Inc.) to enter the abdominal cavity obliquely, thus opening a defect in the anterior fascia, the internal oblique fascia, and the transverse abdominal fascia, each at different levels. The removal of these ports does not result in the escape of carbon dioxide and also does not result in a persistent defect. Therefore, we have not closed these ports in laparoscopic colon resections and other complex laparoscopic procedures for the past 9 months. We have had no evidence of hernia defect or small bowel obstruction in these cases. Our initial data indicate that the surgeon saves 22.5 min on average per case by not closing the fascia at these port sites.

We completed our assessment of this study in March 1995. Since April 1995, we have become participants in the National Cancer Institute study for prospective randomized assessment of the treatment of colon cancer by the laparoscopic approach vs the open approach. We believe that while our results and data are very convincingly positive, it is important to contribute our experiences to the prospective randomized trial to define for the surgical community the objective data which will be convincing to all.

References

1. Reddick EJ, Olsen DO (1989) Laparoscopic cholecystectomy: a comparison with mini-lap cholecystectomy. Surg Endosc 3 : 131–133
2. McKernan JB (1991) Laparoscopic cholecystectomy. Am J Surg 57(5) : 309–312
3. Ramos JM, Beart RW Jr, Goes R, Ortega AE, Schlinkert RT (1995) Role of laparoscopy in colorectal surgery: a prospective evaluation of 200 cases. Dis Colon Rectum 38 : 494–501

4. Wexner SD, Reissman P (1994) Laparoscopic colorectal surgery. A provocative critique. Int Surg 79(3): 233–234
5. Phillips EH, Franklin M, Carroll BJ, Fallas MJ, Ramos R, Rosenthal D (1992) Laparoscopic colectomy. Ann Surg 216(6): 703–707
6. Plasencia G, Jacobs M, Verdeja JC, Viamonte M III (1994) Laparoscopic-assited sigmoid colectomy and low anterior resection. Dis Colon Rectum 37: 829–833
7. Geis WP, Kim HC (1994) Improved efficiency in laparoscopic abdominoperineal resection: the Kim-Geis approach. Int Surg 79: 226–227
8. Hoffman GC, Baker JW, Fitchett CW, Vansant JH (1994) Laparoscopic-assited colectomy: initial experience. Ann Surg 219(6): 732–743
9. Simons, AJ, Anthone GJ, Ortega AE, Franklin M, Fleshman J, Geis WP, Beart RW Jr (1995) Laparoscopic-assisted colectomy learning curve. Dis Colon Rectum 38: 600–603
10. Wishner JD, Baker JW Jr, Hoffman GC, Hubbard GW II, Gould RJ, Wohlgemuth SD, Ruffin WK, Melick CF (1995) Laparoscopic-assisted colectomy: the learning curve. Surg Endosc 9: 1179–1183
11. Geis WP, Coletta AV, Verdeja JC, Plasencia G, Ojogho O, Jacobs M (1994) Sequential psychomotor skills development in laparoscopic colon surgery. Arch Surg 129: 206–212
12. Geis WP, Brennan EJ Jr, Kim HC (1996) Complexity of laparoscopic colon procedures and program development. Proceedings of the International Laparoscopic Colorectal Surgery Workshop, Hamburg. November 27–29, 1995 (this volume)
13. Fidler IJ, Hart IR (1982) Principles of cancer biology: biology of cancer metastasis. In: Devita VT, Hellman S, Rosenberg SA (eds) Cancer: principles and practice of oncology. Lippincott, Philadelphia, pp 80–92
14. Savalgi RS (1995) Mechanism of abdominal wall recurrence after laparoscopic resection of colon cancers. Semin Laparosc Surg 2: 158–162
15. Plaus WJ (1993) Laparoscopic trocar site hernias. J Laparoendosc Surg 3: 567–570

Need for Clinical Trials and Randomized Studies to Assess Laparoscopic Colectomy

F. L. Greene

The technical aspects of laparoscopic colectomy have been reasonably well established and it has been shown that laparoscopic-assited colectomy or total intracorporeal maneuvers are possible in resecting portions of the colon and in achieving appropriate reanastomosis of the gastrointestinal tract [1]. The role of laparoscopic colectomy in the management of patients with cancer remains problematic, however. Several studies have shown that patients may benefit from a reduced stay in hospital and an earlier return to normal activity following laparoscopic colectomy both for benign and malignant disease [2]. These studies have indicated that a reduction in costs to the patient, the insurer, and to society in general may be reduced without compromising short-term cancer control in the patient with colorectal carcinoma. In addition, parameters indicating reasonable cancer operations, such as the number of lymph nodes resected and the length of proximal and distal margin of resection, seem to suggest that the laparoscopic removal of colorectal cancer is similar to that achieved during open celiotomy [3]. The real trouble, however, is that the long-term outcome regarding recurrence rates, both locally and systemically, is completely unknown.

The issues of both cancer control and the overall economic benefit must be studied in a scientific way, and this requires utilization of the randomized prospective trial, which may be performed in one institution or in multiple institutions, studying patients having open traditional operations versus laparoscopic colectomy. The important issues in cancer control that must be studied are the extent of lymphadenectomy, the margin of resection, the potential of port-site recurrence, and overall outcomes regarding anastomotic recurrence and the appearance of metastatic disease. The ability to adequately stage patients with colorectal cancer is important, not only to ensure adequate registry but also data by which to continue stratifying patients into subgroups who may benefit from adjuvant chemotherapy. If inadequate nodal dissection is performed, the pathologist will be unable to provide such data, which may effectively reduce the opportunity for appropriate cancer management. Several studies have noted that lymph node resection may be similar in laparoscopic and open colectomy. While this is an important piece of information, the role of a clinical trial will be to expand this concept and to provide methods of following patients to see the full effect of lymph node harvest (number of nodes removed) versus possible understaging of disease. The power of the randomized clinical trial may be seen in the results reported by Wiggers [4], who compared the "no touch" group and 119 patients in the control group. Complications were equivocal in both groups and survival did not significantly differ between groups. According to this study, early ligation of the regional blood supply of the colon segment containing the cancer may not be necessary in either traditional or laparoscopic approaches for colorectal cancer.

One of the important issues to assess using randomized clinical trials is the true rate of port-site recurrence. Several early reports of tumor implantation, both in trocar sites and in small incisions created for removal of colectomy specimens, have indicated that perhaps we are seeing an increasing rate of port-site recurrence after laparoscopic procedures [5]. The rate of recurrence after open celiotomy has been generally less than 1% [6]. We are hampered currently by not having an adequate denominator by which to judge the overall risk of port-site recurrence after laparoscopic surgery. Early registry information suggests that port-site recurrence after laparoscopic colectomy may be only slightly higher than that noted in the abdominal wound after open celiotomy [7]. These details must be closely recorded during the development of clinical trials in order to accumulate adequate data regarding recurrence patterns. We may learn that recurrence in the abdominal wall is of such importance that the techniques utilized during laparoscopic colectomy contribute directly to tumor implantation.

Well-designed randomized clinical trials comparing the creation of pneumoperitoneum with abdominal wall lift devices need to be performed to ensure that tumor dispersion is not occurring by increased abdominal pressure. Only by well-designed clinical trials can such information be gleaned. Similarly, clinical trials comparing laparoscopic-assisted and traditional open colectomy must be performed to ensure that the counterincision utilized to remove colonic tissue does increase the risk of tumor implantation. These technical concepts must be thought out clearly and incorporated into single and multi-institutional trials.

Well-designed clinical trials must include information relative to the time of the return of bowel function, rates of initiating alimentation, length of hospital stay, postoperative utilization of analgesic agents, and time needed for the return to productive activity. Careful comparison must be performed in order to avoid underestimating the benefit of traditional open procedures. One of the interesting phenomena recently noted is that patients having "open" procedures may in fact achieve a shorter length of stay because of the concepts that we have learned in managing patients with minimal-access techniques. This "reduction creep" in length of stay must be scientifically investigated and can only be understood when groups of patients are compared in a scientific manner.

It is unlikely that laparoscopic colectomy will achieve a survival advantage over "open" techniques for patients with colorectal cancer. The real question to be answered by randomized clinical trials is whether the laparoscopic approach is as efficacious as our traditional methods of colectomy. If minimal-access procedures are associated with less impairment of immune function than open operations [8], then long-term studies may show better survival in patients who undergo minimal-access cancer resection.

It is quite possible that we have yet to recognize all of the potential benefits and drawbacks associated with laparoscopic colectomy from the standpoint of physiology and tumor biology. Through the use of well-performed clinical trials, designed to monitor patterns of cancer recurrence, solid information will be obtained in these areas. Currently, a prospective randomized study comparing laparoscopic-assited to traditional colectomy has been designed under the auspices of the United States National Cancer Institute. Issues of cancer control and cost-effectiveness will be studied in a randomized prospective fashion. Currently, patients may be recruited through one of several cooperative surgical or radiation oncology groups dealing with issues of colorectal cancer. It is hoped that during the next 5 – 10 years adequate outcome data will be obtained which will support the concept that laparoscopic colectomy is indeed appropriate for the management of colorectal cancer.

References

1. Elftmann TD, Nelson H, Ota DM et al. (1994) Laparoscopic-assisted segmental colectomy: surgical techniques. Mayo Clin Proc 69 : 825
2. Phillips EH, Franklin M, Carroll BJ et al. (1992) Laparoscopic colectomy. Ann Surg 216 – 703
3. Falk PM, Beart RW, Wexner SD et al. Laparoscopic colectomy: a critical appraisal. Dis Colon Rectum 36 : 28
4. Wiggers T (1988) No-touch technique in colon cancer: a controlled prospective trial. Br J Surg 75 : 409 – 415
5. Savalgi RS (1995) Mechanism of abdominal wall recurrence after laparoscopic resection of colonic cancers. Semin Laparosc Surg 2 : 158 – 161
6. Berman IR (1995) Laparoscopic colectomy for cancer: some cause for pause. Ann Surg Oncol 2 : 1
7. Ramos JM, Gupta S, Anthone GJ et al. (1994) Laparoscopy and colon cancer: is the port site at risk? Arch Surg 129 : 897
8. Allendorf JD, Bessler M, Kayton ML et al. (1995) Increased tumor establishment and growth after laparotomy vs laparoscopy in a murine model. Arch Surg 130 : 649 – 653

VI Advantages of the Laparoscopic Approach

Laparoscopic Surgery for Carcinoma of the Colon: Does it Come Up to Standard?

P. Buchmann and D. Christen

Standards in colorectal surgery change in line with progress in technology, adjuvant therapy and the consequent long-term results. In the past 10 years, the improvement in results appears to be limited to surgical morbidity and mortality [1]. Apart from this, the results of prospective studies using pre- and postoperative chemotherapy [2, 3] in colon cancer and preoperative radiotherapy in rectal carcinoma [4] demonstrate a favourable effect on the incidence of recurrence and on long-term survival.

The pressure to expand the range of indications is coupled with the irresistable triumphal march of the technique of minimally invasive surgery in the abdomen, led by laparoscopic cholecystectomy. Laparoscopic fundoplication and appendicectomy are already widely practised, and the minimally invasive treatment of a perforated duodenal ulcer is linked to lower morbidity than open surgery (P. Buchmann, unpublished material). With all of these procedures, removal of a specimen is unnecessary or can be done through a trocar. The situation is otherwise with operations on the colorectum. A suggested route for removal of the resected specimen of sigmoid colon and rectum from the abdomen is through the anus. This route is suitable for endoscopic operations on the lowermost part of the bowel [5], but not for the removal of laparoscopically resected segments of colon; the risk of sphincter injury, as observed after manual anal dilatation [6], is too great. For this reason, mini-laparotomy will become the established method for removal of the specimen, and we must therefore use the term "laparoscopically assisted colorectal surgery".

Referring to our own experiences, we investigate below whether laparoscopically assisted surgery of the colon meets modern standards.

Our Experience

Our series comprises 171 patients, 88 women and 83 men, with a mean age of 67 years (range 21–90 years). The diagnoses of patients undergoing colorectal resection are presented in Table 1. A conversion to the open technique had to made in 24 cases for various reasons (Table 2), so that 147 laparoscopically assisted operated patients could be analysed. The operations performed can be seen in Table 2.

The principal reason for changing over to laparotomy was adhesions, division of which appeared too time-consuming or risky ($n = 9$), followed by tumor infiltration in the vicinity ($n = 6$) and haemorrhage which could not be

Table 1. Diagnoses of the 171 patients undergoing laparoscopically assisted operation

Diagnosis	Total	Converted	Completed laparoscopically
	n	n	n
Cancer	82	14	68
Polyp	9	1	8
Diverticulosis,	52	8	44
of which diverticulitis[a]	18	4	
Rectal prolapse and enterocele	26	1	25
Crohn's ileocolitis	1		
Appendicitis with necrosis of ascending colon	1		1
Total	171	24	147

[a] Sigmoid diverticulosis: elective operation for recurrent diverticulitis; diverticulitis: operation immediately after subsidence of a conservatively treated episode, two with rectovesical fistula.

controlled laparoscopically ($n = 3$). Visibility was poor in three cases: with massive obesity, massively dilated colon due to obstruction, and diffuse peritonitis with fibrin deposits and black colouration of the entire pelvis after over-vigorous colonoscopic marking of an adenoma with dye [7]. On two occasions, the tumor was so large that the incision for its removal was almost that of a laparotomy and so it was immediately operated by the open method. The anaesthetist requested conversion because of difficulty in maintaining the patient's blood pressure on only one occasion.

What follows refers to the 147 patients operated on entirely laparoscopically. The mean operation time was 228 min (range 110–445 min). A complication arose in the course of the operation, postoperatively or later in 39 patients (Table 3). Injury to the ureter occurred in the fourth case after the left ureter was separated completely from the wall.

The incidence of wound infection has decreased markedly since we started inserting a wound protector routinely in the removal laparotomy. This is also obligatory in order to prevent implantation of tumor cells in the wound margins. Secondary haemorrhage has become rare since the dangers of the laparoscopic technique were recognized (trocar placement, removal of stapler point, haemostasis during dissection) [8]. The incidence of anastomotic leak, which occurred in 5 of 147, is low in relation to the incidence of 0.4%–11% reported in the literature for the open technique [9]. Only one of there cases should possibly be blamed on the endoscopic operation, in that the splenic flexure was insufficiently mobilized. Of the others, two were in pre-irradiated patients who had a deep anterior

Table 2. Laparoscopically assisted colorectal operations performed (177 procedures in 171 patients)[a]

Type of operation	Total	Converted			Reasons for conversion
		total	Cancer	Benign disease	
	n	n	n	n	
Resection of caecal pole	2				
Ileocaecal resection	3				
Right hemicolectomy	17	3	3		2 Tumorinfiltration 1 Adhesions
Left hemicolectomy	4	2	2		1 Tumor infiltration 1 cardiac intolerance of pneumoperitoneum
Sigmoid resection	36	2	1	1	1 Colon obstruction 1 Adhesions
Rectosigmoid resection	58	12	2		2 Tumor infiltration
			1		1 Tumor size
			1	6	7 adhesions (1 post-irradiation)
				1	1 obesity
				1	1 dye staining (see text)
Deep anterior rectal resection	10	3	3		1 Tumor infiltration 2 Haemorrhage
Rectal excision	10				
Colectomy	1	1	1		1 Tumor size
Hartmann resection	3				
Hartmann reanastomosis	2				
Rectopexy	25	1		1	1 Haemorrhage
	177	24	14	10	

[a] Rectopexy was combined with sigmoid resection in six cases.

resection of the rectum and one in a patient in very poor general condition with a T4 cancer of the ascending colon.

Port-site hernias were a consequence of un-sutured lateral insertions of 12-mm trocars.

The postoperative course is distinguished otherwise by a much faster return to well-being, which is particularly striking in older patients. The wish to eat is a measure of this. The interim results of a prospective study comparing postoperative eating after laparoscopic vs open operation shows a highly

Table 3. Complications encountered in 39 of 147 patients after completed laparoscopically assisted surgery

Complications	Total	Patients with	
		benign disease	cancer patients
	(n = 147)	(n = 79)	(n = 68)
Intraoperative			
Division of ureter	1	–	1
Postoperative			
Wound infection	12	7	5
Perineal abscess	4	–	4
Abscess in pouch of Douglas	1	1	–
Anastomotic leak	5	2	3
Secondary haemorrhage	5	3	2
Pneumonia	6	2	4
Pulmonary embolism	1	–	1
Deep vein thrombosis	–	–	M
Late			
Port-site hernia	2	2	–
Port-site metastases	2	–	2[a]
Anastomotic stenosis	3	3	–
Death	3	–	3[b]

[a] See text.
[b] one of myocardial infarct day of discharge, 1 of influenza on 44th day after Hartmann operation, 1 of liver failure with liver metastases.

significant difference in favour of the minimally invasive technique ($p < 0.001$). Over half of the patients operated on in this way were eating normally on the 2nd postoperative day [10].

Most of the expectations of minimally invasive surgery have been largely fulfilled [11]. The cosmetic result is unquestionably better than after a laparotomy. The postoperative course is pleasanter and the complication rate is not higher. So for, however, the duration of hospitalization has not diminished, as secure healing of the anastomosis can only be assessed on the 7th day and many patients are of advanced age. These patients also do not contribute to the figures for a reduction in the duration of unfitness for work, as they are nearly all retired.

Laparoscopy in Malignant Disease

If one wishes to perform laparoscopically assisted surgery in malignant colorectal disease, further aspects have to be considered. Both the recurrence-free follow-up and survival time must be comparable to those associated with conventional methods. The criteria for cancer surgery must also be met.

Video technology with its four-fold magnification of the picture and ability to see into every corner of the abdomen permits greater precision of resection. The tumor must never be grapsed or squeezed; this cannot be avoided during open operations, especially in the pelvis. Preliminary ligature of the inferior mesenteric artery and vein can be done easily and the subsequent resection can then be undertaken in accordance with the rules of cancer surgery. An important prerequisite is experience of the surgeon in both open cancer surgery and in laparoscopic surgery of benign disease.

We have compared the radicality of resection in 45 laparoscopically assited and 44 open resections of colorectal cancer. The patient groups were comparable with regard to age, sex, tumor stage and grading and site of cancer. There were no differences with regard to the length of the removed segment of bowel, the number of resected lymph nodes or the amount of blood transfusion required [12].

The postoperative course was similar to that after resection for benign illness (Table 3). The late course remains to be discusssed; this will decide the usefulness or otherwise of laparoscopically assisted surgery for colon cancer.

Port-site Metastases

The follow-up time in all series is still too short for comparison of long-term survival, as none of them is yet 5 years old. Many reports are unsettling because they mention implantation metastases at the trocar insertion sites which appear relatively early. We have observed two such metastases, both after palliative resection of a T4 cancer, once at the site of drain exit and once at all port sites. In both cases, the patient died of the underlying illness without symptoms referable to the implantation metastases.

A vigorous controversy is going on with regard to the importance of these reports. Some authors declare a complete ban on laparoscopic surgery in malignant disease [13], while others warn against drawing overhasty conclusions and argue lack of experience on the part of those reporting. As an example, there is one series of 545 colon cancer resections with 10 port-site metastases (1.86 %). These represent the collected statistics of 23 surgeons. The ten metastases were reported by nine of these surgeons, and the remaining surgeons observed none at all during the same period (Cadiere, personal communication). A 1 % incidence of skin metastasis is recognized in open surgery [14, 15]. However, these figures derive from retrospective analyses, which suggests that the figures may well be too low. They are nearly all metastases at a drain exit site. The long-term prognosis after complete excision is a 5-year survival of 30 % [14].

The aetiology of metastases at the trocar sites is still unclear. Correct technique must of course be assumed. A communication suggesting that the cause is squeezing of the specimen and contact with instruments laden with tumor cells is not valid [16]. The only case in the literature of a Dukes stage A cancer giving rise to a cutaneous metastasis relates to an operative mistake in that, while looking for a degenerated polyp, a colectomy was performed and the specimen was drawn through the abdominal wall without a covering bag or wound protector (Bégin, personal communication).

Nonetheless, the problem of port-site metastases merits the closest attention. We have therefore begun a prospective controlled study to compare tumor cell clusters in the irrigation fluid of open and laparoscopically operated patients and will analyse the connection between cytological findings and tumor behaviour in the follow-up. Hitherto, we have found positive irrigation cytology in 16 % of patients with pT3 tumors and 28 % with pT4 tumors. The ration of open to laparoscopic is 3 : 1. No malignant cells were found in tumor stages pT1 and pT2. In a short follow-up period of 1–12 months, no cutaneous metastasis has occurred. Naturally, a conclusion is not yet possible from these observations (P. Buchmann, D. Christen, G. Pedio, and R. Flury, unpublished material).

The lively discussion of port-site metastases has inspired many researchers to investigate the effects of laparotomy and laparoscopy on the human body. It is apparent that both the stress response, as measured by C-reactive protein and interleukin 6 HLA [16], and immune reactions, such as delayed-type hypersensitivity [18] or neutrophil oxidative function, are affected [19]. All investigations indicate that laparoscopy, unlike laparotomy, has less effect or indeed no effect on these systems. The significance for the healing process and long-term survival cannot yet be predicted, however. Nonetheless, a part, at least, of the beneficial effect of levamisole and 5-fluorouracil therapy on the outcome of colon carcinoma treatment can be attributed to the stimulating effect on the immune system [20].

Conclusion

Laparoscopically assisted colon surgery is technically feasible and makes the early postoperative period considerably easier for the patient. The long-term results in cancer patients have not yet been established. For this reason, we demand, as do others, that minimally invasive methods for resection of colon cancer should be used only in centres with great experience and within a prospectively controlled study [21]. It goes without saying that the patient should receive detailed information about the current state of knowledge and be able to give informed consent.

References

1. Sales JP, Parc R (1994) Le stade de diagnostic et la prise en charge chirurgicale des cancers coliques se sont-ils modifiés en 10 ans? A propos de 303 patients. Ann Chir 48 : 591–595
2. Francini G, Petrioli R, Lorenzini L et al. (1994) Folic acid and 5-fluorouracil as adjuvant chemotherapy in colon cancer. Gastroenterology 106 : 899–906
3. Marsh JC (1994) Is there a role for adjuvant therapy in bowel cancer? J Clin Gastroenterol 18 : 184–188

4. Willet CG, Warland G, Hagam MP et al. (1995) Tumor proliferation in rectal cancer following preoperative irradiation. J Clin Oncol 13:1417–1424
5. Buchmann P, Christen D, Rentsch RU (1995) Rektumkarzinom: minimal invasive Verfahren. Chir Gastroenterol 11:380–384
6. MacDonald A, Smith A, McNeill AD, Finlay IG (1992) Manual dilatation of the anus. Br J Surg 79:138–1382
7. Christen D, Bernardi M, Buchmann P (1995) Identifikation von Kolonpolypen bei laparoskopischer Kolorektalresektion mittels präoperativer Tuschemarkierung oder intraoperativer Koloskopie. Schweiz Med Wschr 125 [Supp]: 24 S
8. Christen D, Buchmann P, Klingler K (1994) Probleme beim Einstieg in die laparoskopische Kolonchirurgie. Langebecks Arch Chir Suppl 231–233
9. Christen D, Buchmann P (1996) Gefahrenquellen bei laparoskopischen Kolonoperationen und deren Vermeidung. Swiss Surg (in press)
10. Buchmann P, Bischofberger U, DeLorenzi D, Sartoretti C (1996) Frühe enterale Ernährung nach kolorektalen Resektionen – eine prospektive kontrollierte Studie. Schweiz med Wochenschr 126:Suppl 82:335
11. Buchmann P, Christen D (1995) Pro laparoscopic surgery for colorectal cancer. Dig Surg 12:296–301
12. Buchmann P, Christen D, Bischofberger U, Flury R (1995) Die laparoskopische Chirurgie des Kolonkarzinomes. Ein Vergleich mit der offenen Technik. Langebecks Arch Chir Suppl II:497–500
13. Wexner SD, Cohen SM, Johansen OB, Nogueras JJ, Jagelman DG (1993) Laparoscopic colorectal surgery: a prospective assessment and current perspective. Br J Surg 80:1602–1605
14. Hohenberger W (1995) Weichteilmetastasen. 112th Congress of the Deutsche Gesellschaft für Chirurgie, Berlin, 1995
15. Hughes ESR, McDermott FT, Polglase AL, Johnson WR (1983) Tumor recurrence in the abdominal wall scar tissue after large-bowel cancer surgery. Dis Colon Rectum 26:571–572
16. Nduka CC, Monson JR, Menzies-Gow N, Darzi A (1994) Abdominal wall metastases following laparoscopy. Br J Surg 81:648–652
17. Kloosterman T, von Blomberg BM, Borgstein P, Cuesta MA, Scheper RJ, Meijer S (1994) Unimpaired immune functions after laproscopic cholecystectomy. Surgery 115:424–428
18. Trokel MJ, Bessler M, Treal MR, Whelan RL, Navygrod R (1994) Preservation of immune response after laparoscopy. Surg Endosc 8:1385–1388
19. Carey PD, Wakefield CH, Thayeb A, Monson JRT, Darzi A, Guillon PJ (1994) Effects of minimally invasive surgery on hypochlorous acid production by neutrophils. Br J Surg 81:557–560
20. Holcombe RF, Stewart RM, Betzing KW, Kannan K (1994) Alteration in lymphocyte phenotype associated with administration of adjuvant levamisole and 5-flourouracil. Cancer Immunol, Immunother 38:394–394
21. Cirocco WC, Schwartzman A, Golub RW (1994) Abdominal wall recurrences after laparoscopic colectomy for colon cancer. Surgery 116:842–846

Laparoscopic Colorectal Surgery as Routine in a Community Hospital: Tactics and Results

G. Ehren and J. Konradt

Since 1991 laparoscopic surgery has become the standard technique for cholecystectomy, appendectomy, and hernia repair in our community hospital in Berlin. From April 1993 through October 1995 we performed 131 colorectal operations by minimally invasive technique. The different procedures performed are shown in table 1.

Table 1. Types of laparoscopic colorectal procedures performed

	n
Colostomy	21
Hartmann's operation	1
Side-to-side anastomosis	1
Right colectomy	11
Left colectomy	9
Sigmoid / anterior rectal resection	63
Low anterior resection	17
Abdominoperineal resection	3
Rectopexy	5
Total	131

Colostomy and Hartmann's Operation

Of 21 colostomies, 16 were formed as loop and 5 as end colostomies. The reasons for colostomy are shown in table 2. One patient underwent Hartmann's procedure because of perforated sigmoid diverticulitis. In one patient with an irresectable tumor of the splenic flexure a side-to-side transverso-sigmoidostomy was performed. None of these patients had any severe complications.

Table 2. Reasons for colostomies

	n
Protective for low anterior resection	2
Anastomotic leak	2
Anal incontinence	4
Ileus, obstruction	8
Perforation	2
Rectovaginal fistula	1
Postradiation proctitis	1
Anal carcinoma with ischiorectal abscess	1
Total	**21**

Colectomy and Rectopexy

At the start of our experience with laparoscopic colorectal surgery we operated only on patients with benign disease or on cancer patients for palliation. In July 1995 we started laparoscopic surgery for colorectal cancer with curative intent. Since there were and still are some unanswered questions about the oncological risk of the laparoscopic procedure, we only began after we were able to fulfill the following conditions:

1. Surgeons had to be well trained in laparoscopic colorectal surgery and experienced in conventional cancer surgery.
2. The standards of cancer surgery had to be respected in regard to the following:
   - Adequate margins of resection.
   - En bloc mesenteric/vascular resection.
   - Minimal intraoperative manipulation of the tumor mass.
3. There had to be oncological follow-up of patients and participation in a nationwide multicenter study.

The indications for colectomy are listed in table 3.

Table 3. Indications for colectomy and rectopexy

	n
Diverticulosis, diverticulitis	45
Inflammatory bowel disease	2
Dolichocolon	3
Rectal prolapse	5
Adenoma	8
Stage T1 carcinoma	5
Carcinoma (palliative)	16
Carcinoma (curative)	24
Total	**108**

Procedure and Techniques

After gaining experience in laparoscopic handling of the colon through forming colostomies and in a training workshop using a pig, we began to perform the first resections. The first 100 resections were performed by just two surgeons. The rest of the team changed frequently according to shift and schedule as normally occurs in a community hospital. We standardized our procedures from the beginning in order to minimize technical problems through lack of experience on the part of the operating room team. We now have four surgeons performing colorectal resections. The operating room team is now familiar enough with the procedures for laparoscopic sigmoid resection to be performed during any shift. We have never preselected patients and have started laparoscopically on every patient except where there was a contraindication. We have thus had several conversions, but have also completed some difficult laparoscopic operations, resulting in a strong learning effect.

Right and Left Colectomy

The patient's position and operating room set-up are shown in Fig. 1. Both right and left colectomy are performed as laparoscopically assisted procedures. There are three steps to be performed:

1. Laparoscopic mobilization and dissection of the mesentery, vascular ligation.
2. Extension of one incision, exteriorization of the bowel, and extracorporal resection and anastomosis.
3. Repositioning of the bowel in the abdominal cavity and closure of the incision. Laparoscopic inspection, lavage, and placing of a suction drain.

Fig. 1. Operating room set-up for right colectomy. *O*, Operator; *S*, nurse; *1.A, 2.A*, first and second assistants; *An*, anesthetist

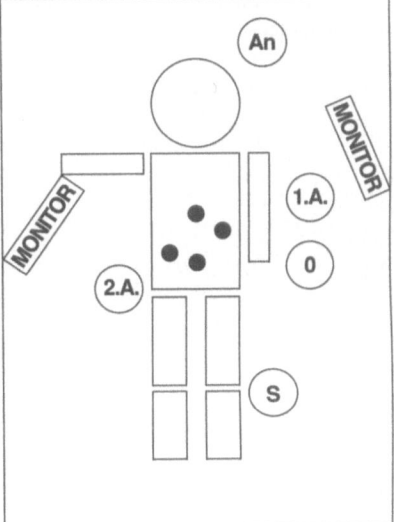

We use four or five 10- to 12.5-mm trocars, one placed next to the umbilicus and the others in a half circle around.

Sigmoid and Anterior Resection

Figure 2 demonstrates the patient's position and the set-up in the operating room for sigmoid and anterior resection. During the operation an extreme Trendelenburg position is often necessary. We use four 10- and 12.5-mm trocars placed as Fig. 2. The anastomosis is performed using a double stapler technique, the specimen being removed through a mini-laparotomy. These are the steps of the procedure:

1. Mobilization of the left colon, sigmoid, and mesentery from its embryonal adhesions; identification of the left ureter.
2. Incision of the peritoneum from the right side of the rectosigmoid and division of either the superior rectal artery or the inferior mesenteric artery (in curative cancer surgery). Division of the sigmoid mesentery and the mesorectum. In low anterior resection, rectopexy and abdominoperineal resection, the rectum and mesorectum have to be mobilized down to the pelvic floor, and the lateral ligaments including the medial rectal arteries have to be dissected.
3. Intracorporal resection of the rectum with a 30- or 60-mm linear cutter.
4. Extension of the trocar incision in the right lower abdomen. Exteriorization of the proximal segment, resection, and insertion of the anvil of a circular stapler. Repositioning into the abdominal cavity and closure of the incision.

Fig. 2. Operating room set-up for sigmoid and anterior resection

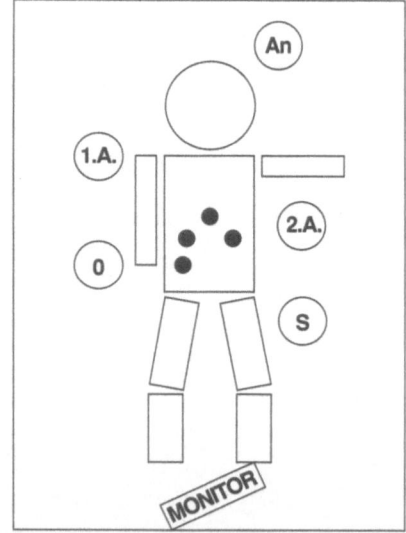

5. Transanal insertion of the circular stapler, attachment to the anvil, and completion of the anastomosis.
6. Check of anastomosis for leakage by rectoscopy and insufflation of air. Lavage and placing of suction drain.

Rectopexy

We prefer the Wells procedure for rectopexy. After mobilization of the rectum down to the pelvic floor, a polypropylene mesh is attached to Waldeyer's fascia with sutures and an endoscopic hernia stapler and then wrapped and fixed to the rectum. In the presence of a dolichocolon the procedure can be combined with a sigmoid resection, and in that case the rectum can be directly attached to the presacral fascia with sutures.

Abdominoperineal Resection

Mobilization and vascular and mesenteric division of the rectosigmoid are performed in the same way as described above. After the rectum is mobilized down to the pelvic floor, the sigmoid is dissected with an Endo-GIA and the proximal end is brought out through the extended incision in the left mid abdomen in order to form the colostomy. The specimen is delivered through the perineal incision, which is performed in a standard manner. After the perineal phase has been completed, the operation is finished by a final laparoscopic inspection.

Results

From April 1994 through October 1995, 108 patients underwent colorectal resection or rectopexy. Of these, 56 patients were female and 52 male. Ages ranged from 21 to 92 years (mean 62 years).

Conversion to laparotomy was necessary in 14 cases (13%), mostly in sigmoid/anterior (8 = 13%) and especially in low anterior resection (6 = 35%), for various reasons, such as adhesions, obesity, narrow pelvis in men, and technical problems. In diverticulitis there were ruptures of the colon wall when introducing the circular stapler. In low anterior resection the rectal wall was sometimes too thick to fit into the linear cutter. Twice there were technical failures with the stapler.

There were no other major intraoperative complications.

Tables 4 shows the mean operative time.

The long initial operative times became shorter an experience grew. A sigmoid resection, for example, is now performed in about 2 h. We have seen no long-term complications connected with long operative times, and the rate of conversion for purely anesthesiological reasons is negligible, although several patients with hypothermia required additional time on the respirator postoperatively.

In the postoperative phase peristaltic action was heard on the 1st or 2nd postoperative day and the first bowel movement took place on the 3rd day (median: range 1–6 days).

Table 4. Operative time: median (range), in minutes

Right colectomy	120	(70–235)
Left colectomy	150	(65–175)
Sigmoid anterior resection	180	(75–400)
Low anterior resection	195	(125–380)
Abdominoperineal resection ($n = 3$)		(225, 315, 480)
Rectopexy	145	(100–325)

Analgesics were used for 5 days (median: range 1–11 days).

The median postoperative stay was 14 days (range 6–38 days). This parameter, however, is dependent on many factors besides the recovery from surgery, such as patient age, the family situation, accompanying diseases, and the current structure of payment of hospital care in Germany.

There were three deaths during the postoperative period (2.7% mortality), all in patients aged 70 or older (one being 92), and all with severe cardiopulmonary problems. All three patients had undergone anterior resection. One patient with postoperative bleeding and reoperation died from circulatory and renal failure and the other two patients from sepsis. One case of anastomotic leakage was proven, in the other one it was the suspected cause of peritonitis.

Complications

There were 12 (11%) severe surgery-related complications. The rate of minor and major complications all together was 34% (37/108 patients). Six patients had to be reoperated on, three because of bleeding, two because of peritonitis due to anastomotic leakage, and one because of an abdominal abscess 4 weeks after surgery. Six additional patients had an anastomotic leak without reoperation. Three of them had no clinical manifestations and the leaks were detected only on routine postoperative X-ray with contrast agent. All but one (left colectomy) of the leakages appeared after sigmoid/anterior ($n = 3$) or low anterior resection ($n = 4$). Table 5 gives an overview of the complications.

Table 5. Complications seen in 37 of 108 patients (34%)

	n	%
Bleeding	3[a]	2.7
Anastomotic leakage without reoperation	6	5.5
Anastomotic leakage, with reoperation	2[a]	1.8
Douglas pouch abscess	1	0.9
Prolonged ileus	3	2.7
Wound infection	10	9.2
Fever for unknown reason	1	0.7
Urinary tract infection	9	8.3
Other cardiopulmonary complications, stroke	2	1.8
Total	37	34

[a] There was one death in this group.

Table 6. Tumor stages (UICC) of patients undergoing curative resection		
Stage 1	5
Stage 2	6
Stage 3	12
No staging (carcinosis)	1
Total	24

Cancer Stage and Number of Lymph Nodes

Twenty-four patients with colorectal cancer have undergone resection for cure. Tumor stages are listed in Table 6.

The median number of lymph nodes found by histopathological analysis was 12, with a range from 0 to 22.

Discussion

We have established laparoscopic colorectal surgery as the standard technique in our community hospital in Berlin. After 3 years' experience in laparoscopic surgery for gallbladders, appendicitis, and hernia we began with operations on the colorectum. In the first phase we used this technique only for benign diseases and palliatively for malginancies. Through early standardization of our technique the operating room team was able quickly to learn the more complicated operative procedure. There were no severe intraoperative complications. The long operative times have decreased to 2 h or less for a sigmoid resection. The postoperative course showed benefits such as early bowel movement, resumption of diet, and mobilization. The rate of complications and mortality did not exceed those after open surgery.

In the following phase we included curative cancer resection in our list of indications. We are careful to respect the standards of cancer surgery. The pathohistological findings showed sufficient tumor resection margins and the number of resected lymph nodes was equal to that in open surgery. All patients are enrolled in a multicenter study and all cancer patients are followed up at 3-month intervals.

There is sufficient evidence that patients benefit from the laparoscopic procedure in colorectal surgery. The question that remains is whether there is a higher long-term oncological risk for patients with malignancies, which is why a careful follow-up is required.

Open Versus Laparoscopic Surgery in Colorectal Surgery: Results

K. Lebrecht, H. A. Richter, A. Franke, and S. Zeyfang

Introduction

After remaining more or less unnoticed for a long time, minimally invasive surgery has entered the mainstream of surgery of the abdominal and thoracic cavities, ever more complex operations can be performed. The continuing development of technology and instruments allows cholecystectomy must be regarded as the pacesetter of video-controlled procedures. It has now become the standard under defined conditions. Minimally invasive operations on the large and small bowel on the other hand, are still at the stage of individual observations. Surgery is dependent on experience and analysis of that experience. Experience in minimally invasive surgery dates back only 6 – 7 years, and in some procedures, e. g. in colorectal surgery, even much less, so we are still in the learning phase. Minimally invasive surgery will enhance and in some cases replace many conventional procedures, but it will not make them superfluous. All new operative procedures are performed in the protective shelter of classic conventional surgery.

Finding a technical solution to various problems was an essential requirement before laparoscopic colorectal procedures could become established. For instance, construction of a secure intra-abdominal anastomosis was only possible once a special set of instruments had been developed. A further basic requirement of the performance of laparoscopic colorectal procedures was delivery of the resected specimen in water-and cellproof bags [5].

The increased technical demands and the markedly higher costs of laparoscopic surgery can only be justified if it can be shown in a prospective study that the new procedure has advantage for the patient. The new operative procedure should be just as safe for the patient as the conventional technique, and more comfortable.

Method and Patients

The aim of the present observation study was to compare the effectiveness and safety of the minimally invasive procedure with those of the conventional operation in patients with various colorectal disorders. After the technical feasibility of laproscopic left-sided colorectal resection was established, the question of improved recovery in the early postoperative phase was investigated. As comparative parameters, we employed analgesic consumption, the beginning of normal micturition, the resumption of bowel activity, the first

Table 1. Distribution of patients according to indication for surgery and type of surgery performed

	Laparoscopic surgery	Conventional surgery
Diverticulitis	31	15
Rectal and sigmoid carcinoma	15	29

postoperative passage of stool, the duration of hospitalisation and post-operative complications.

We divided the patients treated between May 1993 and August 1995 into two groups according to whether they were operated on conventionally or laparoscopically. The procedures performed were resection of the sigmoid colon or upper rectum with restoration of continuity in diverticulitis and carcinoma (Table 1). They were further divided into those with benign (in this case, diverticulitis only) and those with malignant disease; within each patient group, the age distribution and the severity of illness were comparable. Patients with a history of previous abdominal surgery and patients with extensive tumors were ruled out from the laparoscopic operative procedure. In these patients, conventional procedure seemed advisable because of the anticipated adhesions or the extended delivery minilaparotomy.

In the statistical analysis of the results, the χ^2 test or the Fisher test was used to compare frequency and the Mann-Whitney test was used to compare variables. All statistical calculations were performed at the Institute of Theoretical Surgery at the University of Marburg.

Results

Since it appeared impossible to determine analgesic consumption in the patients in precise detail in view of the varying forms of treatment in our intensive care unit and regular wards we have defined analgesic consumption as follows for our purposes:

- "Low consumption" covered oral and parenteral analgesic administration up to the 3rd postoperative day.
- If analgesics were required until the 5th postoperative day, we designated this as "moderate consumption."
- If analgesics were administered beyond the 5th day, consumption was classified as "high."

One the basis of this definition, the low analgesic consumption in the laparoscopically operated diverticulitis patients compared to patients with diverticulitis operated on conventionally was highly singificant (Table 2). In the carcinoma patients, on the other hand, there was no significant difference in analgesic requirement (Table 2).

Table 2. Postoperative analgesic consumption

Operative procedure	Analgesic consumption			p value[a]
	Low	Moderate	High	
Diverticulitis patient				
Laparoscopic	11	11	9	
Conventional	1	0	14	< 0.001
Carcinoma patients				
Laparoscopic	5	6	4	
Conventional	7	6	17	n.s.

[a] Fisher's test.

Table 3. Postoperative resumption of normal mictwition

Operative procedure	Postoperative day			p value[a]
	1	2–4	< 4	
Diserticulitis patients				
Laparoscopic	11	12	8	
Conventional	1	4	10	< 0.03
Carcinoma patients				
Laparoscopic	2	9	4	
Conventional	1	13	15	< 0.05

[a] Mann-Whitney test.

Normal postoperative micturition resumed significantly earlier in both the diverticulitis and the carcinoma patients operated by the minimally invasive method than in the patients who had conventional surgery (Table 3).

Postoperative gut peristalsis occurred significantly earlier in the diverticulitis and carcinoma patients who were operated on laparoscopically than in the conventionally operated patients. In consequence, the laparoscopically operated patients could begin oral fluid intake immediately postoperatively (Table 4).

While the first bowel movement occurrred markedly earlier after laparoscopic surgery than after conventional surgery in diverticulitis patients, no difference in this regard could be established in the carcinoma patients (Table 5).

Although postoperative hospitalisation was shorter among the laparoscopically operated diverticulitis patients than among those operated on conventionally, on significant difference was found. Among the carcinoma patients there was virtually no difference according to operative procedure (Table 6).

Table 4. Postoperative restoration of gut peristalsis

Operative procedure	Postoperative day			p value[a]
	1	2	3–4	
Diverticulitis patients				
Laparoscopic	28	2	1	< 0.001
Conventional	0	2	13	
Carcinoma patients				
Laparoscopic	13	1	1	< 0.001
Conventional	0	5	24	

[a] Mann-Whitney test.

Table 5. Occurrence of first postoperative bowel movement

Operative procedure	Postoperative day			p value[a]
	1–3	4–6	> 7	
Diverticulitis patients				
Laparoscopic	10	18	3	< 0.01
Conventional	2	7	6	
Carcinoma patients				
Laparoscopic	4	11	0	n.s.
Conventional	4	17	8	

[a] Mann-Whitney test.

Table 6. Length of postoperative hospital stay (days)

Operative procedure	Diverticulitis	Carcinoma
Laparoscopic	17	20
Conventional	26	21

Mann-Whitney test, no significant differences.

Occurrence of any of the following postoperative complications was recorded: cardiopulmonary complications, pneumonia, delayed postoperative wound healing, anastomotic leak, secondary hemorrhage, prolonged gastrointestinal atony, ileus, renal failure, liver failure and sepsis. In the diverticulitis group, there was a significantly lower rate of complications in the laparoscopically operated patients than in the patients who had undergone open surgery. No difference could be demonstrated between the two groups of carcinoma patients (Table 7).

Table 7. Occurrence of postoperative complications

Operative procedure	Complications		p value[a]
	Present	Absent	
Diverticulitis patients			
Laparoscopic	9	22	< 0.09
Conventional	10	5	
Carcinoma patients			
Laparoscopic	5	10	n. s.
Conventional	15	14	

[a] χ^2 test.

Discussion

Once we had mastered the technical problems of laparoscopic colorectal resection, the question arose as to whether this method should be offered to patients as an alternative to the conventional procedure. It had become evident in many patients that they had less postoperative pain and that bowel activity started sooner.

On this basis of this controlled but non-randomised study, we were able to show that our results agree with reports in the literature. The low level of postoperative pain [15] and the resulting early mobilisation of the patient are just as much an expression of greater patient comfort as the rapid occurrence of bowel peristalsis [2, 9, 16, 20] and the consequent early oral feeding.

In contrast to the reports in the literature [2–4, 7–9, 11, 12, 13, 15, 17, 18, 21], we did not see a significantly shortened postoperative stay in the laparoscopically operated patients. This discrepancy can be ascribed to the fee system still in force at present. Because of this fee system on the one hand and the high material costs in laparoscopic procedures on the other, we have only been able to more or less offset the financial expense through the hospital charges. In some patients not included in this prospective study, the postoperative hospital stay after laparoscopic procedures was 5 – 8 days. A change in the fee system will result in a marked shortening of postoperative hospitalisation.

There was a clearly lower complication rate among our patients who were operated on laparoscopically [1, 2, 6, 9, 14, 15, 22] than in patients operated conventionally. With increasing operative experience and further improvement in instruments, it will be possible to get past the present learning phase and improve the postoperative results further with regard to complications.

The results achieved by us in this study reinforce our impression that patients should be offered the laparoscopic procedure in colorectal surgery as an alternative to the conventional operation.

References

1. Alexander S, Kerlakian G, Kasper G, Hearn A (1995) Laparoscopic assisted colectomies versus open colectomy. J Laparoendosc Surg 5 : 1 – 6
2. Falk PM, Beart RW Jr, Wexner SD, Thorson AG, Jagelman DG, Lavery IC, Johansen OB, Fitzgibbons RJ Jr (1993) Laparoscopic colectomy: a critical appraisal. Dis Colon Rectum 36 : 28 – 34
3. Franklin ME Jr, Ramos R, Rosenthal D, Schuessler W (1993) Laparoscopic colonic procedures. World J Surg 17 : 51 – 56
4. Franklin ME Jr, Rosenthal D, Norem R (1995) Prospective evaluation of laparoscopic colon resection versus open colon resection for adenocarcinoma. A multicenter study. Surg Endosc 9 : 811 – 816
5. Gastinger J, Köckerling F, Schneider B et al. (1992) Zum Problem der Präparatebergung im Rahmen der laparoskopischen colorectalen Chirurgie. Minim Invasive Chir 1 : 73 – 74
6. Guillou P (1994) Laparoscopic surgery for diseases of colon and rectum – quo vadis? Surg Endosc 8 : 669 – 671
7. Guillou PJ, Darzi A, Monson JRT (1993) Experience with laparoscopic colorectal surgery for malignant disease. Surg Oncol 2 [Suppl 1] : 43 – 49
8. Hoffmann GC, Baker J, Fitchett CW, Vansant JH (1994) Laparoscopic assisted colectomy. Ann Surg 219 : 732 – 743
9. Jacobs M, Verdeja JC, Goldstein HS (1991) Minimally invasive colon resection (laparoscopic colectomy). Surg Laparosc Endosc 1 : 144 – 150
10. Monson JRT, Darzi A, Carey PD, Guillou PJ (1992) Prospective evaluation of laparoscopic-assisted colectomy in an unselcted group of patients. Lancet 340 : 831 – 833
11. Ortega AE, Beart RW, Steele GD, Winchester DP, Greene FL (1995) Laparoscopic bowel surgery registry. Preliminary results. Dis Colon Rectum 38 : 681 – 686
12. Phillips EH, Franklin M, Carrol B, Fallas MJ, Ramos R, Rosenthal D (1992) Ann Surg 216 : 703 – 707
13. Plasencia G, Jacobs M, Verdeja JC, Viamonto M (1994) Laparoscopic-assisted sigmoid colectomy and low anterior resection. Dis Colon Rectum 37 : 829 – 833
14. Puente J, Soza J, Sleeman D, Desai U, Tranakas N, Hartmann R (1994) Laparoscopic assisted colorectal surgery J Laparoendosc Surg 4 : 1 – 7
15. Senagore AJ, Luchtefeld MA, Mackeigan JM, Mazier WP (1993) Open colectomy versus laparoscopic colectomy: are there Differences? Am Surg 59 : 549 – 553
16. Sharpe DR, Redwine DB (1995) Laparoscopic segmental resection of the sigmoid and rectosigmoid colon for endometriosis. Surg Laparosc Endosc 2 : 120 – 124
17. Tucker JG, Ambroze WL, Orangio GR, Duncan TD, Mason EM, Lucas GW (1995) Laparoscopically assisted bowel surgery. Analysis of 114 cases. Surg Endosc 9 : 297 – 300
18. Van Ye TM, Cattey RP, Henry LG (1994) Laparoscopically assited colonresection compare favourably with open technique. Surg Laparosc Endosc 4 : 25 – 31
19. Vara-Thorbeck C, Garcia-Caballero M, Salvi M, Gutstein D, Toscano R, Gomez A, Vara-Thorbeck R (1994) Indications and advantages of laparoscopy-assisted colonresection for carcinoma in elderly patients. Surg Laparosc 4 : 110 – 118
20. Wexner SD, Johansen OB (1992) Laparoscopic bowel resection: advantages and limitations. Ann Med 24 : 105 – 110
21. Wexner SD, Cohen SM, Johansen OB, Nogueras JJ, Jagelman DG (1993) Laparoscopic colorectal surgery: a prospective assessment and current perspective, Br J Surg 80 : 1602 – 1605
22. Zucker K, Pitcher R, Martin D, Ford R (1994) Laparoscopic-assisted colon resection. Surg Endos 8 : 12 – 18

Laparoscopic Diagnosis, Staging, and Follow-Up of Colorectal Malignancies

F. L. Greene and D. A. Dorsay

Introduction

Until the late 1980s, laparoscopic was used primarily as a diagnostic modality except in the field of gynecology, where it was successfully applied to tubal ligation. More complex procedures were hindered by the need to manipulate the laparoscope with one hand and the inability of assistants to visualize the intra-abdominal proceedings. The development of video-laparoscopy freed more hands and enabled increasingly complex manipulations. The first laparoscopic cholecystectomy was performed in 1987 [1], and since then this approach has been widely adopted. The arguments for the laparoscopic approach are strong. Bowel function returns faster and postoperative pain is much less than with a formal laparotomy. Hospital stay is usually shorter and return to baseline functional level is faster. For these reasons, minimal-access techniques are being adapted for all areas of abdominal and thoracic surgery.

This chapter considers their potential application in the diagnosis, staging, and follow-up of colorectal malignances. This is an area that has been little explored; by necessity much of what follows is speculative or extrapolated from the traditional approach to these problems as well as from other applications of laparoscopy. Much will depend on the development of appropriate new techniques and the instrumentation to realize them, tempered by their judicious application.

Diagnosis

As always, the foundation of diagnosis is a thorough history and physical examination. Other then testing a stool sample for the presence of heme, laboratory studies play little part in the diagnosis of colorectal malignancy, although anemia, hypokalemia, or elevated hepatic enzymes may prompt further evaluation. Carcinoembryonic antigen testing is generally felt to be a poor screening modality for colorectal cancer, due to the frequent false-negative results (particularly when a tumor is potentially curable) [2], and the high cost of frequent false-positive results [3]. Its usefulness in the follow-up of colon cancer continues to be debated. Currently the definitive diagnosis depends on radiology and/or endoscopy. These should be considered complementary, and every effort should be made to evaluate the entire colon and rectum thoroughly.

Sigmoidoscopy, either rigid or flexible, engenders little morbidity and only moderate discomfort, and is easily performed without anesthesia. As such, it is usually the first invasive step in the evaluation of complaints attributable to the large bowel. Rigid sigmoidoscopy permits evaluation of the distal 20 cm of the rectosigmoid colon and has been estimated to detect one-third of intraluminal tumors [4]. A flexible sigmoidoscope may consistently reach 55 cm and permit visualization of an additional 30 % of lesions.

Even if sigmoidoscopy is positive, further evaluation of the colon is warranted by the finding of synchronous malignancies in 1.5–7.6 % of known colorectal cancers, and synchronous polyps in another 25–40 %. Colonoscopy and/or air-contrast barium enema may be used to complete this evaluation. Once again, this choice is controversial in that each study has unique advantages and disadvantages. Generally, air-contrast barium enema is the next step and, if of adequate quality, will allow most significant lesions to be discerned and anatomically (localized). If this study is equivocal, inadequate, or negative in the face of sings of symptoms of colonic malignancy, then colonoscopy should be performed. This will permit

- Small polyps to be detected
- Samples to be taken for biopsy
- Extraluminal masses to be distinguished from intraluminal ones

Further information may be obtained from magnetic resonance imaging or computed tomography (CT) with or without biopsy. These scans are particularly useful in staging or in identifying the origin of mural or extrinsic masses.

These steps will provide a diagnosis in the great majority of cases. However, occasionally events may conspire to prevent diagnosis without open exploration. Examples include:

- An extramural mass that cannot be biopsied by CT or ultrasound guidance
- Stricture preventing adequate colonoscopy or barium enema, with non-diagnostic biopsies
- Inadequate visualization of the colon due to redundancy or other anatomic factors
- Obstruction or perforation requiring urgent or emergent exploration

If there is reason to suspect malignancy, this should be followed by celiotomy, exploration, biopsy, and extirpation with curative or palliative intent. It is at this point that laparoscopy becomes a diagnostic option.

In the past, laparoscopic diagnosis would have offered no advantage over an open procedure, because even when colorectal malignancies are unresectable, palliative procedures may provide significant benefits in terms of survival and quality of life. Furthermore, a negative laparoscopic examination would not have completely ruled out disease. Recently, however, "laparoscopically assisted" colectomies [6, 8] and bypass and diverting procedures [9] have been developed which offer significant palliation with greatly shortened recovery times. Therefore, in the narrowly defined group which might avoid laparotomy on the basis of discovery of distant metastases or local spread not amenable to en bloc resection, laparoscopy may be indicated as a diagnostic tool to be followed by palliative laparoscopic colectomy, bypass procedures, or ablative procedures. Laparoscopic colectomy may fail to achieve adequate nodal clearance, which is they key factor in both staging and achieving curability. Until there are studies which indicate that nodal (mesenteric) dissection with laparoscopic techniques is comparable with open methods, laparoscopic colectomy for malignancy must be approached with caution.

Laparoscopic diagnosis, especially in the identification of hepatic metastases, is based on gross appearance and the histologic examination of tissue obtained by fine-needle aspiration, or core-needle, forceps, or excisional biopsy. Two new techniques may prevent the loss of tactile feedback during laparoscopic exploration. The first is the laparoscopic two-dimensional ultrasound probe, which can be used to identify and delineate primary tumors as well as hepatic or nodal metastases. The second is the application of radioimmunolocalization techniques to laparoscopic examination of the abdomen. An example is the development of second-generation monoclonal antibodies directed against the tumor-associated glycoprotein 72 antigen (TAG-72) [10]. Utilizing these highly sensitive and specific markers, laparoscopic localization and staging could be followed by celiotomy for curative resection, or resection of "occult" metastases identified by these techniques.

Staging

Current staging of colorectal cancer requires preoperative, intraoperative, and histopahtologic findings. Each contributes to subsequent decision-making, and the methods and information derived from them overlap. For example, tissue may be obtained for histologic examination during colonoscopy or CT-guided biopsy, during intraoperative excisional biopsy or by examination of the resected specimen. Evidence of distant metastasis may materialize during preoperative evaluation or intraoperatively. The result is an algorithm leading to a limited number of therapeutic options. These options include:

- Doing nothing
- Adopting a palliative approach
- Minimizing tumor load in anticipation of adjuvant therapy
- Resecting for cure, with or without adjuvant therapy

The goal of tumor staging is to determine the optimal therapy while inflicting minimal morbidity at the lowest cost. To stage colorectal carcinoma adequately, one must:

1. Resect the primary tumor and assess the extent of local invasion
2. Harvest tissue from epicolic, paracolic, intermediate, and mesenteric or iliac lymph nodes
3. Inspect the peritoneal surface for metastases
4. Search for evidence of hepatic metastases

All of these are achievable with laparoscopic techniques, and this ability will probably improve along with advances in instrumentation and technology.

The real advantage of preoperative staging may be seen in the management of rectal carcinoma, especially in patients at greater risk with major abdominal exploration and conventional resection. If laparoscopy uncovers hepatic or advanced local regional disease, palliative modalities such as laser ablation, local transanal resection, or intracavity radiation therapy may be viable options.

Techniques

Although diagnostic laparoscopic procedures may be performed with local anesthesia and intravenous sedation, we prefer to use general anesthesia. Careful preoperative assessment and optimization of cardiopulmonary function are mandatory, as carbon dioxide pneumoperitoneum crates severe stresses which may lead to hemodynamic compromise or hypercapnia in the patient with marginal functional reserve. Aggressive mechanical and anti-biotic bowel preparation is essential if therapeutic measures are being considered. In addition, we normally administer a second- or third-generation cephalosporin as prophylaxis.

Surgeon Position and Trocar Placement

Surgeon position and trocar placement depend upon the suspected location of the primary tumor as well as the location of any previous abdominal incisions. In general, trocar placement should allow access to the area of interest from multiple angels and close inspection of the liver, peritoneum, and lymph-node-bearing regions. Additional trocars may be placed as needed for retro-peritoneal nodal or liver biopsies. Although we usually place an infraumbilical 10-mm trocar for the camera following insufflation via a Veress needle, this may be modified in the presence of previous abdominal incisions. In such instances a Hasson trocar may be inserted using an open technique or, if there is a midline scar, the trocar may be inserted in the left iliac fossa lateral to the rectus abdominis muscle. This decision may be aided by preoperative CT or ultrasound which may suggest focal adhesions to the anterior abdominal wall. Initially, two additional trocars (usually 12 mm, to permit application of stapling devices if needed) are inserted parallel to the region of interest under laparoscopic vision. If the lesion involves the ascending or descending colon or cecum, the additional ports are placed cephalad and caudad to the camera port in the linea alba. If we are approaching the transverse colon or rectosigmoid, the trocars ore oriented transversely, just above or below the umbilicus at the linea semilunaris.

It is not uncommon to encounter adhesions in a previously operated abdomen. These are taken down with scissors using unipolar electrocautery. Extensive adhesions may warrant conversion to an open procedure. Generally the patient is in the supine position; however, for procedures such as a laparoscopic abdominoperineal resection, stapled end-to-end anastomosis, pull-through procedure, or intraoperative colonoscopy, the patient should be placed in the dorsal lithotomy position. A fully adjustable operating table is essential and should be used freely to enlist gravity as an ally in obtaining exposure. The surgeon is usually positioned opposite the focus of attention. During diagnostic procedures this focus may change, and the surgeon should reposition him- or herself accordingly.

Lesion Identification and Examination

Upon entering the peritoneal cavity, the primary lesion should first be identified unequivocally. Copies of the barium enema and CT scans should be available for review. If colonoscopy is performed preoperatively ad the lesion is small, it should be tattooed at that time. If doubt exists, the tumor can be definitively identified with intraoperative colonoscopy. Once identified, the serosa is inspected for signs of penetration. If bulky, the region is examined for invasion of adjacent viscera or the abdominal wall. The omentum, peritoneal surfaces, and, in women, the ovaries are then examined for metastatic implants. Biopsies are taken from suspicious lesions and sent for frozen and permanent section. Examination of the liver is performed in conjunction with information derived from preoperative ultrasound or CT scans. Visualization of the diaphragmatic and inferior surfaces is aided by use of a wide retractor and a 300 or 450 laparoscope. The recent introduction of flexible laparoscopes should facilitate the examination. Metastatic lesions may appear as whitish superficial plaques or surface dimpling. Identification of metastatic lesions is aided by remotely palpating the hepatic surface with a blunt-tipped probe. Surface lesions are biopsied with cup forceps and deep lesions with a percutaneous, laparoscopic-guided core-needle biopsy. Laparoscopic ultrasound with a linear array 7.5-MHz probe was introduced in 1984 and used to identify an intrahepatic lesion and guide a needle biopsy [11]. Another group [12] used a 3.5- and 5-MHz probe on the tip of a flexible laparoscope to visualize pancreatic and hepatic malignancies in 20 patients with disease previously diagnosed by CT scanning or extracoroporeal ultrasound. This technique is only now being reintroduced, using phased array technology, and it should greatly enhance the sensitivity of laparoscopic detection of hepatic metastases.

Staging of Rectal Carcinoma

Staging of rectal carcinoma may require the laparoscopic evaluation of pelvic lymph nodes. This is performed with the same (transverse) trocar arrangement and the patient in the Trendelenburg position. An additional 5-mm trocar may be placed in the midline, halfway between the umbilicus and pubic symphysis, to facilitate exposure. The inguinal ligament, pubic tubercle, and internal inguinal ring are identified, and, beginning ventral to the inguinal ligament and just lateral to the medial umbilical ligament, the peritoneum is incised with scissors and unipolar cautery. This incision is then carried dorsally to a point just proximal to the bifurcation of the iliac vessels. The peritoneal edges are grasped medially and laterally and freed up using a blunt dissector, using care to avoid injury to the obturator vessels and nerve. The ureter is carefully identified while the nodal tissue surrounding the hypogastric vessels is grasped and dissected free. Hemostasis is maintained with judicious use of multiple clips and electrocautery. If no further dissection is to be carried out in the pelvis, the peritoneal defect is closed with a running absorbable suture using a "ski" needle. This is then repeated on the opposite side. If resection of the lesion is planned, the lymph node dissection can be carried out in continuity with the specimen.

Occasionally a patient with known colorectal cancer may have CT evidence of para-aortic lymphadenopathy but no other known metastatic disease. In such cases, positive tissue will profoundly affect therapy. In general, laparoscopic access to this region is extremely awkward due to the presence of the small bowel. Despite this, Salky and colleagues [13] obtained a biopsy diagnosis in 16 of 19 patients with retroperitoneal pathology approached laparoscopically, and in 1992 Childers and Surwit [14] reported a laparoscopic para-aortic lymph node biopsy resulting in a diagnosis of non-Hodgkin's lymphoma. Herd and colleagues [15] recently described the development of an elegant technique using a porcine model which may ease this procedure. With the animal in steep Trendelenburg, the retroperitoneum was opened beginning lateral to the right common iliac vessels. After extending the incision cephalad, a pretied o chromic gut ligature is passed through one of the trocars lateral to the umbilicus and secured on the peritoneal edge (Fig. 2). The end of the ligature is maintained under tension extracorporeally and additional ties are placed at short intervals and brought under tension. This is repeated on the left side with the ties brought out through the left lateral trocar. The result is a tenting of the peritoneum which effectively retracts the small bowel. The trocars through which the ligatures pass may still be used introduce instruments, although there may be some loss of pneumoperitoneum. The nodal tissue is then removed using traction and electrocautery with clips placed as needed.

Additional efforts to localize nodal involvement may be realized through the technique of radioimmunolocalization using monoclonal antibodies to colorectal tumor antigens. A 1992 report [16] describes the use of radiolabeled CC49 (a second-generation monoclonal antibody directed against tumor-associated glycoprotein) and a hand-held γ-detecting probe during open abdominal exploration in the detection of primary and recurrent colorectal cancer. The authors succeeded in detecting 18 of 21 primary and 29 of 30 recurrent tumors. In at least 14 specimens the tumor was occult, and in many cases it was discovered in gastrohepatic, iliac, or celiac nodes. Of particular interest, 6 of 15 specimens which were considered CC49 positive and histologically negative were found on re-examination to have tumor foci. In addition, the authors stated that their findings altered management in nearly half of their patients. Application of this technique to laparoscopic staging awaits the development of an appropriately modified gamma probe.

Celiotomy

Following laparoscopic investigation, a variety of situations mandate progressing on to formal celiotomy. The first would be the finding of local invasion by a primary tumor requiring en bloc resection. Another is the identification of potentially resectable hepatic metastases. The third situation arises when laparoscopic staging is completely negative and the primary lesion is easily resectable. This area will remain controversial for several years, since the argument against pursuing laparoscopic resection at this point is the newness of the procedure and the lack of even short-term data on recurrence. On the other hand, if there is laparoscopic evidence of significant hepatic or distal nodal spread, then open resection offers no theoretical benefit, and laparoscopic colectomy may be a reasonable option to achieve palliation.

Results

Although the literature contains no reports of laparoscopic staging of colorectal carcinoma, the technique has been applied with some success to the staging of lymphoma and esophageal, gastric, pancreatic, prostate, and ovarian cancer. In 1989, Watt and coworkers [16] discussed the evaluation of 90 patients who had endoscopically diagnosed carcinoma of the esophagus or gastric cardia. They compared laparoscopy, ultrasound, and CT in the detection of hepatic, nodal, and peritoneal metastases, and found laparoscopy to be superior to imaging studies in identifying hepatic and peritoneal metastases, and equivalent to CT regarding nodal metastases.

In a study of 40 patients with documented gastric carcinoma and negative abdominal ultrasound and CT, Kriplani and Kapur [17] laparoscopically identified 5 patients with metastases and 11 patients whose disease was considered unresectable due to local extension. Twenty-three of the remaining patients were explored; only three had further findings obviating resection.

Warshaw and colleagues [18] evaluated two groups of patients with pancreatic cancer using a laparoscopic approach. In 1986 they reviewed 40 patients deemed resectable following endoscopic retrograde cholangiopancreatography, ultrasound, CT and mesenteric and celiac angiography, and who subsequently underwent laparoscopy. In this manner, they obtained histologic proof of metastasis in 14 (6 hepatic, 7 peritoneal, and 1 omental). Three of the 26 remaining patients who underwent celiotomy were also discovered to have metastases. A second study published in 1990 [19] demonstrated the value of multiple diagnostic modalities in avoiding unnecessary celiotomy. Individually, angiography, CT, and laparoscopy were approximately 50% successful in predicting resectability of a pancreatic malignancy. However, in combination, this rose to 87.5%.

Parra and colleagues [20] compared the results of open and laparoscopic staging pelvic lymphadenectomy in 24 men with prostate cancer and found them to be equivalent in assessing nodal tissue. Rosenhoff and coworkers [21] evaluated seven patients referred to them with ovarian cancer and noted to have disease localized to the pelvis (stage I and II) at diagnostic celiotomy. They performed staging laparoscopy prior to initiating local therapy, and found that six had developed extrapelvic disease.

The utility of laparoscopy in the identification and biopsy of hepatic lesions continues to be debated. Studies have been published supporting all views [22], but all are lacking in objective evidence. Probably the most realistic assessment is that expressed by Fornari et al. [23], who found that a combination of ultrasound-guided fine-needle aspiration followed by laparoscopy resulted in a diagnostic accuracy of 98.4% and a sensitivity of 97.5% in the diagnosis of hepatic lesions. This does not change the fact that there is a very low yield for ultrasound and CT in the primary evaluation of colorectal cancer, and that their routine use is not recommended.

Follow-Up

Despite resection for cure, nearly half of all colorectal carcinomas will recur [26] most frequently within 2 years of operation. Patterns of recurrence differ markedly between colon and rectal carcinomas after "curative" resection. Willett and colleagues [27] discussed recurrence patterns 5 years after curative resection of colon malignancies with a typical distribution of stages. Of 533 patients, 163 (31%) developed recurrence during that period, with metastatic disease in 25% and local disease in 19%. Six percent had local disease only, while 71 patients (31%) had extra-abdominal metastases. Michelassi and colleagues [28] reported an 8% overall local recurrence rate with a median time to diagnosis of 18 months and with all but 16% representing within 5 years. In those patients who underwent resection of a rectal lesion, the incidence of local recurrence was 12%. Metastatic lesions were not addressed in that study. Stipe et al. [29] recently examined recurrence retrospectively in 469 patients who had undergone resection of colorectal cancer with curative intent. At a median follow-up of 42 months, 31.1% showed evidence of relapse (10% local only, 3.4% local and metastatic, and 17.5% metastatic only). Rectal cancers recurred locally with an incidence of 18.3% as opposed to 8.9% for colon cancer. McDermott and coworkers [30] examined a series of 1008 patients following curative resection of rectal carcinomas, of whom 934 were available for analysis. They found relapse in 38% of their subjects (11% local only, 17% metastatic only, and 9% both). It is now recognized that, if identified early, aggressive resection of recurrent local disease, as well as limited metastatic disease, may result in long-term survival [31]. The key word is "early", which opens up the question of what constitutes ideal follow-up.

In the past, patients underwent reoperation only for sings or symptoms of recurrent disease and depending on the aggressiveness of the surgeon. By this time tumors were usually far advanced and surgery was palliative at best. In 1951, Wangensteen and colleagues [32] advocated routine "second-look" abdominal exploration at 6–8 months postoperatively in all patients with gastrointestinal malignancies resected for cure, with repeat laparotomies performed until no residual tumor was found. This led to an unacceptably high number of

negative explorations, with attendant morbidity and mortality. The results were particularly dismal in patients with gastric cancer treated in this manner: only 1 of 22 patients who had a positive second exploration remained cancer-free 31 months after the fourth operation. The results in subjects with rectal tumors were no better, with only 1 of 15 positive second-look subjects free of disease 12 months after the final procedure. The numbers were somewhat better (4/14) for colon lesions. Overall, 52 of 93 initial re-explorations were negative, yet 11 of these patients developed recurrent disease. Thankfully, means have been developed to reduce the number of negative explorations. If these could be eliminated, a salvage rate of 29 % for recurrent colon cancer would be more than acceptable.

Histopathologic stage has been used to identify a population at risk of recurrence. In most studies, Duke's stage A lesions recurred in less than 5 % of cases [26] The percentage increases rapidly with advancing stage. This information, along with a directed history, physical examination, and various diagnostic tests, could theoretically be used to identify patients likely to have recurrent disease early enough to offer the possibility of salvage through second-look laparotomy.

In 1987, Sugarbaker and colleagues [34] published the results of a prospective study begun in 1978 which examined this concept in detail. They studied 66 patients deemed to be at high risk on the basis of stage (Duke's C/TNM stage III), perforation, invasion of adjacent organs, locally recurrent disease, or age less than 30 years). All underwent resection with no apparent residual disease, and were followed for a median of 4 years with all modalities available at the time. Follow-up included:

- A review of symptoms and physical examination at every visit (monthly)
- Carcinoembryonic antigen (CEA) assays (monthly)
- Abdominopelvic CT scanning (monthly)
- Complete lung tomograms (monthly)
- Liver-spleen scintigraphy every 4 months
- Intravenous pyelography (annually)
- Barium enema (annually)
- Bone scintigraphy (annually)

Thirty-one patients (47 %) developed recurrences. A serial increase in CEA levels was the first indication in 22 (67 %), while symptoms or examination provided the first indication in seven (21 %). Abdominal CT uncovered two recurrences and corroborated disease in 17 of 20 cases; however, this record is marred by a 50 % false-positive rate. The other studies were useful only for corroboration and localization of relapse.

Second-Look procedures

Several groups have applied the concept of second-look surgery directed only by an increase in CEA in an attempt to intervene in recurrent cancer at an early (and potentially curable) stage. The best results are those from studies by the Society of Surgical Oncology and a group from Ohio State University in which CEA levels were closely followed and secondary resections were aggressively performed, for the most part by specialists in surgical oncology. In 1985, Martin et al. [25] reported a study of 145 patients who underwent second-look laparotomy on the basic of rising CEA alone. Their criterion for exploration was a steadily rising CEA level greater than 7.5 ng/ml. Of these 139 had demonstrable disease, and recurrence later became evident in 6 of the remaining patients. Resections were considered possible in 81 (65%). Of the 45 patients followed for 5 years or more, 14 (41%) remained alive.

In 1978, Minton et al. [36] began a prospective, nonrandomized study of 400 patients following curative resection of colon or rectal cancer: 130 recurrences were documented (32%), and 75 (19%) underwent second-look laparotomy. A rising CEA level greater than 2.5 ng/ml was the primary indication in 43, and 23 (59%) of the tumors were considered resectable. Of the patients followed for more than 5 years, 37% of those undergoing curative resection because of rising CEA remained alive without disease, compared with 28% of those directed by clinical information.

On a more sobering note, Fucini et al. [37] followed 64 patients prospectively and detected 90% of 22 recurrences with CEA determinations. However, of 12 patients undergoing second-look celiotomy, only one was still alive, with metastases, at the time of publication. Four of the five patients undergoing celiotomy solely for rising CEA levels had no detectable disease and one had unresectable carcinomatosis.

Even in the best circumstances and with thorough preoperative staging, a large number of patients are found to have unresectable disease at second-look laparotomy and suffer needlessly. Laparoscopy may be utilized to reduce this number, and may in the future offer therapeutic benefit as well. It must be remembered that a negative examination in no way rules out recurrence, and therefore it may be followed by celiotomy.

Second-look laparoscopy has been reported in the gynecologic literature. In 1984, Xygakis et al. [38] reported on 46 asymptomatic women who underwent laparoscopy 10–18 months after surgical, radiation or chemical therapy for ovarian cancer. Findings in 20 obviated laparotomy, 16 of remainder underwent laparotomy, at which time 3 were found to have recurrence. No major morbidity was reported.

Marti-Vicente et al. [39] performed 44 second-look and 28 third-look laparoscopies in 52 women with ovarian cancer in clinical remission. Nearly 50% of these examinations demonstrated recurrent tumor, yet a 31% false-negative rate was discovered at laparotomy. Neither of these studies addressed the benefits of surgical debulking in the treatment of this disease.

Currently the indications and opportunities for second-look laparoscopy remain limited. If recurrence is suggested on the grounds of a rising CEA level or clinical finding, evidence of unresectable disease should be sought using roentgenograms, CT, ultrasound, magnetic resonance imaging, and possibly scintigraphy using radiolabeled monoclonal antibodies. The presence of distal metastases, if unresectable, would make further evaluation unnecessary except for histologic confirmation. The extent of locally recurrent disease is difficult to appraise using noninvasive imaging studies, due to scar formation, alteration of the normal anatomy, and possible reactive lymphadenopathy. Therefore the suggestion of recurrence by history, examination, or rising CEA levels, even where imaging has given negative or equivocal results, would justify invasive evaluation. Laparoscopy may represent the next stage in the evolution of the second-look evaluation, with a goal of performing celiotomy only in patients with resectable disease. A major obstacle to this goal is the prevalence of adhesions in the previously operated abdomen. These are frequently present to such a degree as to limit severely or even prevent inspection by this method. However, the careful insertion of trocars using an open technique, followed by patient adhesiolysis, will permit laparoscopic examination in most patients. Visual examination may be augmented by laparoscopic ultrasound and radiomimmunolocalization techniques in the near future. A finding of peritoneal carcinomatosis or unresectable hepatic metastases would obviate further surgical intervention, but other findings may be more difficult to interpret. In general, a finding of potentially resectable recurrence or lack of evidence of unresectable disease would warrant a subsequent celiotomy with aggressive resection of all malignant tissue in the low- or moderate-risk patient.

Concepts for the Future

There may be a therapeutic role for laparoscopy in the near future as well. Several recent studies have demonstrated prolonged remission in as many as 22% of patients with multiple hepatic metastases from colorectal cancers [40] and in 37.5% of patients with unresectable hepatocellular carcinoma [41] following ultrasound-guided hepatic cryosurgery. Instruments are now being developed for the laparoscopic application of this technique.

Conclusion

The treatment of cancer is an emotional issue for all involved, including the surgeon. On the one hand we have a strong desire to do something to offer our patients the chance of a cure; on the other we are reluctant to add what may prove to be unnecessary pain and disability to what the patient is already suffering. In some instances, minimal-access techniques may offer a means of achieving both of these goals.

The diagnosis of colorectal cancer still rests on endosocopic or radiologic demonstration of tumor, and laparoscopy will probably continue to play a very restricted role here. The real strength of laparoscopy in the treatment of this disease lies in its potential ability to stage primary and recurrent malignancy accurately, coupled with a real and growing potential for therapeutic intervention.

References

1. Nagy AG, Poulin EC, Girotti MJ et al. (1992) History of laparoscopic surgery. Can J Surg 35:271–274
2. Moertel CG, O'Fallon JR, Go VLW et al. (1986) The preoperative carcinoembryonic antigen test in the diagnosis, staging and prognosis of cancer. Cancer 58:603–610
3. Lieberman DA (1990) Colon cancer screening: the dilemma of positive screening tests. Arch Intern Med 150:740–744
4. Winnan C, Berci C, Panish J et al. (1980) Superiority of the flexible to the rigid sigmoidoscope in routine proctosigmoidoscopy. N Engl J Med 302:1011–1012
5. Howard ML, Greene FL (1990) The effect of preoperative endoscopy on recurrence and survival following surgery for colorectal carcinoma. Am Surg 56:124–127
6. Schlinkert RT (1991) Laparoscopic-assisted right hemicolectomy. Dis Col Rect 34:1030–1031
7. Corbitt JD Jr (1992) Preliminary experience with laparoscopic-guided colectomy. Surg Laparosc Endosc 2:79–81
8. Phillips EH, Franklin M, Carroll BJ et al. (1992) Laparoscopic colectomy. Ann Surg 216:703–707
9. Shimi S, Banting S, Cuschieri A (1992) Laparoscopy in the management of pancreatic cancer: endoscopic colecystojejunostomy for advanced disease. Br J Surg 79:317–319
10. Arnold MW, Schneebaum S, Berens A et al. (1992) Intraoperative detection of colorectal cancer with radioimmunoguided surgery and CC4, a second-generation monoclonal antibody. Ann Surg 216:627–632
11. Bonhof JA, Linart P, Bettendorf U et al. (1991) Liver biopsy guided by laparoscopic sonography. Endoscopy 16:237–239
12. Okita K, Kodama T, Oda M et al. (1984) Laparoscopic ultrasonography; diagnosis of liver and pancreatic cancer. Scand J Gastroenterol 19 [Suppl 94]:91–100
13. Salky BA, Bauer JJ, Gelernt IM et al. (1988) The use of laparoscopy in retroperitoneal pathology. Gastrointest Endosc 34:227–230
14. Chiders JM, Surwit EA (1992) Laparoscopic para-aortic lymph node biopsy for diagnosis of a non-Hodgkins lymphoma. Surg Laparosc Endosc 2:139–142
15. Herdj, Fowler JM, Shensos D et al. (1992) Laparoscopic para-aortic lymph node sampling: development of a technique. Gynecol Oncol 44:271–276
16. Nabi HA, Doerr RJ (1992) Radiolabeled monoclonal antibody imaging of colorectal cancer: current status and future perspectives. Am J Surg 163:448–456
17. Watt I, Stewart I, Anderson D et al. (1989) Laparoscopy, ultrasound and computed tomography in cancer of the oesophagus and gastric cardia: a prospective comparison for detecting intra-abdominal metastases. Br J Surg 76:1036–1039
18. Kriplani AK, Kapur BML (1991) Laparoscopy for pre-operative staging and assessment of operability in gastric carcinoma. Gastrointest Endosc 37:441–443
19. Warshaw AL, Tepper JE, Shipley WU (1986) Laparoscopy in the staging and planning of therapy for pancreatic cancer. Am J Surg 151:76–80
20. Parra RO, Andrus C, Boulier J (1992) Staging laparoscopic lymph node dissection: comparison of results with open pelvic lymphadenectomy. J Urol 147:875–878
21. Rosenhoff SH, Young RC, Anderson T et al. (1975) Peritoneoscopy: a valuable staging total in ovarian carcinoma. Ann Int Med 83:37–41
22. Brady PC, Peebles M, Goldschmid S (1991) Role of laparoscopy in the evaluation of patients with suspected hepatic or peritoneal malignancy. Gastrointest Endosc 37:27–30
23. Jeffers L, Speigleman C, Reddy R et al. (1988) Laparoscopically directed fine needle aspiration for the diagnosis of hepatocellular carcinoma: a safe and accurate technique. Gastrointest Endosc 34:235–237
24. Gadolfi L, Muratori R, Solmi L et al. (1989) Laparoscopy compared with ultrasonography in the diagnosis of hepatocellular carcinoma. Gastrointest Endosc 35:508–511
25. Fornari F, Rapaccini GL, Cavanna L et al. (1988) Diagnosis of hepatic lesions: ultrasonically guided fine needle biopsy or laparoscopy. Gastrointest Endosc 34:231–234

26. Beahrs OH (1986) Staging and prognostic features of cancer of the colon and rectum. In: Beahrs OH, Higgins GA, Weinstein JJ (eds) Colorectal tumors. Lippincott, Philadelphia, p 115

27. Willett CC, Tepper JE, Cohen AM et al. (1984) Failure patterns following curative resection of colonic carcinoma. Ann Surg 200 : 685–690

28. Michelassi F, Vannucci L, Ayala JJ et al. (1990) Local recurrence after curative resection of colorectal adenocarcinoma. Surgery 108 : 787–793

29. Stipa S, Nicolanti V, Botti C et al. (1991) Local recurrence after curative resection for colorectal cancer: frequency, risk factors, and treatment. J Surg Oncol Suppl 2 : 155–160

30. McDermott FT, Hughes ESR, Pihl E et al. (1985) Local recurrence after potentially curative resection for rectal cancer in a series of 1008 patients. Br J Surg 72 : 34–37

31. Schiessel R, Wunderlich M, Herbst F (1986) Local recurrence of colorectal cancer: effect of early detection and aggressive surgery. Br J Surg 73 : 342–344

32. Wangensteen OH, Lewis FJ, Tongen LA (1951) The "second look" in cancer surgery. Lancet 71 : 303–307

33. Wangesteen OH, Lewis FJ, Arhelger SW et al. (1954) An interim report upon the "second look" procedure for cancer of the stomach, colon, and rectum and for "limited intraperitoneal carcinosis". Surg Gynecol Obstet 99 : 257–267

34. Sugarbaker PH, Gianola FJ, Dwyer A et al. (1987) A simplified plan for follow-up of patients with colon and rectal cancer supported by prospective studies of laboratory and radiologic test results. Surgery 102 : 79–87

35. Martin EW Jr, Minton JP, Hoehn JL, Gerber DM et al. (1985) Results of a 400-patient carcinoembryonic antigen second look colorectal cancer study. Cancer 55 : 1284–1290

36. Minton JP, Hoehn JL, Gerber DM, et al. (1985) Results of a 400-patient carcinoembryonic antigen second look colorectal cancer study. Cancer 55 : 1284–1290

37. Fucini C, Tommasi SM, Rosi S (1987) Follow-up of colorectal cancer resected for cure: an experience with CEA, TPA, Ca19-9 analysis and second look surgery. Dis Colon Rect 90 : 273–277

38. Xygakis AM, Politis CS, Michalas SP et al. (1984) Second-look laparoscopy in ovarian cancer. J Reprod Med 29 : 583–585

39. Marti-Vicente A, Sainz S, Soriano G et al. (1990) Utilidad de la laparoscopia como metodo de second-look en las neoplasias del ovario. Rev Esp Enf Dig 77 : 275–278

40. Onik G, Rubinsky B, Zemel R et al. (1991) Ultrasound-guided hepatic cryosurgery in the treatment of metastatic colon carcinoma. Preliminary results. Cancer 67 : 901–906

41. Zhou X-D, Tang Z-Y, Yu Y-G et al. (1988) Clinical evaluation of cryosurgery in the treatment of primary liver cancer: report of 60 cases. Cancer 61 : 1889–1894

VII   Roundtable

Workshop: Laparoscopic Colorectal Surgery

Summary of Discussion and Opinion Poll

During the workshop the presentations were followed by lively discussions involving both the speakers and the floor. This led to clarification of controversial issues as well as to the identification of areas where the results of research are still lacking. The opinion of the auditorium was polled during the final session. A brief résumé of the discussions and the results of the survey are given below.

Not surprisingly, more than 90 % of the workshop participants intended to perform and/or had personal experience with laparoscopic colorectal surgery. Among colorectal procedures, right hemicolectomy was considered to be most easily performed laparoscopically, followed by sigmoid resection, abdomino-perineal resection, anterior resection, and left hemicolectomy. As for the question of indication in benign conditions, half of the participants felt that a laparoscopic operation should be performed for sigmoid diverticulitis. Other indications were rectal prolapse (38 %), ulcerative colitis (7 %), and Crohn's colitis (6 %).

Throughout the workshop there was ongoing discussion about the place of laparoscopic surgery in the treatment of colorectal cancer. Not surprisingly, no unanimous opinion emerged nor was consensus reached or even aimed at by this workshop. Some interesting points were formulated, however. The factors determining the feasibility of laparoscopic surgery for malignant conditions were felt to be N stage (46.6 %), T stage (31.8 %), M stage (11.4 %) and tumor location (10.2 %). Majority opinion from the floor was that laparoscopic colorectal surgery would eventually replace conventional surgery for benign conditions, whereas this was thought to apply for malignant conditions as well by only a third.

On a general scale, almost 90 % of participants were of the opinion that laparoscopic colorectal surgery, although less invasive, should not be regarded as less risky than conventional surgery. There was a common feeling that technical innovations were highly desirable. This need seemed to relate first to anastomotic techniques and suturing, then to improvements of access, dissection, and application of energy. The present situation, which requires the addition of a mini-laparotomy to most procedures, was considered to be transitional by only a minority; almost 90 % thought that laparoscopically assisted procedures were here to stay.

Looking at the general conditions under which laparoscopic colorectal surgery is performed, it was felt by two-thirds of the participants that the need for cost containment definitely does developments and will continue to do so in the future. Turning to quality of performance and acquisition of the necessary skills for this kind of surgery, the majority expressed a constant need for training courses. The perceived need was more for advanced than for basic courses – a finding which might be interpreted to mean that basic skills in laparoscopic surgery by now are part of regular surgical training.

There was almost unanimous conviction that a continuing need exists for quality assessment of both training and performance of laparoscopic colorectal surgery. Equally important, and an indication of the high scientific level of the workshop, was the fact that 94% of the participants agreed on the necessity of randomized studies to evaluate laparoscopic colorectal procedures.

A sense of uncertainty found its expression in the results of an inquiry into participants' willingness either to perform or to undergo certain laparoscopic colorectal procedures. The fact that without exception individuals were reluctant to undergo procedures that they were willing to perform on their patients points to a dilemma that is till unresolved. The data given in Table 1 permit the conclusion that reservations exist against the performance of laparoscopic surgery for malignant conditions and that this is most pronounced when the advantages of the less invasive approach are less evident, e.g., right hemicolectomy for cecal carcinoma.

Instead of trying to summarize a discussion that continued throughout the workshop within and between plenary sessions and in small groups, the reader is referred to the concluding vote taken on four statements formulated for this purpose by the chairman. They are as follows:

– Available experience has shown that a wide spectrum of colorectal pathology can be approached laparoscopically because this technique is feasible, effective, and safe: Yes = 79.4%; No = 11.8%; Undecided = 7.4%.
– At present, generally accepted indications for open colorectal operations should not be changed because of the possibility of a laparoscopic approach: Yes = 90.5%; No = 9.5%; Undecided = 0%.

Table 1. Would you perform/undergo laparoscopic colorectal surgery for the following conditions?

	perform		undergo	
	Yes/No (%)		Yes/No (%)	
Inflammatory bowel disease	81.4	16.9	63.3	26.7
Sigmoid diverticulitis	87.3	12.7	73.0	20.6
Rectal prolapse	86.2	12.3	72.9	22
Cecal carcinoma	73.8	23.1	33.3	65.2
Sigmoid carcinoma	77.8	20.6	43.3	53.3
Rectal carcinoma	78.8	19.7	61.5	35.4

- Available data from retrospective analyses at present do not allow us to consider the laparoscopic approach for colorectal carcinoma as equivalent to the open approach: Yes = 79.4%; No = 11.8%; Undecided = 7.4%.
- If laparoscopic procedures are used for colorectal carcinoma with curative intent, the established principles of cancer surgery (lymph node resection, margin of clearance, prevention of tumor spillage) must be observed. In addition, complete records and follow-up are indispensable: Yes = 90.5%; No = 3.2%; Undecided = 3.2%.

Springer
and the
environment

At Springer we firmly believe that an international science publisher has a special obligation to the environment, and our corporate policies consistently reflect this conviction.

We also expect our business partners – paper mills, printers, packaging manufacturers, etc. – to commit themselves to using materials and production processes that do not harm the environment. The paper in this book is made from low- or no-chlorine pulp and is acid free, in conformance with international standards for paper permanency.

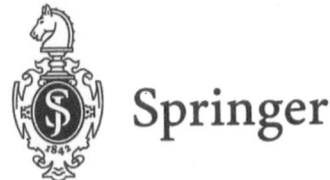